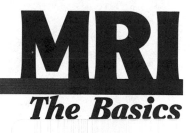

MRI
The Basics

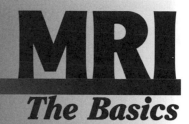

MRI
The Basics

Ray H. Hashemi, M.D., Ph.D.
Director
Bay Harbor MRI and Diagnostic Center
Harbor City, California

William G. Bradley, Jr., M.D., Ph.D., F.A.C.R.
Director, MRI and Medical Research
Memorial MRI Center
Long Beach, California

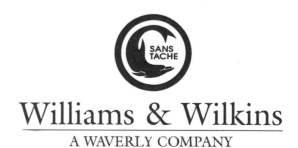

Williams & Wilkins
A WAVERLY COMPANY

BALTIMORE • PHILADELPHIA • LONDON • PARIS • BANGKOK
BUENOS AIRES • HONG KONG • MUNICH • SYDNEY • TOKYO • WROCLAW

Editor: Charles W. Mitchell
Managing Editor: Marjorie Kidd Keating
Production Coordinator: Carol Eckhart
Copy Editor: Kathy Gilbert
Designer: Wilma E. Rosenberger
Cover Designer: Silverchair Science & Communications, Inc.
Typesetter: Bi-Comp, Inc.
Printer and Binder: Vicks Litho

351 West Camden Street
Baltimore, Maryland 21201-2436 USA

Rose Tree Corporate Center
1400 North Providence Road
Building II, Suite 5025
Media, Pennsylvania 19063-2043 USA

Accurate indications, adverse reactions and dosage schedules for drugs are provided in this book, but it is possible that they may change. The reader is urged to review the package information data of the manufacturers of the medications mentioned.

Printed in the United States of America

Library of Congress Cataloging-in-Publication Data

Hashemi, Ray H.
   MRI: the basics/Ray H. Hashemi, William G. Bradley, Jr.
     p. cm.
   Includes bibliographical references and index.
   ISBN 0-683-18240-4
   1. Magnetic resonance imaging.   I. Bradley, William G.
  II. Title.
   [DNLM: 1. Magnetic Resonance Imaging—examination questions.
  2. Physics—problems.   3. Mathematics—problems.   WN 18.2 H348m
  1997]
   RC78.7.N83H44   1997
   616.07′548—dc20
   DNLM/DLC
   for Library of Congress   96-9064
                                       CIP

To purchase additional copies of this book, call our customer service department at **(800) 638-0672** or fax orders to **(800) 447-8438**. For other book services, including chapter reprints and large quantity sales, ask for the Special Sales department.

Canadian customers should call **(800) 268-4178**, or fax **(905) 470-6780**. For all other calls originating outside of the United States, please call **(410) 528-4223** or fax us at **(410) 528-8550**.

Visit *Williams & Wilkins on the Internet:* **http://www.wwilkins.com** or contact our customer service department at **custserv@wwilkins.com**. Williams & Wilkins customer service representatives are available from 8:30 am to 6:00 pm, EST, Monday through Friday, for telephone access.

97 98 99
2 3 4 5 6 7 8 9 10

To our wives, Heidi Hame, DDS, MS and Rosalind Dietrich, MD, for their support in general—but particularly during the writing of this book.

Preface

"Things should be made as simple as possible—but no simpler."

—*Albert Einstein*

MRI has been called "the most important development in medical diagnosis since the discovery of the x-ray" 100 years ago. It has become one of the major new tools of radiology, now being applied to virtually every part of the body. So, one might ask, if this MRI is so wonderful, why are so many radiologists reluctant to "get into" it? In a word: "physics." The physics of MRI can be truly terrifying, particularly for those attempting to enter the explanation halfway through without a proper foundation in the basics. And without a proper understanding of the basics, any MR clinician is merely "faking it," not truly understanding the physical basis for the signal changes in the image. *MRI: The Basics* attempts to rectify that situation.

In this book we have attempted to present this complicated topic in a readable, understandable, and even entertaining fashion without sacrificing the fundamental concepts. The reader will find a comprehensive coverage of MRI physics, from basic principles to more advanced topics such as MR angiography and fast scanning techniques. Some of the latest MR techniques made possible with high performance gradients, e.g., echo planar imaging, are also discussed. Because most of the chapters arose from lectures given by the first author to radiology residents, the language used through most of the text is of an informal or conversational nature that makes it easy to follow.

While attempting to be thorough, this book does not get bogged down in the minor details. An introductory math chapter is designed to introduce the reader to the most fundamental mathematics used in MRI (no knowledge of calculus is required!). Considerable attention is paid to the process of image creation, including the concepts of gradients, signal/image processing, and k-space. One of the distinguishing features of this book is its introduction and treatment of signal/image processing. There are two chapters dedicated to image creation, two to k-space, one to Fourier transform, and one to signal processing, as well as several chapters on fast scanning (fast spin echo, gradient echo, fast gradient echo, and echo planar imaging). There are also chapters that deal in depth with flow and MR angiography as well as MRI artifacts.

More than 400 illustrations provide the reader with a clear visual tool to follow the text. The *key points* of each chapter are summarized at the end of that chapter. In addition, there is a set of *problem solving and multiple choice questions* at the end of each chapter (with answers at the end of the book) to test the reader's knowledge of that chapter. The material presented in smaller print may be skipped because it is intended for the mathematically-oriented reader.

This book is intended primarily for radiologists and radiology residents and fellows as well as radiologic technologists. However, other physicians, medical students, scientists, and professionals dealing with MRI could also benefit from it. It is intended to provide the shortest learning path from the basics through the applications, avoiding the extraneous. This book can be used by radiology residents preparing for the physics portion of the American Board of Radiology exam and by MR technologists preparing for their MR certification exam.

In short, you can find in this book almost everything you always wanted to know about MR physics but were afraid to ask. In addition, this book may not only be read cover to cover as a textbook to learn about all aspects of MR basics, but also may be used as a reference for the fundamentals and advanced technological breakthroughs in MRI. We hope you'll enjoy reading it as much as we did writing it.

RHH
WGB

Acknowledgments

I would like to express my great appreciation to Edward Helmer, MD, at Kaiser Permanente Medical Center, who painstakingly transcribed my physics lectures to the residents. It was his transcriptions that inspired me to write this book. Ed was my mentor in neuroradiology, and he is the kind of teacher that any student would love to have.

RHH

Most of the MR images in the chapter on MRI artifacts are compliments of John E. Jordan, MD, MPP. Thanks to Dar-Yeong Chen, PhD and Dennis Atkinson, MS, for their scientific help. Thanks to Cathy Reichel-Clark for her excellent art work.

RHH/WGB

Contents

Part I Basic Concepts

INTRODUCTION

In this chapter, we will review some of the basic mathematical concepts that are used in MR imaging. We don't want to scare you away so we'll keep things as simple as possible. An understanding of these basic concepts will help the reader a great deal to comprehend the subtleties of MR imaging and obtain the necessary tools for manipulating the scan parameters to improve the quality of the images.

It is not that important to memorize these mathematical formulas; what's crucial is the understanding of the **concepts** behind these formulas. In this chapter, we hope to emphasize the most important mathematical concepts of MRI physics.

SINUSOIDALS

Consider a **right triangle** (having a right angle) with sides a and b and hypotenuse c and angle x formed by a and c (Fig. 1-1). We can define $\sin x$ (read *sine* of x), $\cos x$ (read *cosine* of x), $\tan x$ (read *tangent* of x), $\cot x$ (read *cotangent* of x), and $\arctan x$ (read *arc-tangent* of x) in terms of a, b, and c:

$$\sin x = b/c$$
$$\cos x = a/c$$
$$\tan x = \sin x/\cos x = b/a$$
$$\cot x = 1/\tan x = \cos x/\sin x = a/b$$
$$\arctan b/a = \arctan (\tan x) = x \qquad \text{(Eqn. 1-1)}$$

The variable x can be represented in degrees, i.e., 45°, 90°, and 180°, or it can be represented in radians, i.e., $\pi/4$, $\pi/2$, and π, where $\pi = 180°$. Table 1-1 shows x vs. $\sin x$, $\cos x$, and $\tan x$, where $\sqrt{2} \cong 1.4$ so $\sqrt{2}/2 \cong .7$ and $\sqrt{3} \cong 1.7$ so $\sqrt{3}/2 \cong .85$.

Let's plot x vs. $\sin x$ (Fig. 1-2). This is called a sinusoidal function. What about $\cos x$? (Fig. 1-3). Let's now draw $\cos x$ and $\sin x$ on a single graph (Fig. 1-4). We can appreciate the symmetry between $\sin x$ and $\cos x$. The difference between the two functions is that $\sin x$ is shifted to the right of $\cos x$ by 90°. Later, when we talk about phase and phase shifts, this mathematical concept will become more important. We can think of $\sin x$ as being $\cos x$ with a phase difference of 90°.

Now, let's go back to Figure 1-1. What is c in terms of a, b? According to the Pythagorean Theorem:

$$c^2 = a^2 + b^2 \text{ or } c = \sqrt{(a^2 + b^2)}$$

By Eqn. 1-1

$$(\sin x)^2 + (\cos x)^2 = b^2/c^2 + a^2/c^2$$
$$= (a^2 + b^2)/c^2$$
$$= c^2/c^2 = 1$$

So,

$$(\sin x)^2 + (\cos x)^2 = 1.$$

If we go back to our graph of $\sin x$ and $\cos x$ (Fig. 1-4) we can see graphically that because of the **phase difference** between the $\cos x$ and $\sin x$, the sum of their squares will always equal 1. Another way of looking at *sine* and *cosine* is to consider a circle with a radius of 1 (Fig. 1-5). To understand this concept, it is necessary to bring up the concepts of vectors, imaginary numbers, and exponentials.

Vector

We'll designate a vector by using a letter such as **v** with an arrow above it ($\vec{v}$). This concept will become important later on in the understanding of resonance of spins and dephasing. A vector is a mathematical entity that has both a magnitude and a direction. For example, speed is not a vector—it only has magnitude. Velocity,

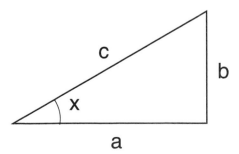

Figure 1-1. A right triangle with sides *a* and *b* and hypotenuse *c* and angle *x* formed by *a* and *c*.

Table 1-1

	0	$\pi/6$	$\pi/4$	$\pi/3$	$\pi/2$	π
x	0°	30°	45°	60°	90°	180°
sin x	0	1/2	$(\sqrt{2})/2$	$(\sqrt{3})/2$	1	0
cos x	1	$(\sqrt{3})/2$	$(\sqrt{2})/2$	1/2	0	−1
tan x	0	$1/(\sqrt{3})$	1	$\sqrt{3}$	∞	0

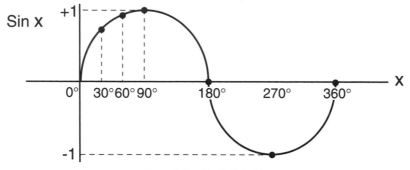

Figure 1-2.   Graph of sin (x).

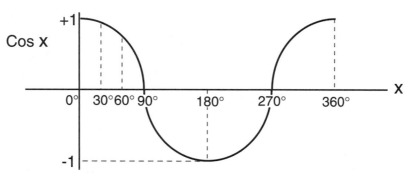

Figure 1-3.   Graph of cos (x).

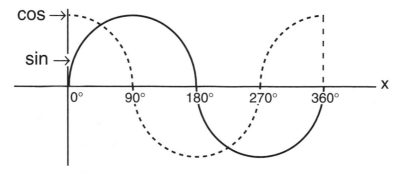

Figure 1-4.   Sin (x) and cos (x) plotted on the same graph.

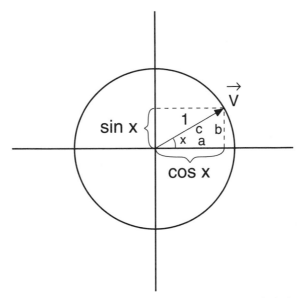

Figure 1-5. A vector **v** with magnitude 1 and angle x to the horizontal. cos x and sin x are the horizontal and vertical components of this vector, respectively.

however, is a vector—it has both magnitude and direction. Another example of a vector is *force* that describes a magnitude (*weight*) and a direction (direction where the force is applied).

The vector that we've drawn in the circle (Fig. 1-5) has a magnitude of 1. The angle between the vector and the horizontal axis is denoted x. If we draw perpendiculars from the vector both horizontally and vertically, we'll get two components of the vector:

(a) The horizontal component of the vector would correspond to cos x. (Remember that the ratio a/c in Figure 1-1 is cos x.)
(b) The vertical component of the vector would correspond to sin x. (Remember that the ratio b/c in Figure 1-1 is sin x.)

Imaginary Numbers

A positive number n^2 has two square roots, $+n$ and $-n$. For example,

$$3^2 = 9$$
$$(-3)^2 = 9$$

so (3) and (−3) are the square roots of 9.

It is impossible to square a real number and have a negative product. Therefore, we shall make up an entity and call the number $\sqrt{-n}$ an **imaginary number**. Any of the following would be

imaginary numbers:

$$(\sqrt{-9}), (\sqrt{-37}), (\sqrt{-1}), (\sqrt{-18})$$

Imaginary numbers can be manipulated in the following way:

$$(\sqrt{-9}) = \sqrt{[(9)(-1)]} = (\sqrt{9})(\sqrt{-1}),$$

Any imaginary number can be written as a positive number times $(\sqrt{-1})$. The expression $(\sqrt{-1})$ is designated by the letter "i". (Mathematicians use the symbol i to denote an imaginary number, whereas engineers use the symbol "j" in lieu of i because i is reserved to symbolize electric current!). The symbol i is then known as the **imaginary unit**. In other words, $i \times i = -1$.

EXAMPLES:

$$\sqrt{-16} = \sqrt{(16)(-1)} = \sqrt{16}\sqrt{-1} = i\sqrt{16} = 4i$$

So i is an **imaginary** number. It doesn't exist. When you take a square root of a number, it has to be a positive number. However, in this case, if we multiply i by i, we get (−1). Therefore, i is an imaginary number that doesn't exist.

Complex Numbers

A **complex** number is a number that has both a **real** and an **imaginary** component:

Complex = real + imaginary

EXAMPLE:

Let's say a complex number has two components: 2 and 3. The imaginary component is multiplied by (*i*), where $i = \sqrt{-1}$ is the imaginary unit. Then,

$$c = (2) + i(3)$$

If you draw this complex number on an x-y plane (Fig. 1-6), the vector (2,3) illustrates the complex number 2 + 3i. Usually you only care about the real part of a complex number, but it makes life easier to deal with the complex number and carry all the computations using complex numbers or vectors and then, at the end, just keep the real part.

Magnitude, Angle

Sometimes, however, the imaginary part is also helpful. For example, consider Figure 1-6. In this diagram, if we take the tangent of the **angle** between the vector and the x-axis, we get

$$tan\ \theta = 3/2 = imaginary/real$$

In other words, the ratio of imaginary part to the real part gives us the *tangent* of the **angle**. The **magnitude** of the vector (sometimes called the **modulus**) is given by the **Pythagorean**

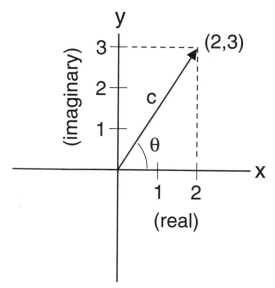

y

3 ┄┄┄┄┄ (2,3)

(imaginary)

2

c

1

θ

————————————— x

1 2

(real)

Figure 1-6. Representation of a complex number 2 + i 3 as a point in a two-dimensional (Cartesian) coordinate system and the relationship between a complex number, its angle *θ*, and its real and imaginary components.

Theorem

$$c = \sqrt{(a^2 + b^2)}$$

Thus,

vector magnitude
$$= \sqrt{[(imaginary\ part)^2 + (real\ part)^2]}$$
$$= \sqrt{[(3)^2 + (2)^2]} = \sqrt{13} \cong 3.6$$

When you're dealing with a complex number, if you take the ratio of the imaginary part to the real part, you get some sort of measure of the **angle** of the vector. If you sum the squares of the imaginary and real part, you get the **magnitude** of the vector (squared).

Function

A mathematical function, designated as $f(x)$, is an entity that varies with respect to a variable, x. For example, *sin x* is a function that varies with respect to x in a sinusoidal manner, as we saw earlier in the chapter.

Signal

A signal is a time-varying function, i.e., something that varies over time, usually milli-volts versus time. If the x-axis is time, and the y-axis is magnitude, then a signal is a **waveform** that varies in magnitude with time.

In an electrical system, a signal is a time-varying current or voltage that can be measured. In MRI, the signal is just a current or voltage that is induced by an oscillating magnetic field. Some signals are periodic—they *repeat* themselves-as the *sine* wave or *cosine* wave repeats itself.

Frequency, Period, Cycle

Let's now introduce the concepts of **frequency** and **period**. Every periodic function has a frequency which we will call *f*. If we measure the time interval between two peaks (or where the signal crosses zero), this interval is called a **period**, and we'll denote this by *T*. Now, frequency = 1/period = 1/T:

$$f = 1/T$$

A **cycle** in a periodic function is any part of the function over one period. For example, let's

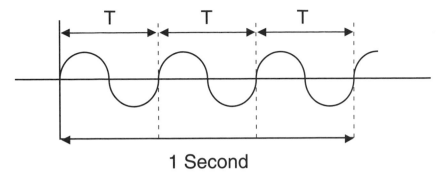

Figure 1-7. An example of a periodic signal spanning three cycles in 1 second. The period is thus one-third of 1 second (1/3 sec).

say that we have three complete cycles occurring in 1 second (Fig. 1-7). In this case,

$$3 \text{ periods take 1 second}$$
$$3\,T = 1 \text{ second}$$
$$T = 1/3 \text{ seconds}$$
$$\text{Frequency} = f = 1/T = 3$$
$$\text{cycles/second} = 3 \text{ Hertz}$$

The unit we use to describe frequency is Hertz or Hz (for cycles/second). There are 2π radians in one cycle. That is to say,

f = frequency when we refer to **linear frequency** in cycles/sec;

ω = frequency when we refer to **angular frequency** in radians/sec; angular frequency (in radians/seconds) = $\omega = (2\pi) \times$ linear frequency (in Hz)

where $\pi = 3.1415927 \cong 3.14$. In short,

$$\omega = 2\pi f \qquad \text{(Eqn. 1-2)}$$

EXAMPLE:
If the vector in the circle makes 3 revolutions/second, then the vector has a frequency of 3 Hz. Therefore, $\omega = (2\pi)(3) = 6\pi = 18.85$ radians/second.

Sometimes a signal (such as a *sine* wave) is represented in the following way:

$$S(t) = \sin(\omega t) = \sin(2\pi f t)$$

Here we can say that the signal is a *sine* wave with a frequency of ω. So, frequency $= f = \omega/2\pi$.

EXAMPLE:
Draw the signal *sin* (ωt) versus time t assuming $f = 1$ Hz (i.e., $T = 1$ sec or $\omega = 2\pi$ radians/sec). Thus, $\sin(\omega t) = \sin(2\pi t)$. This equation is illustrated in Figure 1-8:

when $t = 0$, then $\omega t = 0$, resulting in
$\sin \omega t = \sin 0 = 0$;
when $t = 1/4$, then $\omega t = (2\pi)(1/4) = \pi/2$,
resulting in $\sin \omega t = \sin \pi/2 = 1$;
when $t = 1/2$, then $\omega t = (2\pi)(1/2) = \pi$,
resulting in $\sin \omega t = \sin \pi = 0$; etc.

Phase

Now, let's talk about **phase**. Consider two *sine* waves, with one shifted slightly compared with the other (Fig. 1-9). The two sinusoids have the same frequency—they oscillate at the same rate—but one of them is **shifted** just a little

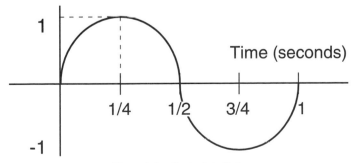

Figure 1-8. Graph of sin $(2\pi t)$.

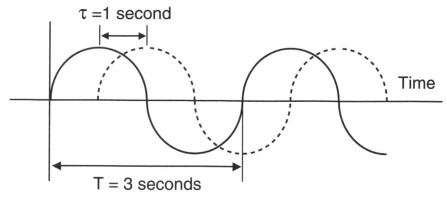

Figure 1-9. Two similar sinusoidal signals with a phase offset.

from the other. Suppose they are shifted apart from each other by a time interval $= \tau = 1$ second. Suppose further that the period of 1 cycle $= T = 3$ seconds (Fig. 1-10).

$T = 1$ period $= 360°$ in 3 seconds
$\tau = 1$ second $= 1/3$ of the total time of 1 period

Thus, $1/3$ of $360° = 120°$. This measurement is the **phase offset** or **phase shift** of the two sinusoidals.

EXAMPLE:

What is *sin* $(x + 90°)$?
Here we have the *sine* wave and a phase offset of 90°. Let's figure out what this looks like on a circle diagram (Fig. 1-10). If *x* is the angle, *sine* of vector *x* is the initial component

perpendicular to vector. Take a phase offset of 90°. This offset causes the original vector to be rotated counterclockwise by 90°, as can be seen in Figure 1-10. Now, drop a vertical perpendicular from this new vector. Because the *vertical* component of a vector is equal to the *sine* of its angle, then the vertical component of the new vector (with its new angle *x + 90°*) *is sine* of (x + 90°). Now, by the law of *congruent triangles*, this new vertical component (which is longer than the horizontal component in Figure 1-10) is equal to the longer horizontal component of the original angle *x*, which is, in fact, *cos x*. In other words,

$$sin\ (x + 90°) = cos\ x \qquad \text{(Eqn. 1-3)}$$

From this we see that *sine* and *cosine* of any given vector have a phase difference of 90°.

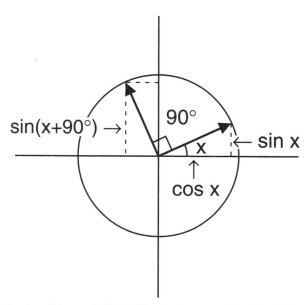

Figure 1-10. Two vectors with a phase difference of 90°. This difference demonstrates the relationship between cos (x) and sin (x + 90°).

EXPONENTIALS

With **exponential functions** (e^x), the letter e is the base of the natural logarithm with a numerical value of

$$e = 2.7182818 \cong 2.72$$

First, let's consider the values of e^x for various values of *x*:

for $x = 0$, $e^0 = 1$ (anything to the power of $0 = 1$)
for $x = 1$, $e^1 = 2.72$.
for $x = 2$, $e^2 = (2.72)(2.72) = 7.4$.
for $x = \infty$, $e^\infty = \infty$
for $x = -1$, $e^{-1} = 1/e = 1/2.72 = 0.37$.
for $x = -2$, $e^{-2} = 1/e^2 = 1/(2.72)(2.72)$
                        $= 0.14$
for $x = -3$, $e^{-3} = 0.05$
for $x = -\infty$, $e^{-\infty} = 0$

If we graph e^x, we see that it is an exponentially growing function (Fig. 1-11). From this graph,

we can see that the function e^x *grows* exponentially from $-\infty$ to $+\infty$.

Now let's consider a decaying function by drawing (e^{-x}) (Fig. 1-12):

for $x = 0$, $e^0 = 1$
for $x = 1$, $e^{-1} = 0.37$
for $x = 2$, $e^{-2} = 0.14$
for $x = 3$, $e^{-3} = 0.05$
for $x = \infty$, $e^{-\infty} = 0$
for $x = -1$, $e^{-(-1)} = e^1 = 2.72$
for $x = -2$, $e^{-(-2)} = e^2 = 7.4$

This represents an exponentially *decaying* function. Let's change *x* to *t* and look at a time-varying function e^{-t} (Fig. 1-13). This now becomes a decaying function of time. Table 1-2 shows the values of e^{-t} for various values of t.

How about a graph of $(1 - e^{-t})$?

for $t = 0$, $(1 - e^{-t}) = 1 - 1 = 0$
for $t = 1$, $(1 - e^{-t}) = 1 - (2.7)^{-1} = 1 - 1/2.7$
                    $= 1 - 0.37 = 0.63$

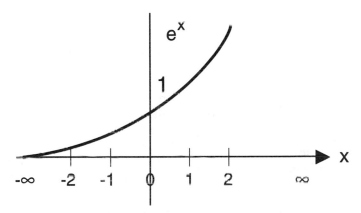

Figure 1-11. Graph of an exponentially growing function e^x.

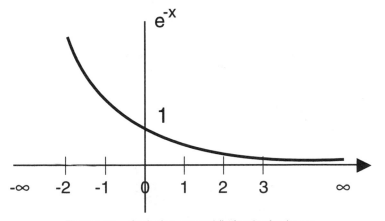

Figure 1-12. Graph of an exponentially decaying function e^{-x}.

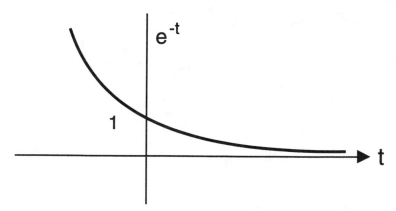

Figure 1-13. Graph of an exponentially decaying function of time e⁻ᵗ.

Table 1-2

t	0	1	2	3	4	5	...	∞
e^{-t}	1	.37	.14	.05	.02	.01	...	0
$1 - e^{-t}$	0	.63	.86	.95	.98	.99	...	1

for t = 2, $(1 - e^{-t}) = 1 - (2.7)^{-2} = 1 - 1/(2.7)$
$$(2.7) = 1 - 0.13 = 0.86$$

As *t* gets larger, e^{-t} gets much smaller, so that $(1 - e^{-t})$ approaches 1. Therefore, a graph of $1 - e^{-t}$ (Fig. 1-14) is the reverse of the exponential curve for e^{-t} (Fig. 1-13).

Time Constant or Decay Constant

In the graph of $(1 - e^{-t})$, the value gets close to 1 after about four to five **time constants**. Let's make the exponential function a little more complicated. Consider

$$e^{-t/\tau}$$

where τ is a **time constant**. So when t = τ, then

$$e^{-t/\tau} = e^{-1} = 0.37$$

If we draw a **tangent** at t = 0 (where the function equals 1 on the vertical axis) along the exponential decay curve $e^{-t/\tau}$, the point of intersection on the time line (i.e., the horizontal axis) is the time constant τ (Fig. 1-15). At this point, the value of $e^{-t/\tau} = e^{-1} = 0.37 \cong 1/3$. This means that at the time of one time constant, we have about one-third of the original signal left. The other interesting thing about this decaying function is that after two time constants (2τ), we are left with one-third of the signal that remained

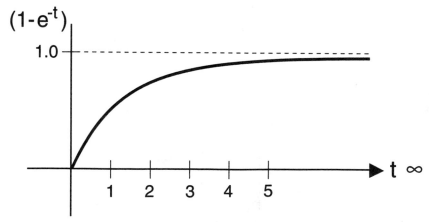

Figure 1-14. Graph of an exponentially growing function of time $1 - e^{-t}$.

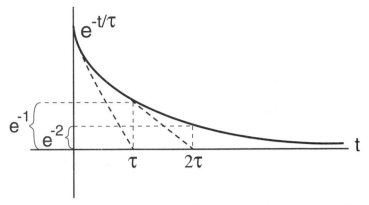

Figure 1-15. Graph of an exponentially decaying function $e^{-t/\tau}$, where τ is the time constant (decay rate).

after one time constant, which is $(e^{-2}) = e^{-1} \times e^{-1} \approx 1/3 \times 1/3 = 1/9$.

The nice thing about this exponentially decaying function is that you can stop anywhere on the curve and the same equation will apply. No matter how many time constants you extend out along the decay curve, you still end up with a calculable percentage value of the original signal.

On the recovery curve $(1 - e^{-t/\tau})$, things are just the opposite (Fig. 1-16). If you draw a tangent at the origin along the exponential recovery curve $(1 - e^{-t/\tau})$, the point of intersection on the maximum line corresponding to complete recovery occurs at one time constant (τ). At this point, we have recovered 63% of the original signal:

$$\text{for } t = \tau, (1 - e^{-t/\tau}) = 1 - e^{-1} \cong 1 - .37$$
$$- 0.63$$

At two time constants, (2τ), we will have recovered 63% of the remaining signal, which comes to 86%.

EXPONENTIALLY DECAYING SINUSOIDALS

We've talked about a *sine* wave ($\sin \omega t$). We've also talked about an exponential function ($e^{-t/\tau}$). What happens if we multiply these functions together?

$$(e^{-t/\tau}) \cdot (\sin \omega t)$$

The first function is a sinusoidal. The second function is a decaying curve. If you multiply the two together, you'll get a graph as in Figure 1-17. The sinusoidal function will have the same frequency but it's contained between the "**envelopes**" of the decaying exponential curve and its mirror image, causing the **magnitude** of the *sine* wave to decrease exponentially with time.

Sinc FUNCTION

There is another function that looks somewhat like Figure 1-17. It is called a *sinc* function

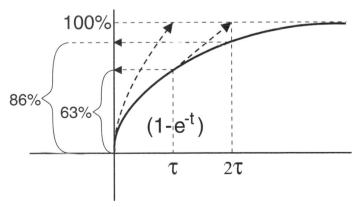

Figure 1-16. Graph of an exponentially growing function $1 - e^{-t/\tau}$, where τ is the time constant (growth rate).

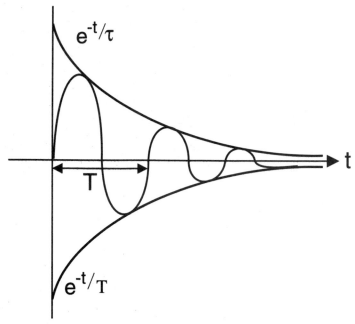

Figure 1-17.   Graph of $e^{-t/\tau} \times \cos \omega t$. This is a sinusoidal function with angular frequency ω whose "envelope" is given by $e^{-t/\tau}$ and $-e^{-t/\tau}$.

and is expressed as $(\sin t)/t$:

$$\frac{\sin(t)}{t} = sinc(t) \qquad \text{(Eqn. 1-4)}$$

Question: What is sinc t at time $t = 0$,?
Answer: $sinc (0) = \sin (0)/0 = 0/0$ which is **indeterminate**. However, using the principles of differential equations and limits, it can be shown than $sinc (0) = 0/0 = 1$ (refer to Problem 1-3). From here on, sinc (t) is an oscillating wave

of t (Fig. 1-18). However, the envelope of this wave is not an exponential function. This is what an **RF (Radio Frequency) pulse** generally looks like. (The **frequency** or **Fourier transform** [FT] of this pulse is a rectangle. More about this later.)

Having been introduced to the concepts of vectors, imaginary numbers, and exponentials, let's again go back to the vector in Fig. 1-5 and introduce a new equation called "Euler's equation." (The importance of this equation will be-

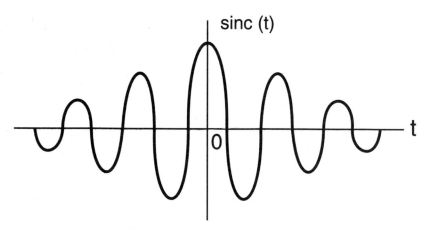

Figure 1-18.   Graph of sinc (t) = sin (t)/t.

come clear later when the concept of "spinning protons" is addressed.)

EULER'S EQUATION:

$$e^{i\theta} = \cos\theta + i\sin\theta \qquad \text{(Eqn. 1-5)}$$

This equation describes the vector that we saw in Figure 1-5 with an angle $= \theta$ and a magnitude $= 1$. The symbol i is the imaginary unit $\sqrt{-1}$. Equation 1-5 expresses a complex exponential function of an imaginary number $(i\theta)$ in terms of the *sine* and *cosine* functions of the angle θ.

Now consider the Euler's equation for the complex signal $e^{i\omega t}$ (using ωt instead of θ):

$$e^{i\omega t} = \underbrace{\cos\omega t}_{\text{real}} + i\underbrace{\sin\omega t}_{\text{imaginary}}$$

This formula has a "real" part and an "imaginary" part. The real part ($\cos\omega t$) is what we are interested in because it corresponds to the measured signal. We use the imaginary part ($\sin\omega t$) because it makes the mathematics simpler (believe it or not!). At the end, we ignore the imaginary part and keep the real component corresponding to the actual signal.

Each value of ($e^{i\omega t}$) is a **vector** that spins around at an angular frequency of ω (Fig. 1-19). It is important to understand the concept of angular frequency because, later when we talk about proton precession, we'll see that the principle of precessional frequency (which is an angular frequency) is used frequently.

LOGARITHMS

The logarithm (log) is sort of the inverse of an exponential, i.e.,

$$\log(e^x) = x$$

The base of log is usually 10. However, a logarithm can have any base. Let's say that the *log* of a number y with base a is equal to x:

$$\log_a y = x$$

Then, taking the exponential of both sides, we obtain

$$a^x = y$$

Thus,

$$\log_a y = x \Leftrightarrow a^x = y$$

That is, if the *log* of y with base a equals x, this implies that a to the power of x equals y.

EXAMPLE:

$$\log_2 8 = 3 \Rightarrow 2^3 = (2)(2)(2) = 8$$

The *log* of a number x to base e is also denoted as the *ln* of that number, or "the natural *log*" of x.

$$\log_e x \equiv \ln x$$

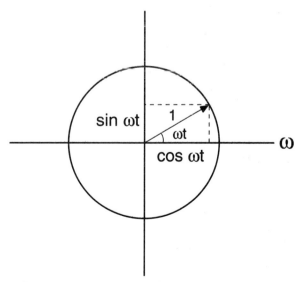

Figure 1-19. Representation of $e^{i\omega t}$ in terms of a rotating vector.

(*ln*) is just the notation for *log* to the base e (e is the base of the natural logarithm, e = 2.71...).

$$ln\ e = log_e\ e = 1$$

This means *log* of e to its own base is 1.

PROPERTIES OF EXPONENTIALS

Mathematical operations done with exponentials include: (e^x is e to the power of x)

(a)   Multiplying exponentials

$$(e^x) \cdot (e^y) = e^{x+y}$$

(b)   Negative exponentials

$$e^{-x} = 1/e^x$$

(c)   Dividing exponentials

$$e^x/e^y = e^{x-y}$$

DERIVATION:
Equation (c) is derived from the first two equations (a) and (b) in the following way:

$e^x/e^y = (e^x)(e^{-y})$ derived from the statement
about negative exponentials;
$(e^x) \cdot (e^{-y}) = e^{x-y}$ derived from the statement
about multiplying exponentials.

Therefore, $e^x/e^y = (e^x)\ (e^{-y}) = e^{x-y}$

PROPERTIES OF LOGARITHMS

(a)   The logarithm of the product of two numbers (A and B) is equal to the sum of their logarithms.

$$log\ (A \cdot B) = log\ A + log\ B$$

This holds for *any base*. So,

$$ln\ (A \cdot B) = ln\ A + ln\ B$$

(b)   The *log* of x to a power *a* is

$$log\ x^a = a\ log\ x$$

This also holds for any base, so:

$$log_b\ x^a = a\ log_b\ x$$
$$ln\ x^a = a\ ln\ x$$

EXAMPLE:
Let's solve the equation: $1/2 = e^{-t/T2}$ for *t*. (This would be the formula for finding the time *t* when a function [with a first-order decay constant T2] decays to half of its initial value.)

1. take *ln* of both sides:
$$ln\ (1/2) = ln\ e^{-t/T2}$$

2. Remember that $1/2 = 2^{-1}$, so
$$ln\ (1/2) = ln\ (2^{-1}) = -ln2$$

3. Now from (b) above,
$$ln\ (e^{-t/T2}) = -t/T2\ ln\ (e)$$
so
$$-ln2 = -t/T2\ ln\ (e)$$

4. Remember that $ln\ (e) = log_e e = 1$ (*log* of a number to its own base = 1), so
$$-ln2 = -t/T2\ (1)\ \text{or}$$
$$-ln2 = -t/T2$$

5. Multiply both sides by −1:
$$ln2 = t/T2\ \text{or}$$
$$log_e2 = t/T2\ \text{or}$$
$$.693 = t/T2\ \text{or}$$
$$t = .693\ (T2).$$

This formula also calculates the half-time (or $t_{1/2}$) in nuclear medicine.

Key Points

Understanding a few mathematical concepts will help you a great deal in understanding of MR physics.

1. Four sinusoidal functions were discussed:
$$sin\ x, cos\ x, tan\ x, cotan\ x$$
$$tan\ x = sin\ x/cos\ x$$
$$cotan\ x = 1/tan\ x$$

2. The angle (or *arc*) on which the above sinusoidal wave is applied is defined as:
$$arcsin, arccos, arctan, arccotan$$
For example,
$$arctan\ (tan\ x\ ) = x\ , arcsin\ (sin\ x) = x\ , etc.$$

3. A *vector* possesses magnitude and direction. *Force*, for example, has magnitude (*weight*) and direction. Another example of a vector is *velocity,* which has a *speed* and a direction.

4. *Imaginary numbers* are represented by a *real* and an *imaginary* component:

$$c = a + ib$$

where i is the imaginary unit $\sqrt{-1}$.

5. A *function f* of a variable x is designated $f(x)$ and represents variations in f as x is varied.

6. A *signal* is a function of time.

7. A *periodic signal* is a function of time that repeats itself after a certain *period T.*

8. The (linear) *frequency* of a periodic signal is defined as $f = 1/T$, where T is the period.

9. The *angular frequency* ω is defined as $\omega = 2\pi f$.

10. A periodic signal over one period represents one *cycle.*

11. An example of a periodic signal is $\cos \omega t = \cos (2\pi ft)$.

12. *Phase* represents the offset between two periodic signals of the same frequency. For example, $\cos (\omega t)$ and $\cos (\omega t + \theta)$ have the same frequency (ω) but are *out of phase* by θ.

13. The function e^t is an *exponential* function of time. It is actually an exponentially *growing* function. It is 1 at $t = 0$ and ∞ at $t = \infty$. At $t = 1$, $e^1 = e = 2.7182818 \cong 2.72$.

14. The function e^{-t} is also an exponential function of time. It is an exponentially decaying function. It is 1 at $t = 0$ and 0 at $t = \infty$. At $t = 1$, $e^{-1} = 0.37$.

15. The function $e^{-t/\tau}$ is an exponentially decaying function with a *time constant* or *decay constant* τ. The value of the signal at time constant τ is 37% ($e^{-1} = 0.37$) of its previous value. The signal is practically zero after five time constants ($e^{-5} \cong 0$).

16. The function $e^{i\omega t}$ is given by *Euler's equation* as

$$e^{i\omega t} = \cos \omega t + i \sin \omega t$$

which represents a vector of radius 1 spinning at an angular frequency ω (in radians/sec).

17. The *sinc* function is defined as

$$\text{sinc } t = \sin t/t$$

which is 1 at $t = 0$. An ideal RF pulse is a sinc wave because its *Fourier Transform* (as we will see later) has a perfect rectangular shape.

18. A *logarithm* (base 10) of a variable y is represented as *log y* and is related to an exponential as

if $\log y = x$ then $10^x = y$

19. The *natural logarithm* (base e) of y is designated *ln y.* Therefore,

if $\ln y = x$ then $e^x = y$.

Having understood the above mathematical concepts, the reader can now read and understand the remainder of this book with greater ease. As mentioned previously, it is not that important to memorize the formulas, but rather to understand the *concepts* behind them.

Questions

1-1. Draw the following functions versus x (from $-\infty$ to $+\infty$)
(a) $\tan x$ (b) $e^{-x} \sin x$ (c) $\sin x/x \equiv \text{sinc } (x)$

1-2. Prove the following equalities
(a) $\cos (x + y) = \cos x \cdot \cos y - \sin x \cdot \sin y$
(b) $\sin (x+y) = \cos x \cdot \sin y + \sin x \cdot \cos y$

Hint: Make use of the Euler equation $e^{ix} = \cos x + i \sin x$ and note that $i \times i = i^2 = -1$

1-3. It can be shown that for certain functions

$$f(0)/g(0) = \lim_{x \to 0} [f(x)/g(x)]$$
$$= \lim_{x \to 0} [f'(x)/g'(x)]$$

where f and g are functions of x and f' and g' are their derivatives, i.e.

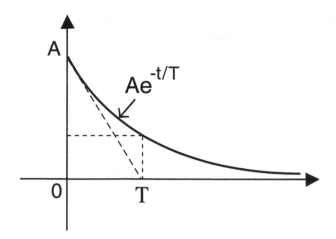

Figure P1-1a

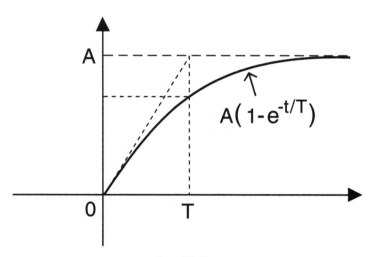

Figure P1-1b

[f′(x) = d/dx f(x)]; "lim" denotes the "limit" as x approaches 0.

Using the above fact, show that

$$\text{sinc}\,(0) = \sin\,(0)/0 = \lim_{x \to 0} (\sin x)/x = 1$$

Hint: d/dx (sin x) = cos x and d/dx (x^n) = n x^{n-1} (n = any integer)

1-4.   (a)   What is the value of an exponential function e$^{-t/T}$ at one time constant T.
(b)   How about at two time constants 2T.
(c)   What is the ratio of (b) to (a).

1-5.   Take the exponentially decaying function $f(t) = A\,e^{-t/T}$ as shown in Fig. P1-1a.
(a)   Prove that if a tangent is drawn at point A, it will cross the t-axis at t = T (T = decay constant).
(b)   Demonstrate the same principle for A (1−e$^{-t/T}$) as shown in Fig. P1-1b.
Hint: The derivative d/dt (e$^{\alpha t}$) = α e$^{\alpha t}$, where α = a constant.

1-6.   Solve the equation e^x = 4 for x. Note: *ln* 2 = 0.693.

2 Basic Principles of MRI

INTRODUCTION

In this chapter, we will discuss the basic principles behind the physics of *magnetic resonance imaging* (MRI). Some of these principles are explained using **Newtonian physics**, and some using **quantum mechanics**, whichever can convey the message more clearly. Although this might be confusing at times, it seems to be unavoidable. In any case, we'll try to keep it straightforward.

Nuclear magnetic resonance (NMR) is a chemical analytical technique that has been used for over 50 years. It is the basis for the imaging technique we now call MRI. (The word *nuclear* had the false connotation of the use of nuclear material; thus, it was discarded from the MR lexicon and "NMR tomography" was replaced by the phrase *magnetic resonance imaging* [MRI].)

ELECTROMAGNETIC WAVES

To understand MRI, we first need to understand what an electromagnetic wave is. Table 2-1 demonstrates the characteristics of a variety of electromagnetic waves, including X-ray, visible light, microwaves, and radio waves. All electromagnetic waves have certain fundamental properties in common:

1. They all travel at the speed of light $c = 3 \times 10^8$ meters/second.
2. By Maxwell's wave theory, they all have two components—an **electric field** E and a **magnetic field** B—that are perpendicular to each other (Fig. 2-1). We will designate the sinusoidal wave, which is drawn in the plane of the paper, the electrical field E. Perpendicular to it is

Table 2-1. The Electromagnetic Spectrum Illustrating the Windows for Radiowaves, Microwaves, Visible Light, and X-rays.

	Frequency (Hz)	Energy (eV)	Wavelength (m)
Gamma rays and X-rays	10^{24}	10^{10}	10^{-16}
	10^{23}	10^9	10^{-15}
	10^{22}	10^8	10^{-14}
	10^{21}	10^7	10^{-13}
	10^{20}	10^6 (1 MeV)	10^{-12} (1 pm)
	10^{19}	10^5	10^{-11}
	10^{18}	10^4	10^{-10}
Ultraviolet	10^{17}	10^3 (1 keV)	10^{-9} (1 nm)
	10^{16}	10^2	10^{-8}
Visible light	10^{15}	10^1	10^{-7}
Infrared	10^{14}	10^0 (1 eV)	10^{-6} (1 μ)
	10^{13}	10^{-1}	10^{-5}
Microwaves	10^{12} (1 GHz)	10^{-2}	10^{-4}
	10^{11}	10^{-3}	10^{-3} (1 mm)
	10^{10}	10^{-4}	10^{-2} (1 cm)
	10^9	10^{-5}	10^{-1}
MRI	10^8 (100 MHz)	10^{-6}	10^0 (1 m)
	10^7	10^{-7}	10^1
Radiowaves	10^6 (1 MHz)	10^{-8}	10^2
	10^5	10^{-9}	10^3 (1 km)
	10^4	10^{-10}	10^4
	10^3 (1 kHz)	10^{-11}	10^5
	10^2	10^{-12}	10^6

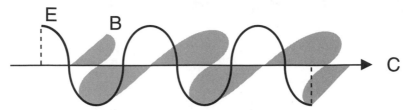

Figure 2-1.   Two components of an electromagnetic wave, the electric component *E* and the magnetic component *B*. These two component are perpendicular with each other, are 90° out of phase, and travel at the speed of light (*c*).

another sinusoidal wave, the magnetic field *B*. They are perpendicular to each other and both are traveling at the speed of light (*c*). The electric and magnetic fields have the same frequency and are 90° *out of phase* with each other. (This is due to the fact that the *change* in the electric field generates the magnetic field and the *change* in the magnetic field generates the electric field. For this reason, electromagnetic waves are self propagating once started and continue out to infinity.)

3. If we think in terms of vectors, the vectors *B* and *E* are perpendicular to each other, and the propagation factor *C* is perpendicular to both (Fig. 2-2). Both the electrical and magnetic components have the same frequency ω. So what we get is a vector that is spinning (oscillating) around a point at angular frequency ω. Remember, the angular frequency ω is related to the linear frequency f:

$$\omega = 2\pi f$$

4. We are interested in the magnetic field component—the electric field component is undesirable because it generates heat.

Table 2-2 summarizes the important electromagnetic windows in nature. In this table, the

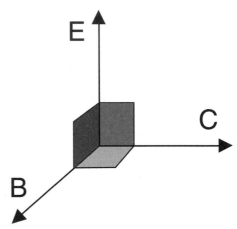

Figure 2-2.   The vector representation of *B, E,* and *c.*

following notations are used:

keV = 10^3 eV = kilo electron volts;
pm = 10^{-12} m = picometer;
nm = 10^{-9} m = nanometer;
MHz = 10^6 Hz = mega Hertz;
meV = 10^{-3} eV = milli electron volts.

In MRI, we deal with much lower energies than X-ray or even visible light. We also deal with much lower frequencies (the energy of an electromagnetic wave is directly proportional to its frequency, $E = h\,\nu$). The wave lengths are also much longer in the radio frequency (RF) window. Table 2-3 contains a few examples of frequency ranges in the electromagnetic spectrum.

Table 2-2

	Frequency (Hz = Hertz)	Energy (eV = electron volts)	Wave Length (m = meters)
X-ray	1.7-3.6 × 10^{18} Hz	30-150 keV	80-400 pm
Visible Light (Violet)	7.5 × 10^{14} Hz	3.1 eV	400 nm
Visible Light (Red)	4.3 × 10^{14} Hz	1.8 eV	700 nm
MRI	3-100 MHz	20-200 meV	6-60 meters

Table 2-3

AM radio frequency	0.54-1.6 MHz (540-1600 kHz)
TV (Channel 2)	slightly over 64 MHz
FM radio frequency	88.8-108.8 MHz
RF used in MRI	3-100 MHz

This is why the electromagnetic pulse used in MRI to get a signal is called an RF (radio frequency) pulse—it is in the **radio frequency** range. It belongs to the radio frequency *window* of the electromagnetic spectrum.

SPINS, ELECTROMAGNETIC FIELD

One of the pioneers of NMR theory was Felix Bloch of Stanford University, who won the Nobel prize in 1946 for his theories. He theorized that any **spinning charged particle** (like the hydrogen nucleus) creates an **electromagnetic field** (Fig. 2-3). The magnetic component of this field causes certain nuclei to act like a **bar magnet**; i.e., a magnetic field emanating from the South pole to the North pole (Fig. 2-4). In MRI, we are interested in **charged nuclei**, like the **hydrogen nucleus**, which is a single, positively charged proton (Fig. 2- 5).

The other thing that we know from quantum theory is that atomic nuclei each have specific **energy levels** related to a property called "**spin quantum number S**." For example, the hydrogen nucleus (a single proton) has a spin quantum

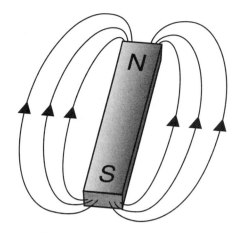

Bar Magnet

Figure 2-4. A bar magnet with its associated magnetic field.

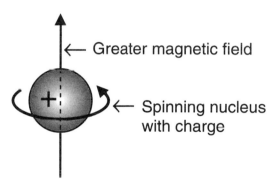

Figure 2-5. A spinning charged hydrogen nucleus (i.e., a proton) generating a magnetic field.

number S of ½:

$$S(^1H) = ½$$

The number of energy states of a nucleus is determined by the formula:

$$\text{\# of energy states} = 2S + 1$$

For a proton with a spin $S = ½$, we have

$$\text{\# of energy states} = 2(½) + 1 = 1 + 1 = 2$$

Therefore, a hydrogen proton has two energy states denoted as $-½$ and $+½$. This means that the hydrogen protons are spinning about their axis and creating a magnetic field. Some hydrogen protons spin the opposite way and have a magnetic field in just the opposite direction. The pictorial representation of the direction of proton

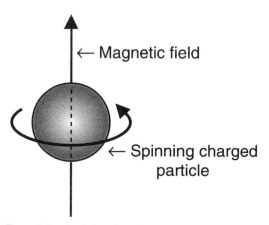

Figure 2-3. A spinning charged particle generates a magnetic fields.

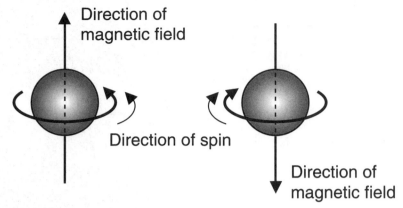

Figure 2-6.   The direction of the generated magnetic field depends on the direction of rotation of the spinning protons.

spins in Figure 2-6 represents the two energy states of the hydrogen proton. Each one of these directions of spin has a different energy state.

Other nuclei have different numbers of energy states. For example:

$$^{13}Na \text{ has a spin } S = \tfrac{3}{2};$$
$$\text{\# of energy states of } ^{13}Na = 2(\tfrac{3}{2}) + 1 = 4.$$

The 4 energy states of ^{13}Na are denoted as $(-\tfrac{3}{2}, -\tfrac{1}{2}, \tfrac{1}{2}, \tfrac{3}{2})$.

The important fact about all this is that in the hydrogen proton, we have one proton with two energy states that are aligned in opposite directions, one pointing north ("parallel"), the other pointing south ("anti-parallel"). (If there were an **even** number of protons in the nucleus, then every proton would be *paired*: for every proton spin with magnetic field pointing up, we'd have a paired proton spin with magnetic field pointing down [Fig. 2-7]. The magnetic fields of these paired protons would then cancel each other out, and the net magnetic field would

be zero.) When there is an **odd** number of protons, then there always exists one proton that is *unpaired*. That proton is pointing either north or south and gives a net magnetic field (Fig. 2-8) or a "**magnetic dipole moment**" (MDM) to the nucleus. Actually, a MDM is found in any nucleus with an *odd* number of protons, neutrons, or both. **Dipole-dipole interactions** refer to interactions between two protons or between a proton and an electron.

The nuclei of certain elements, such as Hydrogen (^1H) and Fluorine (^{19}F), have these properties (Table 2-4). Every one of these nuclei with

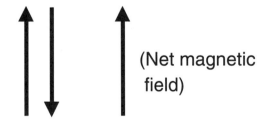

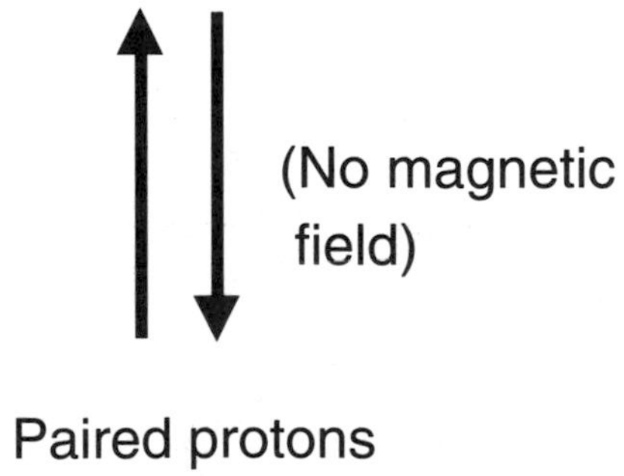

(Net magnetic field)

Unpaired protons

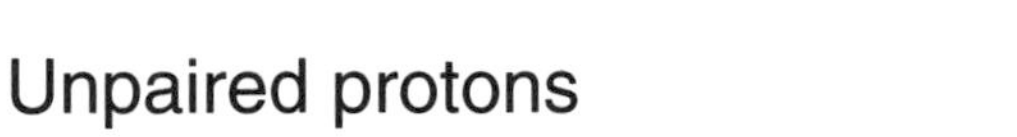

Figure 2-8.   Unpaired protons yield a net magnetic field.

Table 2-4

Nucleus	Spin Quantum Number (S)	Gyromagnetic Ratio* (MHz/T)
^1H	1/2	42.6
^{19}F	1/2	40.0
^{23}Na	3/2	11.3
^{13}C	1/2	10.7
^{17}O	5/2	5.8

(No magnetic field)

Paired protons

Figure 2-7.   The magnetic fields of paired protons (rotating in opposite directions) cancel each other out, leaving no net magnetic field.

an **odd** number of protons or neutrons can be used for imaging in MR. However, there is a reason why we stay with hydrogen. We use *hydrogen* for imaging because of its *abundance*. Approximately 60% of the body is *water*. We find hydrogen protons (^1H), for example, in water (H_2O) and fat ($-CH_2-$). Later on we'll find out how we use the spin of the hydrogen proton and avoid the spins of all the other nuclei with odd numbers of protons.

MAGNETIC SUSCEPTIBILITY

All substances get magnetized to a degree when placed in a magnetic field. However, the degree of magnification varies. The **magnetic susceptibility** of a substance (denoted by the Greek symbol χ) is a measure of *how* magnetized they get. In other words, χ is the measure of magnetizability of a substance.

To develop a mathematical relationship between the applied and induced magnetic fields, we first need to address the confusing issue regarding the differences between the two symbols encountered when dealing with magnetic fields: B and H. We caution the reader that the following is merely a simplification and that the interested reader should refer to an advanced physics textbook on the theory of electromagnetism. The field B is referred to as the **magnetic induction field** or **magnetic flux density**, which is the net magnetic field effect caused by an external magnetic field. The field H is referred to as the **magnetic field intensity**. These two magnetic fields are related by the following:

$$B = \mu H \text{ or } \mu = B/H$$

where μ represents the **magnetic permeability**, which is the ability of a substance to concentrate magnetic fields. The magnetic susceptibility χ is defined as the ratio of the induced magnetic field (M) to the applied magnetic field H:

$$M = \chi H \text{ or } \chi = M/H$$

Furthermore, χ and μ are related by the following:

$$\mu = 1 + \chi$$

making sure that the units used are consistent.

There are three types of substances—each with a different magnetic susceptibility—commonly dealt with in MRI: paramagnetic, diamagnetic, and ferromagnetic. These are described below.

Paramagnetism, Diamagnetism, Ferromagnetism

1. Diamagnetic substances have no unpaired orbital electrons. When such a substance is placed in an external magnetic field B_0, a weak magnetic field (M) is induced in the *opposite* direction to B_0. As a result, the effective magnetic field is *reduced*. Thus, diamagnetic substances have a small, negative magnetic susceptibility χ (i.e., $\chi < 0$ and $\mu < 1$). They are basically nonmagnetic. The vast majority of tissues in the body have this property. An example of diamagnetic effect is the distortion that occurs at an air-tissue interface (such as around paranasal sinuses).

2. **Paramagnetic** substances have unpaired orbital electrons. They become magnetized while the external magnetic field B_0 is on and become demagnetized once the field has been turned off. Their induced magnetic field (M) is in the *same* direction as the external magnetic field. Consequently, their presence causes an *increase* in the effective magnetic field. They therefore have a small positive χ (i.e., $\chi > 0$ and $\mu > 1$) and are weakly attracted by the external magnetic field. In such substances, **dipole-dipole** (i.e., proton-proton and proton-electron) interactions cause T1 shortening (bright signal on T1-weighted images). The element in the periodic table with the greatest number of unpaired electrons is the rare-earth element **gadolinium** (Gd) with seven unpaired electrons, which is a strong paramagnetic substance. Gd is a member of the **lanthanide** group in the periodic table. The rare-earth element **dysprosium** (Dy) is another strong paramagnetic substance that belongs to this group. Certain breakdown products of hemoglobin are paramagnetic: deoxyhemoglobin has four unpaired electrons, and methemoglobin has five. Hemosid-

erin, the end-stage of hemorrhage, contains, in comparison, more than 10,000 unpaired electrons. Hemosiderin belongs to a group of substances referred to as **superparamagnetic**, which have magnetic susceptibilities 100 to 1000 times stronger than paramagnetic substances.

3. **Ferromagnetic** substances are strongly attracted by a magnetic field. They become *permanently* magnetized even after the magnetic field has been turned off. They have a large positive χ, even larger than that of superparamagnetic substances. Three types of ferromagnets are known: iron (Fe), cobalt (Co), and nickel (Ni). Examples include aneurysm clips and shrapnel.

As stated earlier, the majority of tissues in the body are diamagnetic. For example, bulk water is diamagnetic. This may be surprising to hear because the protons that make up the water are the basis for NMR. It is true that the individual protons in a water molecule exhibit a magnetic moment (referred to as **nuclear magnetic moment** or **nuclear paramagnetism**), but bulk water is diamagnetic and its net induced magnetization is in the direction opposite to the main magnetic field. This has to do with the fact that NMR depends on nuclei (protons and neutrons) whereas bulk magnetism depends on electrons

(note that electrons demonstrate a magnetic moment much higher than that of protons due to their much larger mass).

HOW DO WE ACTUALLY PERFORM MR IMAGING?

Let's review a few examples of different types of imaging.

(a) In **photography**, there is an object and a light source that emits light. The light is reflected off the object and is then received by a photographic plate within a camera (Fig. 2-9). This, of course, is utilization of the visible light window of the electromagnetic spectrum. Visible light does not penetrate the object, but instead is reflected off of it.

(b) In **X-ray** imaging, we have an X-ray source that emits radiation which penetrates the object. This penetrating radiation is then received by a photographic (X-ray) plate (Fig. 2-10).

(c) In **MRI**, low frequency radiowaves penetrate the tissue and reflect back off magnetized spins within the object (Fig. 2-11).

RF and MR Signal

If spinning, unpaired protons are placed in an external magnetic field, they will line up with

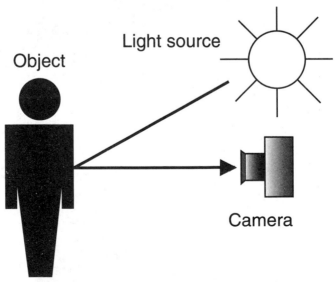

Figure 2-9.   In photography, light is reflected off the object and is received by a photographic plate in a camera.

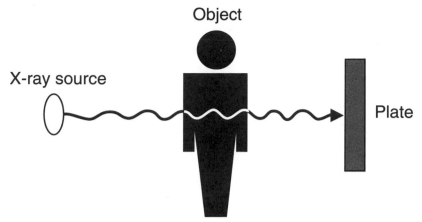

Figure 2-10. In X-ray, radiation penetrates the object and reaches a photographic plate behind the object.

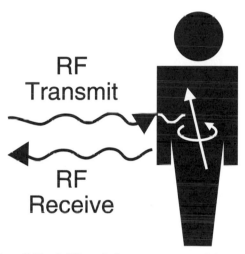

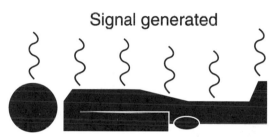

Figure 2-12. After the RF pulse, spins in the patient generate a signal which can be measured by a receiver.

Figure 2-11. In MRI, a radio-frequency wave, or a radiofrequency (RF) pulse, is transmitted into the patient, and a signal is received from magnetized spins (protons) in the body.

that magnetic field. If a radio frequency (RF) wave of a very specific frequency is then sent into the patient, some spins will change their alignment as a result of this new magnetic field. After the RF pulse, they generate a signal as they return to their original alignment. This is the MR signal that we measure (Fig. 2-12).

Spatial Encoding

If we generate a signal from the entire body, how do we differentiate whether the signal is coming from the head or the foot of the patient? This is the process of **spatial encoding** which is used to create an image. It requires the use of **gradient coils**, which will be discussed later in this chapter.

B_0 Field

The external magnetic field is denoted B_0. In MRI, B_0 is on the order of one Tesla (1T). One Tesla is equal to 10,000 Gauss. To appreciate the strength of this field, the earth's magnetic field, in comparison, is only about 0.5 Gauss (30,000 times weaker than a 1.5T scanner!). This field is not uniform in reality. These non-uniformities are usually caused by improper shimming or environmental distortions. The required standards for magnetic uniformity is on the order of 6-7 ppm (parts per million). Proper **shim coils** (see later text) can help minimize this problem.

TYPES OF MAGNETS

First of all, magnets can be categorized in terms of their field strength; five types exist:

1. Ultra high field (3.0 to 4.0 T): these are mainly used for research and MR Spectroscopy (MRS).
2. High field (1.0 to 2.0 T)
3. Midfield (0.3 to 1.0 T)

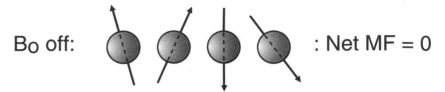

Figure 2-13. In the absence of an external magnetic field B_0, no net magnetization is produced by protons.

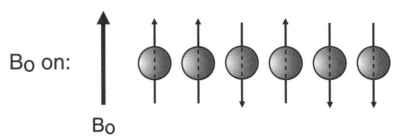

Figure 2-14. In the presence of an external magnetic field B_0, net magnetization is produced.

4. Low field (less than 0.1 to 0.2 T)
5. Ultra low field (less than 0.1 T)

Next, we can categorize magnets in terms of their design; three main types exist:

1. Permanent magnets
2. Resistive magnets
3. Superconducting magnets

(1) **Permanent magnets** (such as Fonar, Toshiba Access, and Hitachi MRP-5000) always stay on and cannot be turned off. They have the advantage of lower cost and lower maintenance (they require no cryogens for cooling).

(2) **Resistive magnets** (such as Siemens OPEN and Picker OUTLOOK) are based on the electromagnetic principle that electric current running through a coil produces a magnetic field. These magnets can be turned off and on.

(3) **Superconducting magnets** are a form of electromagnets. These magnets operate near absolute zero temperature (e.g., 4.2° Kelvin or −270° C). Consequently, there would be almost no resistance in their wires. This in turn allows us to use very strong electric currents to generate a high magnetic field without generating significant heat (hence the name superconducting). To achieve these ultra low temperatures, cryogens (such as liquid nitrogen and/or liquid helium) are required (which are very expensive). The majority of the available scanners today are superconducting magnets.

MAGNETIC DIPOLE MOMENT (MDM)

From now on, we will just talk about protons of hydrogen nuclei. We won't discuss any other nuclei. Let's take a number of protons. They all have their own small magnetic fields and they are all spinning about their own axes. Each one of the magnetic fields is called a **magnetic dipole moment (MDM)** and is denoted by the symbol μ. The axes of the magnetic dipole moments are arranged in a random way and they all cancel each other out. If we add up all the dipole moments, the **net** magnetic field will be zero (Fig. 2-13). This result occurs in the absence of any external magnetic field (B_0).

What happens if we turn on an external magnetic field? What would happen to the proton spins? They will act like bar magnets and line themselves up with the large magnetic field, much like compass needles in the earth's magnetic field (Fig. 2-14). But they don't all line up in the same direction. Approximately half point north and half point south. Eventually, enough extra spins point north (about one in a million[a])

---

[a] This number might appear insignificant. However, according to Avogadro's Law, there are over 10^{23} molecules per gram of tissue. Thus, in each gram of tissue, there will be 10^{17} (i.e., $10^{23}/10^6$) excess hydrogen protons pointing north.

to make the net magnetization point in the direction of B_0.

Let's examine how this happens. At time $t = 0$, proton spins are distributed randomly and the net magnetic field at $t = 0$ is zero. Immediately after being placed in a magnetic field, half the spins are lined up in the direction of the magnetic field and half are lined up in the reverse direction. Over time, more spins line up in the direction of the magnetic field, creating net magnetization (Fig. 2-15). If we graph the net magnetization versus time, it will look like the curve in Fig. 2-16. This increase in magnetization follows an *exponentially growing* curve that we talked about earlier (see Chapter 1). The time constant of this curve depends on the following:

1. the kind of tissue we are imaging
2. the strength of the magnet

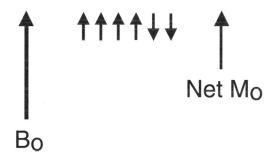

Net M$_O$

B$_0$

Figure 2-15. Vector representation of net magnetization M_0 a certain amount of time after introduction of the external magnetic field B_0.

T_1 RELAXATION TIME

The time constant of the curve in Figure 2.16 is denoted T_1. Therefore, the growth of magnetization M occurs with a time constant T_1 described by the equation $1 - e^{-t/T1}$. Usually, when we talk about T_1, we're talking about **recovery** of magnetization along the axis of the B_0 field. As time goes by, more and more spins are going to line up with the external magnetic field. The net magnetization keeps growing exponentially until it reaches a limit (Fig. 2-17). Remember how with an exponential growth curve we would draw a tangent at the beginning of the curve to establish T_1, and then we would draw a tangent from the curve at that time to establish $2\ T_1$? After about four or five T_1 times, we almost reach the plateau of the exponential growth curve.

If we were to change the *strength* of the magnetic field, what would happen to T_1? If B_0 decreases, the T_1 of the tissue also decreases:

$$\downarrow B_0 \rightarrow\ \downarrow T_1$$

For instance, biologic tissues have shorter T_1 values at 0.5 Tesla than at 1.5 Tesla.

PROTON (SPIN) DENSITY

Magnetization also depends on the *density* of the protons (or "**spins**"), i.e., how many protons per unit volume there are in the tissue. Certain tissues have more protons per unit volume than other tissues. For example, air doesn't have a large number of protons in it, so it has a very

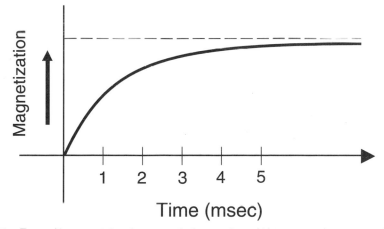

Figure 2-16. The graphic representation of net magnetization over time, which turns out to be an exponential function.

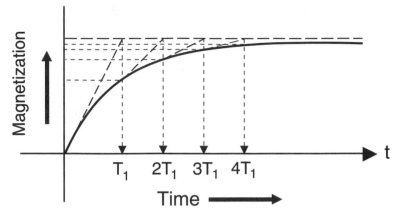

Figure 2-17. Net magnetization is described by the recovery curve $1 - e^{-t/T1}$, where T1 is the time constant (recovery rate).

small **proton density (spin density)**. We denote proton density or spin density by $N(H)$. It isn't just the *absolute number* of protons in the tissue that's important; it is also the number of protons that are **mobile** enough to be able to change direction and line up with the external magnetic field.

$$N(H) = \text{density of \textbf{mobile} protons}$$

The **net magnetization** at a particular time is based both on the T_1 of the tissue and on the mobile proton density:

$$\text{Magnetization} \propto N(H)\,(1 - e^{-t/T1})$$

If we redraw the T_1 growth curve, the x axis would be time, and the y axis would be:

$$M = N(H)\,(1 - e^{-t/T1}).$$

PRECESSION

When a proton is placed in a large magnetic field, it begins to "wobble" or **precess**. When we take a single proton spinning about its axis, but not in an external magnetic field, it will generate its own small magnetic field (Fig. 2-18). When we turn the external magnetic field *on*, the proton behaves like a spinning top, which not only spins about its own axis but also "**wobbles**" about the vertical axis as a result of gravity (Fig. 2-19). The proton, likewise, not only spins about its own axis, but also rotates or "precesses" about the axis of the external magnetic field (B_0).

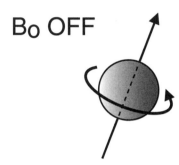

Figure 2-18. In the absence of an external magnetic field B_0, a proton rotating about its own axis generates a magnetic field.

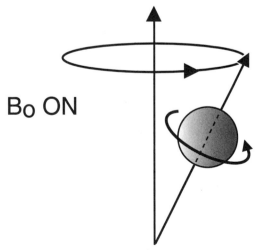

Figure 2-19. In the presence of an external magnetic field B_0, a proton not only rotates about its own axis but also "wobbles" about the axis of B_0.

Each proton spins much faster about its own axis than it rotates or precesses around the axis of the external magnetic field.

LARMOR EQUATION

The rate at which the proton precesses around the external magnetic field is given by an equation called the **Larmor equation**:

$$\omega = \gamma\, B_0 \qquad \text{(Eqn. 2-1)}$$

where ω = angular precessional frequency of proton, γ = gyromagnetic ratio, and B_0 = strength of external magnetic field.

The angular frequency ω can be expressed in Hertz (Hz) or radians per second, depending on the units used for γ. If γ is in terms of MHz/Tesla, then ω (or, actually, the linear frequency f) is expressed in terms of MHz. The gyromagnetic ratio γ is a proportionality constant that is fixed for the nucleus that we're dealing with. For hydrogen protons,

$$\gamma\,(H) = 42.6 \text{ MHz/Tesla}.$$

EXAMPLE:
If the magnetic field strength is 1 Tesla, the precessional frequency of hydrogen is

$$(42.6)\,(1) = 42.6 \text{ MHz}.$$

As the external magnetic field strength increases, the precessional frequency of the hydrogen proton also increases, i.e., at 1.5 Tesla the precessional frequency of hydrogen is

$$(42.6)\,(1.5) \cong 64 \text{ MHz}.$$

Remember that MRI involves the radio frequency portion of the electromagnetic spectrum, in the range of 3-100 MHz. This range is caused by the precessional frequency ranges of the hydrogen protons for the magnetic field strengths we use clinically, i.e.,

for B_0 from 0.064 T → 2 T,
$$\omega = 2.8 \text{ MHz} \to 85 \text{ MHz}.$$

COILS

A coil is an electrical device generally composed of multiple loops of wire (Fig. 2-20) that can either generate a magnetic field (**gradient coil**) or detect a changing (oscillating) magnetic

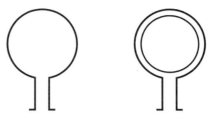

Figure 2-20. A coil is an electrical device generally composed of multiple loops of wire.

field as an electric current induced in the wire (**RF coil**). Several types of coils are used in MRI, including the following:

1. Gradient coils
   (a) imaging gradient coil
   (b) shim coil
2. Transmit and/or Receive RF Coils
   (a) single phase or quadrature (receive or transmit)
   (b) surface or volume (Hiemholtz or solenoid)
   (c) single or phased-array

Transmit/Receive Coil

A transmitter coil sends or transmits an RF pulse. A receiver coil receives an RF pulse. Some coils are both transmitters and receivers (such as body coils and head coils). Others are just receivers (e.g., surface coils). These coils act in much the same way as do radio or television antennas.

The body coil is a fixed part of the magnet that surrounds the patient and is used in a variety of applications as a transmitter and/or receiver. A head coil is a helmet-like device that surrounds the patient's head and may act as both a transmitter and receiver or just as a receiver. There are a variety of surface coils (e.g., coils used in imaging the joints) that serve as receivers, with the body coil employed as the transmitter. Even when a surface coil is placed over the area of interest, the received signals come from the entire body (this situation again differs from CT imaging); however, the signals received in the region of the surface coil have a higher magnitude, i.e., a higher signal-to-noise ratio (SNR). In other words, surface coils improve SNR in the region of interest.

Gradient Coils

Gradient coils cause an intentional *perturbation* in the magnetic field homogeneity (usually in a linear fashion), which allows one to decipher *spatial information* from the received signal and localize it in space. This perturbation or variation in magnetic field is several orders of magnitude smaller than the external magnetic field but is significant enough to allow spatial encoding. To achieve this, three orthogonal gradient coils are used (Fig. 2-21) corresponding to the axes x, y, and z in a three-dimensional coordinate system. This then allows encoding (or deciphering) of data in three coordinates. These gradients are referred to as:

1. the **slice-select** gradient
2. the **phase-encoding** gradient
3. the **frequency-encoding** or **readout** gradient

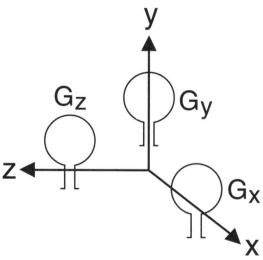

Figure 2-21. Three gradient coils exist in MRI, one along each direction (x, y, and z).

For an axial image, these would correspond to G_z, G_y, and G_x, respectively. They are discussed at length in chapters to come.

Shim Coils

These coils are used to create a more uniform external magnetic field B_0. Keep in mind that inhomogeneities in the external field are undesirable and can cause artifacts, especially when a gradient-echo or a chemical fat suppression technique is used. Shim coils help minimize (although not totally eliminate) such variations.

Quadrature Coils

In quadrature coil design, two receivers are present 90° to one another, capable of distinguishing *real* and *imaginary* components of the received signal. This design can increase the signal-to-noise ratio (SNR) by a factor of $\sqrt{2}$.

Solenoid Coils

These coils can be wrapped around the patient and increase SNR. These coils are usually used in lower field magnets (e.g., open scanners) which have a vertical magnetic field orientation (rather than a horizontal orientation in higher field scanners).

Phased-array Coils

These coils contain multiple small surface coils that are positioned on either side of the anatomy of interest. These coils allow faster scanning with finer details. An example is the pelvic array coil that allows exquisite visualization of pelvic structures.

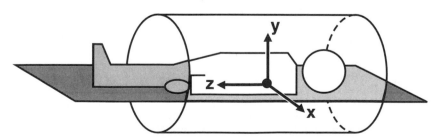

Figure 2-22. An arbitrary designation of x, y, and z for a patient in the scanner.

PLANE OF IMAGING

Selection of the gradient coils along x, y, or z axes is arbitrary. Imaging in different (axial, sagittal, coronal, or oblique) planes in MRI is different from CT and is possible simply by appropriate assignment of the gradient coils while the patient is always positioned in the magnet with his or her long axis along the long axis of the scanner (Fig. 2-22). For instance, assuming the z axis to be along the long axis of the magnet in the craniocaudal (CC) direction, y axis to be in the posteroanterior (PA) direction, and x axis to be from right to left (R-L)[b], then axial images

Table 2-5

	Slice-Select Gradient	Phase-Encoding Gradient	Frequency-Encoding Gradient
Axial	z	y	x
Sagittal	x	y	z
Coronal	y	x	z

are obtained by allowing the slice-select gradient to be along the z axis. The possibilities are summarized in Table 2-5. **Oblique** planes are obtained by combining the previously mentioned gradients in a linear fashion.

Key Points

In this chapter, we have discussed the basic principles behind MR. We have talked about electromagnetic waves, proton spins, external magnetic fields, and longitudinal magnetization. We briefly introduced the parameter T_1 that is an inherent property of a tissue. Let's summarize:

1. Electromagnetic waves (as the name applies) have two components: an electric component (E) and a magnetic component (H or B). These two components are perpendicular to each other and 90° out of phase.

2. The propagation component C is perpendicular to both the E and B components, all traveling at the speed of light (c = 3 × 10^6 m/sec).

3. In MRI, it is the magnetic component that interests us. The electric component merely generates heat.

4. Electromagnetic waves are periodic functions of time, oscillating at a frequency of

$$\omega = 2\pi f$$

where ω is the angular frequency (in radians/sec) and f is the linear frequency (in cycles/sec or Hz).

5. Many types of electromagnetic waves exist throughout the electromagnetic spectrum: X-rays, visible light, microwaves, radiofrequencies, etc.

6. The frequencies used in MRI fall in the radiofrequency (RF) range (3-100 MHz). They are therefore called RF pulses.

7. Spinning charged particles generate an electromagnetic field.

8. An example of the previous point is in the body is the hydrogen proton (^{1}H).

9. The magnetic component of hydrogen protons behave like bar magnets. This behavior is referred to as an MDM (Magnetic Dipole Moment).

10. In general, all particles with an odd number of electrons in their covalent orbit have this property (i.e., can generate a magnetic field).

11. Although many different protons exist in the body, hydrogen protons are dealt with in MRI because they are the most prevalent in the body (particularly in H_2O, which composes 60% of the body).

12. The main magnetic field in MRI is denoted B_0.

13. When a patient is placed in a magnetic field B_0, a portion of the protons are

---

[b] This is in fact the convention used throughout this book for simplicity.

aligned parallel to B_0 and a portion anti-parallel to it, but more parallel than anti-parallel, producing a net magnetization (longitudinal magnetization).

14. These protons also oscillate or *precess* about the axis of the external magnetic field.

15. The frequency of precession of protons is described by the *Larmor equation*

$$\omega_0 = \gamma \cdot B_0$$

where γ is the gyromagnetic ratio (in MHz/T). Therefore, the stronger the magnetic field, the faster protons precess about it.

16. Magnetic susceptibility refers to the ability of a substance to get magnetized when placed in a magnetic field.

17. Three types of substances with different magnetic susceptibility effects were discussed: diamagnetic, paramagnetic, and ferromagnetic.

18. There are five types of magnets based on field strength: ultra low field, low field, midfield, high field, and ultra high field.

19. There are three types of magnets based on design: permanent magnets, resistive magnets, and superconducting magnets.

20. Most existing scanners are high-field, superconducting magnets (these require liquid cryogens like liquid helium and nitrogen for cooling).

21. Most "open" type MR scanners are permanent or resistive magnets; they require no cryogens and thus have low maintenance. However, they usually have lower field strengths and thus generate less signal.

22. To create an image, RF pulses are transmitted into the patient. These pulses flip the longitudinal magnetization and generate a signal from the patient.

23. RF pulses flip the longitudinal magnetization Mz away from the z axis: 90° pulses flip Mz by 90°; 180° pulses by 180°; and partial RF pulses by α, which is less than 90°.

24. The received signal has no spatial information. Three types of gradient coils (slice-select, readout or frequency-encoding, and phase-encoding gradients) are employed for the purpose of spatial discrimination.

25. Different types of coils are used: body coil, head coil, surface coil.

26. Surface coils are used for smaller body parts (e.g., joints) to increase the signal and reduce the noise (thus increasing the signal-to-noise ratio).

27. The rate at which the longitudinal magnetization recovers from the transverse plane (after having been flipped by a 90° pulse) is given by the time parameter T1. This parameter also describes the rate at which protons are magnetized when placed in an external magnetic field.

28. The equation for this recovery at any time t is given by

$$1 - e^{-t/T1}$$

which is an exponential growth curve.

What do we need to create an image from the information received from the patient? This process is initiated by the use of a radio frequency (RF) pulse and is discussed in the next chapter.

Questions

2-1. Calculate the Larmor frequency of a proton at the following magnetic field strengths:
(a) 0.35T   (b) 0.5T   (c) 1T
(d) 1.5T   (e) 2T
(the gyromagnetic ratio, γ, of a proton $\cong$ 42.6 MHz/T)

2-2. T/F The T1 of a tissue is larger at a stronger magnetic field environment.

2-3. T/F Proton density represents the density of *all* the protons in the tissue.

2-4. T/F The rate at which protons precess about the main magnetic field is faster than that about their own axes.

2-5. T/F   In MRI, imaging plane is determined by proper assignment of the x, y, and z gradients.

2-6. T/F   Electromagnetic waves travel at the speed of sound.

2-7. T/F   Hydrogen protons are used in MRI because of their abundance.

2-8. T/F   When placed in a magnetic field, protons will line up with that field immediately.

2-9. T/F   When placed in a magnetic field, *all* the protons in the body will line up with the field.

2-10. T/F   The main purpose of x, y, and z gradients is for slice selection and spatial encoding.

2-11. T/F   The rate at which protons are magnetized when placed in a magnetic environment is the same as the rate of recovery of longitudinal magnetization.

3 Radio Frequency Pulse

INTRODUCTION

In the last chapter, we discussed the concept of longitudinal magnetization. However, we have not yet addressed the issue of receiving a signal from the patient. We can only transmit and receive signals that oscillate (like an AC voltage). In addition, we're only sensitive to oscillations along certain axes. Because the longitudinal magnetization is *not* an oscillating function (like a DC voltage), it cannot be read by a receiver. In addition, we're not sensitive to oscillations along the z axis. Consequently, this magnetization needs to be "flipped" into the transverse x-y plane (where it can oscillate or "precess" about the z axis) to generate a readable signal. This is the purpose of the RF (radio-frequency) pulse.

RADIO FREQUENCY (RF) PULSE

Suppose that a patient is in the magnet. Then we transmit an **RF pulse**. What happens? Remember that an **RF pulse** is an **electromagnetic wave**. Initially all the spins are lined up along the axis of the external magnetic field B_0 about which they are precessing (Fig. 3-1). Then we transmit an RF pulse. In a 3-dimensional (x, y, z) coordinate system, the direction of the external magnetic field always points in the z direction. Thus, the net magnetization vector M_0 will also point in the z direction (Fig. 3-2).

One point of clarification about the **magnetization vector M_0**: even though all of the individual spins are precessing around the external magnetic field axis, the **net magnetization**

(which is made up of the *vector sum* of all the individual spins) does *not* precess. The reason for this is that all the individual spins are precessing, but they are all *out of phase* with each other. Therefore, if we add them all up, they'll have a large component along the z axis; however, because of their phase differences, they all cancel each other out and are left with no component along the x or y axis (Fig. 3-3a and b) (Note that in Figure 3-3b, while the two protons are precessing at the same rate, one is pointing towards the right while the other is pointing towards the left). Thus, the *net vector* of *magnetization* does not precess (at least initially—it only precesses in response to the RF pulse—see later text).

Now, let's transmit an RF pulse along the x axis *perpendicular* to the magnetization vector M_0, i.e., the axis of B_0. (The RF pulse would be along the axis "C" in Figure 2-2.) Any proton that is subjected to any sort of magnetic field starts to precess about the axis of that magnetic field at a frequency ω_0 given by the Larmor equation ($\omega = \gamma B$), where B is the strength of that magnetic field. Protons precess about the axis of B_0 at a frequency $\omega_0 = \gamma B_0$. Now we introduce a magnetic field (namely, the magnetic component of the RF pulse) into the system with a direction along the x axis. The protons that were previously aligned with the external magnetic field B_0 in the z direction will now also begin to *precess* about the x axis, i.e., about the axis of the new (RF) magnetic field.

At what rate will these protons precess around this new magnetic field? The new precessional

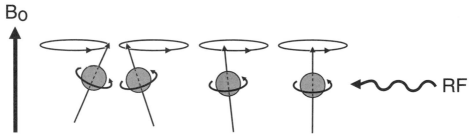

Figure 3-1. An RF pulse is transmitted after the protons have been exposed to the external magnetic field B_0.

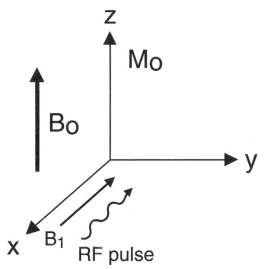

Figure 3-2. The net magnetization vector $\mathbf{M_0}$ has the same direction as the external magnetic field B_0.

frequency will be

$$\omega_1 = \gamma\, B_1 \qquad \text{(Eqn. 3-1)}$$

where B_1 is the weaker magnetic field associated with the RF pulse.

We are now dealing with two different magnetic fields:

B_0 = *a very strong external magnetic field (e.g., 1.5 T)*

B_1 = *a very weak magnetic field generated by the RF pulse (e.g., 50 mT).*

B_0 is a *fixed* magnetic field (much like a DC voltage). B_1, however, is an **oscillating** magnetic field (much like an AC voltage). It oscillates because it is derived from the magnetic component of an oscillating electromagnetic wave.

Because the magnetic field strength of B_1 is much weaker than the external magnetic field B_0, the frequency of precession ω_1 of the spins around the axis of B_1 is much *slower* than the precessional frequency ω_0 of the spins around the axis of the external magnetic field B_0.

So, since $\quad B_1 \ll B_0$,

then $\quad \omega_1 \ll \omega_0$

The protons are precessing about the B_0 field (z axis) at frequency ω_0 and about the B_1 field

(x axis) at frequency ω_1 at the same time. This results in a **spiral motion** of the net magnetization vector from the z axis into the x-y plane. This spiral motion is called "**nutation**."

Another thing to remember about the RF pulse is that, referring back to Chapter 1, the RF pulse has a *cos* (ωt) wave form. The frequency ω of the RF pulse should be identical to the Larmor frequency of the precessing protons. Otherwise, the protons will not precess around the B_1 axis of the RF pulse. This point might be clarified if we first discuss the concept of "resonance."

Resonance

If the frequency ω of the RF pulse *matches* the frequency of precession of the protons, then **resonance** occurs. Resonance results in the RF pulse adding energy to the protons. A simple example of resonance is the frequency of a child on a swing. Based on the length of the swing and the weight of the child, a natural mechanical resonance frequency exists. If the child is pushed faster or slower from this frequency, the effort will be inefficient. If the child is pushed at his or her resonance frequency, energy is added and he or she swings higher. Similarly, if the proton precesses at frequency ω_0 and the frequency of the RF pulse is not ω_0 (say it is ω_2 instead), then the magnetic field B_1 is oscillating at a different frequency than the protons, and the two frequencies won't be matched. If the RF frequency does not match the precessional frequency of the spins, the system won't resonate and no energy will be added.

Consider this in the x-y plane. The protons are spinning at frequency ω_0. If we then have the B_1 magnetic field oscillating at a frequency = ω_2 different from the proton precessional frequency ω_0, then the system won't resonate, i.e., the protons won't "flip" into the x-y plane. A point of clarification: the RF pulse is characterized by two parameters: strength (B_1) and frequency (ω_2). The *frequency* of the RF pulse must match the proton precessional frequency ω_0 in order for resonance to occur—and for the RF pulse to have any effect on the protons at all. If the frequency ω_2 is correct, then the *strength* of the RF pulse (B_1) results in precession of protons

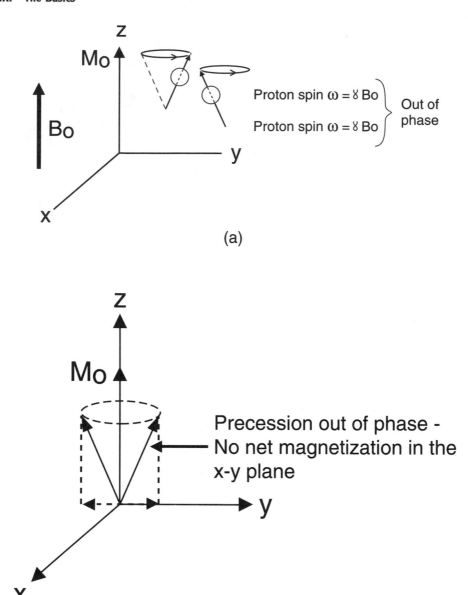

Proton spin $\omega = \gamma\, Bo$ ⎫
Proton spin $\omega = \gamma\, Bo$ ⎭ Out of phase

(a)

Precession out of phase -
No net magnetization in the
x-y plane

(b)

Figure 3-3. Two protons rotating out of phase **(a)** will lead to a net longitudinal magnetization but no component in the x-y plane **(b)**.

about the x axis at frequency ω_1 (according to the Larmor equation $\omega_1 = \gamma\, B_1$).

If ω_0 and ω_2 match (i.e., $\omega_2 = \omega_0$), then the system resonates and the protons flip into the x-y plane. In doing so, the protons precess around the axis of the B_1 magnetic field at a much lower frequency (ω_1), corresponding to the Larmor frequency associated with the RF magnetic field B_1 and not with the larger magnetic field B_0.

Another point of clarification: remember that before the RF pulse, the protons precess about the z axis but they are **out of phase** and hence have no net transverse component. After the RF pulse, the protons are introduced to a *new* magnetic field B_1 (also oscillating at frequency ω_0). Consequently, they will also tend to line up with the *new* magnetic field and will then be **in phase**. This in effect creates transverse magnetization. As more and more protons line

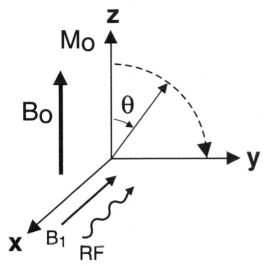

Figure 3-4.   A certain amount of time after the application of the RF pulse, the magnetization vector is partially "flipped" towards the x-y plane forming an angle θ with the z axis.

According to Equation 3-2, the flip angle is proportional to:

1. τ = the duration of the RF pulse
2. B_1 = the strength of the RF magnetic field, i.e., the strength of the RF pulse
3. γ = the gyromagnetic ratio.

We could have a very strong RF pulse applied over a short period of time, or we could have a weak RF pulse applied over a longer time, and still attain the same **flip angle**. The relationship between the flip angle (θ) and frequency (ω_1) is:

$$\theta = (\omega_1)\,(\tau) \qquad \text{(Eqn. 3-3)}$$

Thus,

flip angle = (frequency of RF precession) × (duration of RF pulse)

up, **phase "coherence"** increases as does transverse magnetization. Simultaneously, as previously discussed, the B_1 field also causes a spiral downward motion of the protons. These two factors explain the process of flipping.

Going back to the 3 dimensional coordinate system (Fig. 3-4), the vector M_0 (the net magnetization in the direction of the protons aligned along the external magnetic field) begins to precess about the x axis in the z-y plane. Depending on the *strength* of the RF pulse B_1, and its *duration* τ, we can determine the **flip angle** (i.e., the fractional angle of a single precession):

$$\theta = \gamma\,B_1\,\tau \qquad \text{(Eqn. 3-2)}$$

ROTATING FRAME OF REFERENCE

To simplify the concept of "flipping," consider a new reference frame that rotates at the Larmor frequency ω_0. (If you wanted to study the motion of someone riding a carousel, wouldn't it be easier to be *on* the carousel than to watch it from outside?)

Suppose there were someone who was not in this coordinate system, but rather on the *outside* looking in (Fig. 3-5). To this person, the protons would be precessing simultaneously about the z axis of the B_0 field at frequency ω_0, and about the x axis of the B_1 field at frequency ω_1. This outside observer would witness a rapid precession around the z axis that would slowly *spiral*

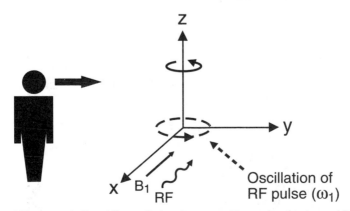

Figure 3-5.   An outside observer looking at the coordinate system sees rapid precession of protons and B_1 about the z axis.

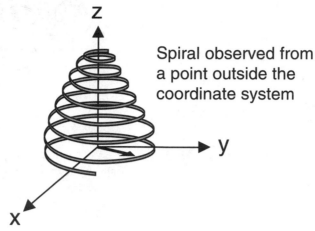

Figure 3-6. The outside observer sees a spiral motion of the magnetization vector towards the x-y plane.

down into the x-y plane (Fig. 3-6). This nutational motion is the result of the two precessional motions happening simultaneously.

If, however, the observer is located within the rotating coordinate system, and moving at the same frequency as one of the oscillating systems (B_1 or B_0), then she will see *only* the movement of the second system. If, for example, she is rotating at the oscillation frequency of the spins in the external magnetic field ω_0, then she will only notice the slow precession of the protons from the z axis into the x-y plane as if they were moving in a simple arc (Fig. 3-7). The above occurs if and only if $\omega_0 = \omega_2$, i.e., when the RF pulse frequency ω_2 matches the precessional frequency of the protons ω_0. This condition will put the system in *resonance*.

If we go back for a moment to the spiral motion of the protons seen from an outside observation point (Fig. 3-6), the consecutive circles around the z axis represent the oscillation frequency ω_0 of the spins in response to the external magnetic field B_0, and the slow downward progress of the spiral to the x-y plane represents the oscillation frequency of the spins in response to the magnetic field of the RF pulse, B_1. If the observer herself is oscillating within the system at a frequency $= \omega_0$, then all she will see is the slow downward arc of the protons precessing in response to the RF pulse. Because the magnetic field created by the RF pulse (B_1) is much smaller than the fixed external magnetic field (B_0), the precessional frequency around the z-y plane is much slower than is the precessional frequency around the z axis.

90° RF Pulse

In response to a strong magnetic field in the z direction, the spins line up. This results in net magnetization, M_0. Next, we apply an external RF pulse that **flips** the magnetization vector 90°

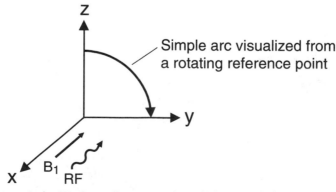

Figure 3-7. If the observer stands within the coordinate system, she would then see a simple arc motion rather than a spiral motion.

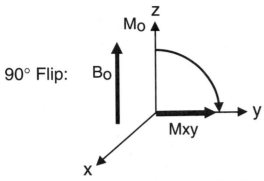

Figure 3-8. When the entire magnetization vector is flipped into the x-y plane, it is called a 90° flip.

into the x-y plane. When the **magnetization vector** is in the x-y plane, we call this M_{xy}.

M_{xy} = component of M_0 in the x-y plane

If the entire vector flips into the x-y plane, then the **magnitude** of M_{xy} equals the magnitude of the vector M_0. This is called a **90° flip** (Fig. 3-8). The pulse that causes the 90° flip is called a **90° RF pulse**.

The protons that are aligned with the external magnetic field are in two energy states (Fig. 3-9). Those in the lower energy state (E_1) are lined up with (i.e., parallel to) the magnetic field B_0, and those in the higher energy state (E_2) are aligned in the opposite direction. After a 90° RF pulse, some of the protons from the lower energy state are boosted to the higher energy state. This happens only at the **Larmor frequency**.

MATH: The Larmor equation can be derived from the following principle. The energy difference between E_1 and E_2, denoted ΔE, is given by:

$$\Delta E = E_2 - E_1 = (2\mu)\,(B_0) \qquad \text{(Eqn. 3-4a)}$$

where μ is the **magnetic dipole moment** (MDM). In other words, to go from one energy state to another, the energy required depends on the magnetic dipole moment of the proton and the strength of the magnetic field B_0. By Planck's law:

$$E = hc/\lambda = h\nu = hf = \hbar\omega \qquad \text{(Eqn. 3-4b)}$$

where $\nu = f$ denotes the linear frequency (in cycles/sec or Hz), ω denotes the angular frequency (in radians/sec), h is Planck's constant (6.62×10^{-34} joules/second or 4.13×10^{-18} keV.sec), and $\hbar = h/2\pi$. Then combining Eqn. 3-4a and 3-4b, we can deduce that

$$\hbar \cdot \omega = 2\mu \cdot B_0 = E$$

and thus

$$\omega = (2\mu/\hbar) \cdot B_0$$

which is the Larmor equation, with

$$\gamma = 2\mu/\hbar \text{ (in radians/Tesla)}$$

or, alternatively,

$$f = (2\mu/h) \cdot B_0$$

with

$$\gamma = 2\mu/h \text{ (in Hz/Tesla)}$$

where

$$\hbar = h/2\pi \text{ and } f = \nu = \omega/2\pi$$

At equilibrium after the protons are placed in the magnetic field, the number of protons in the low energy state (north-pointing) is greater than the number in the high energy state (south-pointing), resulting in the longitudinal magnetization vector M_0 (Fig. 3-10a). As energy is added by the RF pulse to flip the north-pointing pro-

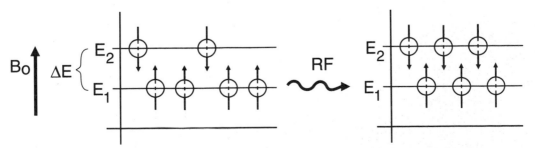

Figure 3-9. When placed in a magnetic field B_0, protons will fall into one of two energy states: in the lower energy state, protons are lined parallel to B_0, whereas in the higher energy state they are antiparallel to it.

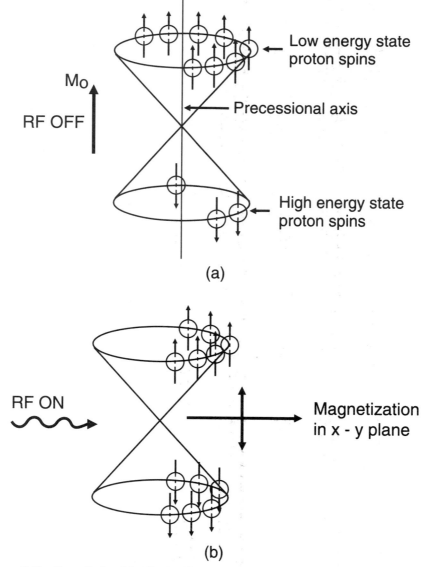

Figure 3-10.   The application of the RF pulse (b) can equalize the number of north- and south-pointing protons.

tons to the higher energy state, the number of protons in both states can be equalized. When this occurs, a measurable longitudinal magnetization vector no longer exists. In addition, the RF pulse causes the spins to begin precessing *in phase* with each other. The vector sum of the in-phase north- and south-pointing, precessing protons lies in the transverse plane (Fig. 3-10b). This transverse magnetization precesses at the Larmor frequency.

The angular frequency at which the protons rotate 90° about the x axis is given by the Larmor equation:

$$\omega_1 = \gamma B_1$$

where, again, B_1 is the magnetic field associated with the RF pulse. As stated previously, the phase, i.e., the number of degrees of precession, is related to the frequency ω_1 and the duration τ of the RF pulse:

$$\theta = \omega_1 \tau = \gamma B_1 \tau \qquad \text{(Eqn. 3-5)}$$

From this we can calculate the time τ it would take to precess the protons 90° ($\pi/2$), i.e., the time it would take for an RF pulse to "flip" the spins 90° into the x-y plane at a given RF strength B_1. Setting

$$\theta = 90° = \pi/2 = \gamma B_1 \tau_{\pi/2},$$

then we obtain

$$\tau_{\pi/2} = (\pi/2)/\gamma B_1 \qquad \text{(Eqn. 3-6)}$$

This equation shows that if we keep the RF pulse on for time $\tau_{\pi/2}$, the magnetization vector is flipped 90°.

180° PULSE

A 180° pulse has twice the power (or twice the duration) of a 90° pulse as shown in Equation 3-5. After a 180° RF pulse, the longitudinal magnetization vector is inverted and the spins begin to recover from $-\mathbf{M}_0$. After a 180° RF pulse, the excess north-pointing spins are boosted from the low energy state to the high energy state. A 180° pulse exactly reverses the equilibrium northward-pointing excess without inducing phase coherence, i e , transverse magnetization.

Using Equation 3-5, we can calculate the RF time duration required for a 180° RF pulse at a given RF strength B_1

$$180° = \pi = \gamma B_1 \tau_\pi$$

resulting in

$$\tau_\pi = \pi/\gamma B_1 \qquad \text{(Eqn. 3-7)}$$

To recapitulate, to obtain a 180° RF pulse, we can use either an RF pulse having the same strength as the 90° pulse but twice as long in duration, or an RF pulse that's twice as strong for the same duration.

PARTIAL FLIP

In the case of a **partial flip** (less than 90°), the component of magnetization ending up in the x-y plane (i.e., M_{xy}) is less than the magnitude of the original magnetization vector $\mathbf{M}_0$ (Fig. 3-11). In fact,

$$M_{xy} = M_0 . \sin \theta$$

A partial flip is achieved by either decreasing the strength or the duration of the RF pulse, according to Equation 3-5. Such flip angles are common in **gradient echo** (GRE) imaging, as will be discussed in later chapters.

AUTO RF (PRESCAN)

Prescan is the process of preparing the scanner for a specific patient. This process is done via an **auto RF pulse** which automatically does the following:

1. It sets transmit gain (which determines the RF power and thus the flip angle). In fact, the flip angle α is proportional to the square root of the transmit power:

$$\alpha \propto \sqrt{\text{power}}$$

2. It sets the receive gain.
3. It sets the optimum ω_0.

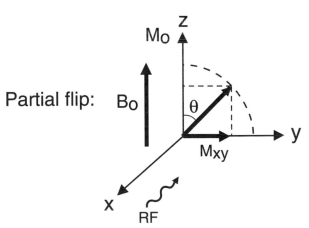

Figure 3-11. In a partial flip, transverse magnetization is smaller than the original longitudinal magnetization. In fact, $M_{xy} = M_0 \sin \theta$.

Key Points

1. An RF (radio frequency) pulse is a brief electromagnetic burst with frequencies in the radiofrequency spectrum.

2. Like all electromagnetic waves, an RF pulse has associated magnetic and electric fields. It is the magnetic component B_1 that we are interested in. (The electric component causes tissue heating.)

3. The purpose of the RF pulse in MRI is to flip the longitudinal magnetization.

4. This flip is done by first causing the protons to precess in phase about the axis of the external field (B_0), as well causing them to precess about the axis of the RF field (B_1). The result is a spiral motion of spins towards the x-y plane, called "nutation".

5. The flip angle is a function of the RF strength (B_1) and its duration (τ) and could be 180°, 90°, or a fraction thereof (i.e., a partial flip less than 90°), depending on the clinical application.

Questions

3-1.   T/F   An RF pulse has a magnetic component.

3-2.   T/F   The function of the RF pulse in MRI is to magnetize the protons.

3-3.   T/F   The immediate action of the RF pulse is to cause the protons to precess in phase.

3-4.   T/F   The flip angle is determined by the duration of the RF pulse and its power.

4 T_1, T_2, and T_2^*

INTRODUCTION

We have already introduced relaxation times T_1, T_2, and T_2^*. In this chapter, we will discuss the physical properties behind them and see what conditions cause them to be increased or decreased. As we have discussed before, T_1 and T_2 are *inherent* properties of tissues and are thus fixed for a specific tissue (at a given magnetic field strength). The parameter T_2^*, however, also depends on inhomogeneities in the main magnetic field, but again is fixed for a specific tissue within a given external magnetic environment.

T_1 RELAXATION TIME

The term "**relaxation**" means that the spins are relaxing back into their lowest energy state or back to the equilibrium state. (Equilibrium by definition is the lowest energy state possible.) Once the **RF** pulse is turned **off**, the protons will have to realign with the axis of the B_0 magnetic field and give up all their excess energy.

T_1 is called the **longitudinal** relaxation time because it refers to the time it takes for the spins to realign along the longitudinal (z) axis. T_1 is also called the **spin-lattice** relaxation time because it refers to the time it takes for the *spins to give the energy they obtained from the RF pulse back to the surrounding lattice* in order to go back to their equilibrium state.

T_1 = *longitudinal relaxation time*
= *spin-lattice relaxation time*

Immediately after the 90° pulse, the magnetization M_{xy} precesses within the x-y plane, oscillating around the z axis with all protons rotating *in phase* (Fig. 4-1). After the magnetization has been flipped 90° into the x-y plane, the RF pulse is turned off. A general principle of thermodynamics is that every system seeks its lowest energy level. Therefore, after the RF pulse is turned off, two things will occur:

1. the spins will go back to the lowest energy state.

2. the spins will get out of phase with each other.

These events result from two simultaneous but separate processes occurring after the RF pulse is turned off (Fig. 4-2):

1. the M_{xy} component of the magnetization vector decreases rapidly; and
2. the M_z component slowly recovers along the z axis.

Question: *What time constant characterizes the rate at which the M_z component recovers its initial magnetization M_0?*
Answer: *The T_1 relaxation time.*

When we first discussed magnetization, we said that the protons start to line up with the external magnetic field at a rate given by T_1. (Because T_1 is a time [in sec], the rate is $1/T_1$ [in sec^{-1}]). The same phenomenon occurs when we flip the magnetization $\mathbf{M_0}$ away from the longitudinal z axis and then allow it to realign with the main magnetic field after an RF pulse. The rate at which M_z recovers to M_0 is also given by T_1.

Immediately after a 90° pulse, all magnetization is in the x-y plane. The M_z component then starts to grow at a rate characterized by T_1 (Fig. 4-3):

$$M_z(t) = M_0 (1 - e^{-t/T1}) \qquad \text{(Eqn. 4-1)}$$

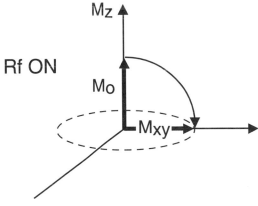

Figure 4-1. After the RF pulse, the longitudinal magnetization vector is flipped into the x-y plane.

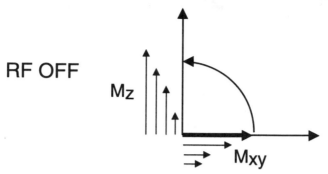

Figure 4-2.   Once the RF is turned off, the transverse magnetization vector begins to decay while the longitudinal component begins to recover.

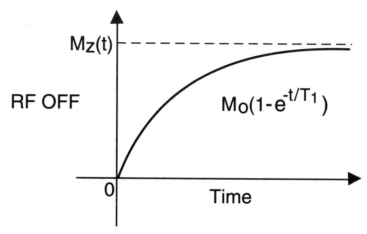

Figure 4-3.   The graph of recovery of longitudinal magnetization with the growth rate of T1.

T_2 RELAXATION TIME

Figure 4-2 also shows rapid decay of the M_{xy} component after the RF pulse is turned off.

Question: *What time constant characterizes the rate at which the M_{xy} component decays?*
Answer: *The T_2 relaxation time.*

As the longitudinal magnetization vector M_z recovers, the transverse vector M_{xy} decays at a rate characterized by T_2 (Fig. 4-4):

$$M_{xy}(t) = M_0\ e^{-t/T2} \qquad \text{(Eqn. 4-2)}$$

Realize that the recovery of magnetization along the z axis and the decay of magnetization within the x-y plane are two independent processes occurring at two different rates (Fig. 4-5). Take a simple exponential process. We would expect the rate at which this process decays in the x-y plane to be the same as that at which it grows along the z axis (Fig. 4-6). This is *not* the

same in the MR system we are discussing because this system involves a much more complicated process. T_2 decay occurs 5 to 10 times more rapidly than T_1 recovery (Fig. 4-7). To understand this, we need to understand the concept of dephasing.

Dephasing

After the 90° **RF** pulse is turned **off**, all spins are **in phase**; they are all lined up in the same direction and spinning at the same frequency ω_0. There are two phenomena that will make the spins get out of phase: interactions between spins and external field inhomogeneities.

(1) INTERACTIONS BETWEEN INDIVIDUAL SPINS

When two spins are next to each other, the magnetic field of one proton affects the proton next to it. Assume one proton is aligned with

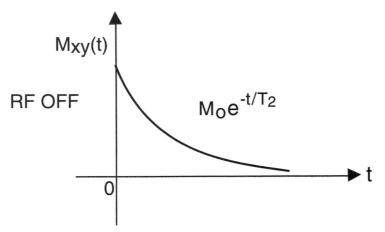

Figure 4-4. The graph of decay of transverse magnetization with the decay rate of T2.

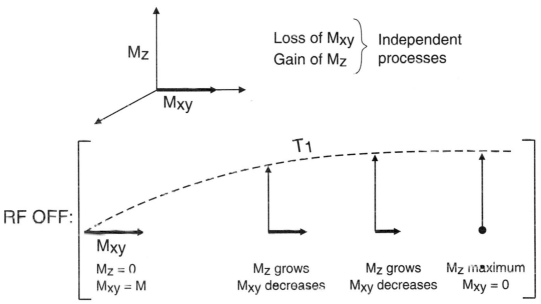

Figure 4-5. The recovery of longitudinal magnetization and the decay of transverse magnetization occur at the same time but are independent of each other.

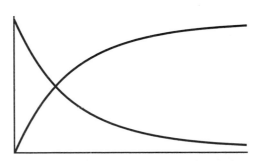

Figure 4-6. The rate of growth and decay of a simple exponential process is expected to be similar.

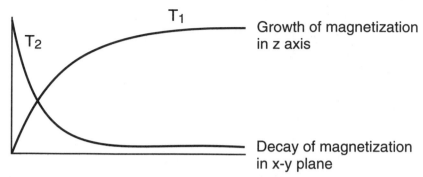

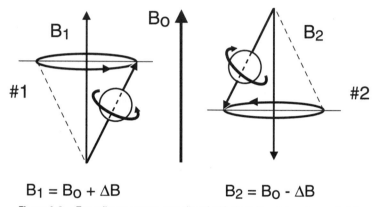

Figure 4-7. Contrary to the previous figure, the rate of decay of transverse magnetization is several times that of the recovery of longitudinal magnetization.

Figure 4-8. Two adjacent protons, one aligned with the field and the other against it.

the field and the other is against it (Fig. 4-8). The proton aligned with B_0 creates a slightly higher magnetic field for its neighbor so that proton #1 is exposed to the magnetic field B_0 plus a small magnetic field created by the other proton (ΔB). The precessional frequency of the proton then will increase slightly as

$$\omega(\text{proton \#1}) = (B_0 + \Delta B)$$

On the other side, the other proton is exposed to a slightly weaker magnetic field because the other proton points against B_0. Therefore, its overall magnetic field strength exposure will be slightly less. The precessional frequency of proton #2 then will decrease slightly as

$$\omega(\text{proton \#2}) = (B_0 - \Delta B)$$

The difference in the magnetic environment created by these proton–proton interactions may be very small, but it makes a difference in the overall homogeneity of the magnetic field to which the spins are exposed. Thus, the first cause of dephasing is *inherent* in the tissue. It is called

a **spin-spin interaction.** This interaction is an inherent property of every tissue and is measured by T_2.

T_2 = *transverse relaxation time*
   = *spin-spin relaxation time*

---

(2) EXTERNAL MAGNETIC FIELD INHOMOGENEITY

This is the second phenomenon that makes spins get out of phase. No matter how good a system we have, no matter how stable the external magnetic field is, some variation in the homogeneity of the magnetic field still exists (usually measured in parts per million).

External magnetic field inhomogeneity makes protons in different locations precess at different frequencies because each spin is exposed to a slightly different magnetic field strength. These varying frequencies are very close to each other, and very close to the true Larmor frequency;

however, these tiny differences in frequency result in spin **dephasing**.

The two causes of spin dephasing are:

1. *spin-spin interactions (internal inhomogeneities)*
2. *external magnetic field inhomogeneities*

These two phenomena together cause protons to spin at slightly different frequencies. Imagine that we have three protons:

1. one is precessing at the true Larmor frequency = ω_0.
2. one, exposed to slightly higher magnetic fields, is precessing at a frequency slightly faster than the Larmor frequency = ω_0^+.
3. one, exposed to slightly weaker magnetic field, is precessing at a frequency slightly slower than the Larmor frequency = ω_0^-.

If we wait long enough, the three protons in the x-y plane will get completely out of phase. The net magnetic field within the x-y plane will then go to zero.

Therefore, at time = 0, all spins are in phase, and their vector sum will be at maximum magnitude. As the spins begin getting out of phase

with each other, their summation vector will become smaller and smaller. When all the spins are completely out of phase with each other, their vector sum will be zero. The effect of spin-spin interaction depends to a degree on the proximity of the spins to each other. For example, in water (H$_2$O), the protons are separated more widely than they are in a solid tissue. Hence, the dephasing effect of spin-spin interaction might not be as prominent in H$_2$O as it is in a solid tissue.

THE RECEIVED SIGNAL

Let's go back to the x-y plane with the RF aligned along the x axis. The RF coil (e.g., head or body coil) is often both a **transmitter** and a **receiver**. The signal is received at the same location at which it is transmitted. Remember that a moving charged particle generates a magnetic field. The reverse is also true. A magnetic field causes movement of charged particles, i.e., electrons. If we have a wire with electrons running in one direction (away from us), the direction of the magnetic field (according to the Right Hand Rule) can be determined (in this case, it is pointing up) (Fig. 4-9a). Similarly, if we have a straight wire, and we have an oscillating mag-

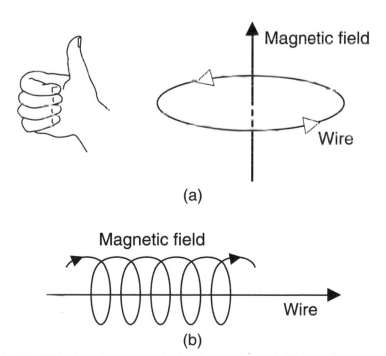

(a)

(b)

Figure 4-9. The right-hand rule determines the direction of generated magnetic field by an electric current in a wire.

netic field about this wire, the magnetic field will induce a voltage and current in the wire (Fig. 4-9b).

The measured current is what we mean by a **signal**. Remember that after a 90° pulse, the magnetization rotates in the x-y plane at frequency ω_0. This magnetization reflects a group phenomenon of multiple precessing protons. Associated with each proton is a magnetic field that is also precessing. Immediately after a 90° pulse, the protons precess in phase. When the magnetic field of each spin (or each group of spins) is in the same direction as the RF coil receiver, a very large signal is induced in the RF receiver coil.

Thus, at time $t = 0$ (in Fig. 4-10a), all the protons are lined up in the direction of the RF coil. As the spins rotate 90° at time $t = t_1$, there will be no component of the magnetization vector along the x direction. All magnetization points in the y direction. But this RF coil can only detect the component of magnetization along the x axis. So at time t_1, there is no signal. After another 90° rotation (at time t_2), a signal exists, but it is the negative of the original signal. At

time t_3, there is again no magnetization in the x direction, and, therefore, no signal. At time t_4, spins are again lined up with the receiver coil and signal is maximal. A graph of the received signal will then look like a sinusoidal curve (Fig. 4-10b). The frequency of the received signal is ω_0 because the protons are spinning at frequency ω_0.

However, is this really the received signal, or is there more to it?

FREE INDUCTION DECAY (FID)

In an ideal situation, if we had a perfectly uniform magnetic field, the received signal would, in fact, have looked like Fig. 4-10b. But this is not what's really happening. What really happens is the following (Fig. 4-11): We start at time $t = 0$ in the x direction. However, because of spin **dephasing** (namely, spin-spin interactions and external magnetic field inhomogeneities), by the time the spins reach t_4, they will have dephased slightly and the signal coming from the spins will be slightly less than it was originally. The signal becomes weaker and

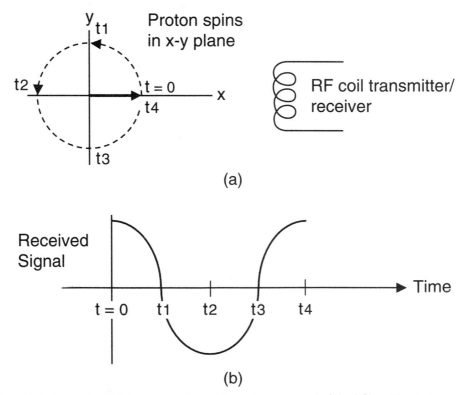

(a)

(b)

Figure 4-10. The relationship between transverse magnetization **(a)** and the received signal **(b)** at different points in time.

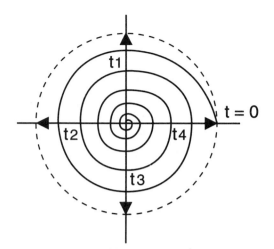

Figure 4-11. The spiral-like decay of transverse magnetization.

weaker as time goes by, and it spirals to the center of the x-y plane.

The signal vector is continuously decaying in magnitude as it is precessing around the x-y plane. How would the signal look to the RF receiver? The answer lies in Figure 4-12. This figure shows the shape of the signal picked up by the receiver; it is an oscillating, decaying signal. It is called an **FID** (free induction decay) because, after we turn off the RF pulse:

1. the spins begin to precess *freely*,
2. the signal starts to *decay* with time, and
3. the spins *induce* a current in the receiver coil.

Thus, the FID results from an oscillating magnetic field generated by the oscillating spins which induces a current in a receiver coil. This decaying oscillating signal is described mathe-

matically as

$$M_{xy}(t) = M_0 e^{-t/T_2^*} (\cos \omega_0 t) \quad \text{(Eqn. 4-3)}$$

We've seen these terms before (refer to Chapter 1):

1. $(\cos \omega_0 t)$: this is the formula for an oscillating wave, with a frequency of ω_0
2. $(e^{-t/T2^*})$: because the signal is decaying we have to include an exponential function. The time constant of this exponential function is given by T_2^*.

Therefore, the general form of the received signal is based on:

1. an *oscillating signal* which varies as $\cos \omega_0 t$;
2. a *decaying signal* which decays with time constant T_2^* as given by the exponential $e^{-t/T2^*}$.

Differences between T_2 and T_2^*

T_2^* decay depends on both:

1. External magnetic field.
2. Spin-spin interactions

T_2 decay depends primarily on:

1. Spin-spin interactions[a]

T_2 of a tissue, because it depends only on spin-spin interactions, is *fixed*—we have no control over what the spins do to each other. T_2^*

---

[a] T_2 also depends on **diffusion** (i.e., how rapidly spins spread out and leave the lattice); however, this is a minor factor in comparison to spin-spin interactions.

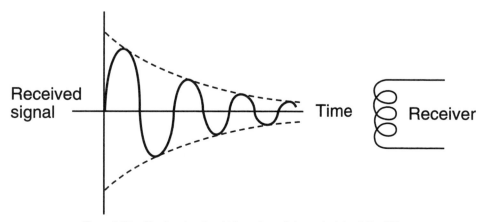

Figure 4-12. The decaying sinusoidal waveform of the received signal (the FID).

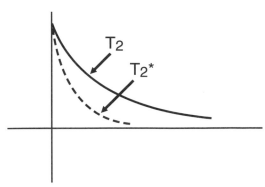

Figure 4-13. T_2 and T_2^* decay curves.

depends on the homogeneity of the external magnetic field, so it is *not fixed*. It varies depending on how uniform the main magnet is.

T_2^* is always less than T_2. T_2^* decay is always faster than T_2 decay (Fig. 4-13). The following equation relates the two together:

$$1/T_2^* = 1/T_2 + \gamma \, \Delta B \qquad \text{(Eqn. 4-4)}$$

The term $1/T$ is the **relaxation rate** with units of sec^{-1} (recall that $1/T$ is a frequency). The relaxation rate $(1/T_2^*)$ depends on the relaxation rate of the tissue $(1/T_2)$ plus the magnetic field inhomogeneity of the external magnet. If we have a perfect magnet that does not introduce any inhomogeneity, then $\Delta B = 0$ and $T_2^* = T_2$. The newer systems have less magnetic field inhomogeneity, thus making the T_2^* effects less strong; however, complete homogeneity is not possible. Hence, there will always be some T_2^* effect.

Key Points

1. The rate of recovery of the longitudinal magnetization is given by T_1.

2. The rate of decay of the transverse magnetization is given by T_2.

3. The rate of decay of the FID is given by T_2^*.

4. T_1 is 5 to 10 times greater than T_2.

5. T_2^* is always less than T_2.

Questions

4-1.   True/false questions:
(a) T_2^* depends on T_2.
(b) T_2 depends on T_2^*.
(c) T_2 depends on the external magnetic field inhomogeneity.
(d) T_2^* depends on the external magnetic field inhomogeneity.

4-2.   The recovery of longitudinal magnetization is proportional to:
(a) $e^{-t/T1}$ (b) $1 - e^{-t/T2}$
(c) $1 - e^{-t/T1}$ (d) $e^{-t/T2}$
(e)   none of the above

4-3.   The decay of transverse magnetization is proportional to:
(a) $e^{-t/T1}$ (b) $1 - e^{-t/T2}$
(c) $1 - e^{-t/T1}$ (d) $e^{-t/T2}$
(e)   none of the above

4-4.   T/F   The rate of decay of the FID is given by T2.

4-5.   Which one of the following equations is correct?
(a) $T2 > T2^* > T1$
(b) $T1 > T2 > T2^*$
(c) $T1 > T2^* > T2$
(d) $T2^* > T2 > T1$

5 TR, TE, and Tissue Contrast

INTRODUCTION

In previous chapters, we discussed the roles of T_1 and T_2, longitudinal and transverse magnetization, and the RF pulse. Obviously, by doing the procedures described in the previous chapters only once, we won't be able to create an image. To get any sort of spatial information, the process must be repeated multiple times, as we shall see shortly. This is where TR and TE come into play. The parameters TR and TE are related intimately to the tissue parameters T_1 and T_2, respectively. However, unlike T_1 and T_2, which are inherent properties of the tissue and therefore fixed, TR and TE can be controlled and adjusted by the operator. In fact, as we shall see later, by appropriate setting of TR and TE, we can put more "weight" on T_1 or T_2, depending on the type of clinical application.

How do we actually measure a signal? With the patient in a large magnetic field (Fig. 5-1a), we apply a 90° RF pulse, and the magnetization vector flips into the x-y plane (Fig. 5-1b). Then, we turn off the 90° RF pulse, and the magnetization vector begins to grow in the z direction and decay in the x-y plane (Fig. 5-1c). By convention, we apply the RF pulse in the x direction, and for that reason, in a rotating frame of reference, the vector ends up along the y axis (Fig. 5-1b).

After a 90° RF pulse, we have decaying transverse magnetization M_{xy} (which is the component of the magnetization vector in the x-y plane) and recovering longitudinal magnetization M_z

(which is the component of the magnetization vector along the z axis). Remember that the received signal can be detected only along the x axis, i.e., along the direction of the RF transmitter/receiver coil. The receiver coil only recognizes oscillating signals (like AC voltage) and not non-oscillating voltage changes (like DC voltage). Thus, rotation in the x-y plane induces a signal in the RF coil, whereas changes along the z axis does not.

At time t = 0, the signal is at a maximum. As time goes by, because of dephasing (see Chapter 4), the signal becomes weaker in a sinusoidal manner (Fig. 5-2). The decay curve of the signal is given by the following term:

$$e^{-t/T2^*}$$

The sinusoidal nature of the signal is given by the equation

$$\cos \omega t$$

Therefore, the decaying sinusoidal signal is given by the product

$$(e^{-t/T2^*})(\cos \omega t)$$

When t = 0:

$$\cos \omega t = \cos \omega(0) = \cos 0 = 1$$
$$e^{-t/T2^*} = e^0 = 1$$

When t = 0, $(e^{-t/T2^*})(\cos \omega t) = 1$. Thus, at time = 0, the signal is maximum (i.e., 100%). As time increases, we are multiplying a sinusoidal func

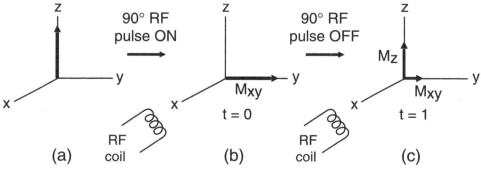

Figure 5-1. **(a)** Longitudinal magnetization before the RF pulse. **(b)** Immediately after the RF pulse, the magnetization vector is flipped into the x-y plane. **(c)** After a certain time period, M_z has recovered by a certain amount while M_{xy} has decayed by a different amount.

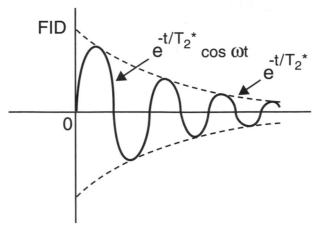

Figure 5-2.   The received signal (the FID) has a decaying sinusoidal waveform.

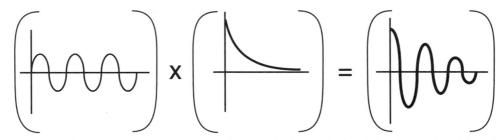

Figure 5-3.   The product of a sinusoidal signal and an exponentially decaying signal results in a decaying sinusoidal signal.

tion (*cos*ωt) and a decaying function ($e^{-t/T2^*}$), which eventually decays to zero (Fig. 5-3).

When we put a patient in a magnet, he or she becomes temporarily magnetized as his or her protons align with the external magnetic field along the z axis. We then transmit an RF pulse at the Larmor frequency and immediately get back an FID (Fig. 5-4). This process gives one signal—one FID—from the entire patient. It doesn't give us any information about the location of the signal. The FID is received from the

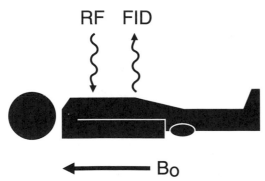

Figure 5-4.   Immediately after transmission of the RF pulse, an FID is formed.

ensemble of all the different protons in the patient's body with *no* spatial discrimination. To get spatial information, we have to somehow specify the x, y, and z coordinates of the signal. Here, **gradients** come into play. The purpose of the **gradient coils** is to **spatially encode** the signal.

To spatially encode the signal, we have to apply the RF pulse multiple times while varying the gradients and, in turn, get multiple FIDs or other signals (e.g., spin echoes). When we put all the information from the multiple FIDs together, we get the information necessary to create an image. If we just apply the RF pulse once, we only get one signal (one FID), and we cannot make an image from one signal. (An exception to this statement is echo-planar imaging [EPI] which is performed after one RF pulse—see Chapter 26.)

TR (THE REPETITION TIME)

After we apply one 90° pulse (the symbol we'll use for a 90° RF pulse is in Figure 5-5) we'll apply another. The time interval between

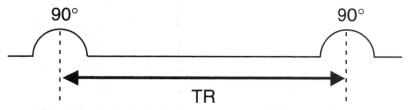

Figure 5-5. The time interval between two successive 90° RF pulses is denoted TR.

applications is called TR (the Repetition Time).

What happens to the T_1 recovery curve during successive 90° pulses (Fig. 5-6)?

1. Immediately before time t = 0, the magnetization vector points along the z axis. Call this vector $\mathbf{M_0}$ **with magnitude** $\mathbf{M_0}$.
2. Immediately after t = 0, the magnetization vector $\mathbf{M_{xy}}$ lies in the x-y plane, without a component along the z axis. $\mathbf{M_{xy}}$ has magnitude M_0 at t = 0^+.
3. As time goes by and we reach time t = TR, we gradually recover some magnetization along the z axis, and lose some (or all) magnetization in the x-y plane. Let's assume at time TR the transverse magnetization M_{xy} is very small. What happens if we now apply another 90° RF pulse? We flip the existing longitudinal magnetization vector (M_z) back into the x-y plane. However, what is the magni-

tude of the magnetization vector M_z at the time TR? Because

$$M_z(t) = M_0 (1 - e^{-t/T1})$$

then at t = TR,

$$M_z(TR) = M_0 (1 - e^{-TR/T1}) \qquad \text{(Eqn. 5-1)}$$

As we see in the T_1 recovery curve, the magnetization vector (M_z) at time TR is less than the original magnetization vector M_0 because the second 90° RF pulse was applied before complete recovery of the magnetization vector M_z.

4. After the magnetization vector is flipped back into the x-y plane, it will begin to grow again along the z axis (according to the T_1 recovery curve) until the next TR, when it will again be flipped into the x-y plane. We now have a *series* of

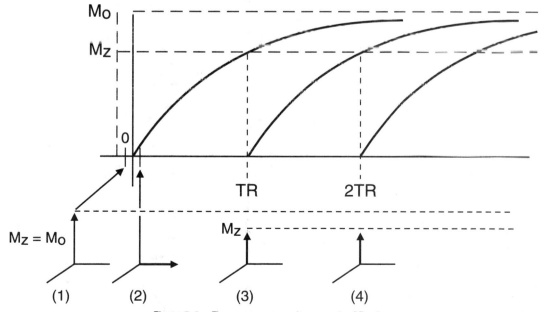

Figure 5-6. The recovery curves after successive RF pulses.

exponential curves that never reach full magnetization.

RECEIVED SIGNAL

Let's now take a look at the signal we are receiving (S). Because we are only applying a series of 90° pulses, the signal will be a series of FIDs:

1. At time $t = 0$, the initial signal will be a strong FID similar to that shown in Fig. 5-7a.
2. At time $t = TR$, the signal will be slightly less in magnitude, but will also be an FID (Fig. 5-7b).
3. At time $t = 2TR$, the signal will be equal in magnitude to that in b (Fig. 5-7c).

Because the T_1 recovery curve is given by the formula $1 - e^{-t/T1}$, if we could measure the signal immediately after the RF pulse is given with no delay, then each FID signal would be proportional to:

$$1 - e^{-TR/T1}$$

(This cannot really happen in practice.) Up to now, the signal S is given by the formula:

$$S \propto 1 - e^{-TR/T1}$$

Remember that the word "signal" is really a relative term. The signal that we get is a number without dimension; i.e., it has no units. If we are dealing with a tissue that has many mobile protons, then, regardless of what the TR and T_1 of the tissue are, we'll get more signal with more mobile protons (see Chapter 3). Thus, when considering the signal, we must also consider the number of **mobile protons** N(H).

$$S \propto N(H)(1 - e^{-TR/T1}) \qquad \text{(Eqn. 5-2)}$$

For a given tissue, the T_1 and the proton density are constant, and the signal received will be according to the above formula. If we measure the FID at time TR immediately after the application of the second 90° RF pulse, it will measure maximal and be equal to $N(H) (1 - e^{-TR/T1})$. Therefore, the FIDs, which are acquired at TR intervals (i.e., 1TR, 2TR) are maximal if they can be measured right after the 90° pulse, i.e., right at the beginning of the FID. However, in reality, we have to wait a certain period until the system electronics allow us to make a measurement.

TE (ECHO DELAY TIME)

TE stands for **Echo Time** (or Echo Delay Time). Instead of making the measurement immediately after the RF pulse (which we could not do anyway), we wait a short period of time and *then* make the measurement. This short time period is referred to as TE.

Let's go back to the T_2* decay curve and see what happens. In the x-y plane, the FID signal decays at a very rapid rate because of two factors:

1. external magnetic field inhomogeneities
2. spin-spin interactions.

The signal decays at rate T_2* according to the decay function:

$$e^{-t/T2*}$$

From this we see that if we take the signal measurement right away, before there is any chance for signal decay, the signal will be equal to the original magnetization (M_0) flipped into the x-y plane (point 1 in Fig. 5-8). However, if we wait a short time period (TE) before we make a mea-

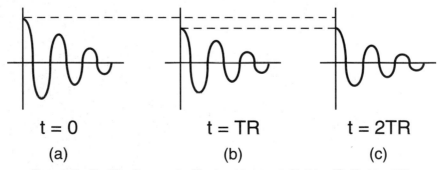

$t = 0$ $t = TR$ $t = 2TR$

(a)   (b)   (c)

Figure 5-7. The FIDs after successive RF pulses: (a) at $t = 0$; (b) at $t = TR$; (c) at $t = 2TR$.

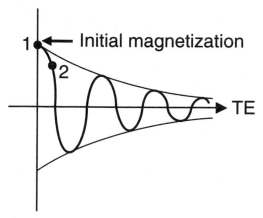

Figure 5-8. The value of the FID at time 0 is M_0, whereas at time TE it is $M_0 \cdot e^{-TE/T2^*}$.

surement, the signal will look like point 2 in Figure 5-8:

$$M_0 \cdot (e^{-TE/T2^*}) \qquad \text{(Eqn. 5-3a)}$$

Now we have to put the two curves together because both T_1 recovery and T_2 decay processes are occurring simultaneously (Fig. 5-9).

Let's go back to the T_1 recovery curve. After the 90° RF pulse, the spins are flipped into the x-y plane. After a time interval TR, the amount of received longitudinal magnetization is

$$M_0 (1 - e^{-TR/T1}) \qquad \text{(Eqn. 5-3b)}$$

Superimposed on this T_1 recovery curve, we'll draw another curve, which is the T_2^* decay curve, with two new axes. The T_2^* decay curve starts out at the value of $M_0 (1 - e^{-TR/TE})$ on the

T_1 recovery curve, and then decays very quickly. The decay rate of the new curve is given by T_2^* according to the formula

$$e^{-t/T2^*}$$

After a period of time TE, we can measure the signal. The value of the signal at TE will be a fraction of the maximum signal intensity on the T_1 recovery curve. In other words, it will be the product of Equations 5-3a and 5-3b:

$$\text{Signal} = S \propto M_0(1 - e^{-TR/T1})(e^{-TE/T2^*})$$

The confusing thing about the diagram is that there are two sets of axes (Fig. 5-9):

1. the first set of axes is associated with TR;
2. the second set of axes is associated with TE.

If we draw them to scale, the T_2 decay curve (time scale TE) will be decaying much faster than the T_1 curve is recovering (time scale TR). However, the graph does give us a visual concept of what the final signal intensity is going to be. Because the initial longitudinal magnetization M_0 is proportional to the number of mobile protons, i.e.,

$$M_0 \propto N(H)$$

then, in general, the signal intensity we measure is given by:

$$\text{Signal Intensity} = SI \propto N(H)(e^{-TE/T2^*})(1 - e^{-TR/T1})$$
$$\text{(Eqn. 5-4)}$$

(The difference between T_2 and T_2^* is the correction for external magnetic field inhomogeneity achieved with spin-echo techniques.)

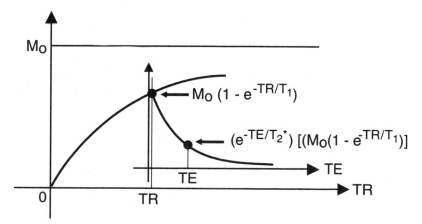

Figure 5-9. The recovery and decay curves plotted on the same graph.

TISSUE CONTRAST (T$_1$ AND T$_2$ WEIGHTING)

Let's see what happens when we deal with two different tissues. So far we have been dealing with a single tissue, but now we'll consider two tissues: tissue A and tissue B.

Question: *Of the two tissues in Figure 5-10a, which one has the longer T$_1$?*
Answer: *Tissue A has the longer T$_1$ (it takes longer to recover).*

If we draw just a tangent along each curve at the origin, tissue A has a longer T$_1$ than tissue B. But just by looking at the curves, it takes tissue A longer to reach equilibrium than tissue B. Let's say we have two different TRs:

1.   short TR = TR$_1$
2.   long TR = TR$_2$

Question: *Which one of the TRs in Figure 5-10b gives better tissue contrast?*
Answer: *TR$_1$ gives the better contrast.*

Let's go back to Equation 5-4 and see if this answer makes sense:

$$SI = N(H)(e^{-TE/T2*})(1 - e^{-TR/T1})$$

where *SI* stands for signal intensity. If TR goes to infinity, then $1 - e^{-TR/T1}$ becomes 1. If TR → ∞, then $1 - e^{-TR/T1} \to 1$ and SI → $N(H)(e^{-TE/T2*})$. If TR is very long, we can get rid of the T$_1$ component in the equation. What this means in

practice is that we eliminate (or, more realistically, reduce) the T$_1$ effect by having a very large TR.

Long TR reduces the T$_1$ effect.

We can't really achieve a long enough TR in practice to totally eliminate the T$_1$ effect 100%, but we can certainly *minimize* the T$_1$ effect with a TR of 2000 to 3000 msec (in general, if TR is 4 to 5 times T$_1$, then the T$_1$ effect becomes negligible). Let's go back to Figure 5-10b and see what happens at TR = TR$_1$. At this point, the TR is not long enough to eliminate the T$_1$ term in the equation $(1 - e^{TR/T1})$. So we have:

$$\text{signal intensity (tissue A)/signal intensity (tissue B)} = (1 - e^{-TR1/T1(tissue A)})/(1 - e^{-TR1/T1(tissue B)})$$

Because the T$_1$'s of tissue A and tissue B are different, the short TR brings out the difference in contrast between tissue A and tissue B. Thus, for short TR, the two tissues can be differentiated on the basis of different T$_1$'s. In other words, we get T$_1$ tissue contrast with short TR.

Short TR enhances the T$_1$ contrast.

We don't want TR to be very long when we're evaluating T$_1$ because, as we've already learned, when TR → ∞, then $(1 - e^{-TR/T1})$ approaches 1, thus eliminating the T$_1$ effect. However, we

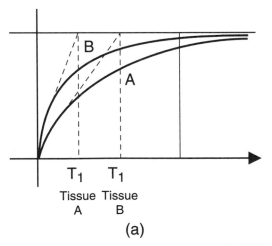

(a)

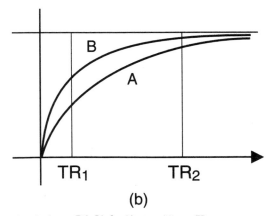

(b)

Figure 5-10.   **(a)** Two tissues A and B with different T1s. Which tissue has the longer T1? **(b)** Consider two different TRs on a recovery curve. Which TR provides better tissue contrast between A and B?

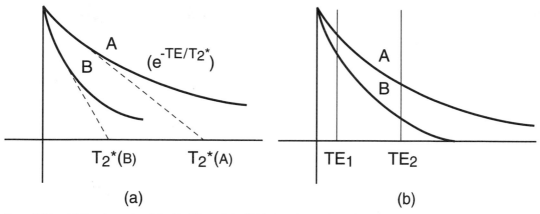

Figure 5-11. **(a)** Two tissues A and B with different T2*s. Which tissue has the longer T2? **(b)** Consider two different TEs on a decay curve. Which TE provides better tissue contrast between A and B?

also don't want TR to be too short. If TR is close to zero, then

$$e^{-0/T1} = e^0 = 1$$

and

$$1 - e^{-TR/T1} = 1 - 1 = 0$$

In this situation, with very short TR, we end up with no signal. Ideally, we would like to have a TR that is not much different than the T_1 of the tissue under study.

T_2^* TISSUE CONTRAST

Let's consider T_2^* contrast between two tissues.

Question: *In Figure 5-11a, which tissue has a longer T_2^*?*
Answer: *Again, if we graphically draw a tangent at t = 0 for each curve, we see that tissue A has a longer T_2^*. Put differently, it takes the signal from Tissue A longer to decay than that from tissue B.*

Let's pick two different TEs (Fig. 5-11b). Here we have two TEs:

1.   short TE = TE_1
2.   long TE = TE_2

Question: *Which one of the TEs in Figure 5-11b results in more tissue contrast between tissue A and tissue B?*

Answer: *TE_2 gives us more contrast.*

Let's again look at the formula for signal intensity (Eqn. 5-4):

$$SI = N(H)(e^{-TE/T2^*})(1 - e^{-TR/T1})$$

If TE is very short (close to zero), then $e^{-TE/T2^*}$ approaches 1.

$$TE \to 0 \Rightarrow e^{-TE/T2^*} \to e^0 = 1$$

Then

$$\begin{aligned} \text{signal intensity} &= N(H)(1)(1 - e^{-TR/T1}) \\ &= N(H)(1 - e^{-TR/T1}). \end{aligned}$$

This means that, with a very short TE, we get rid of the T_2^* effect in the equation. Therefore, we eliminate (or, again, in reality, reduce) the T_2^* effect by having a very short TE.

Short TE reduces the T_2^* effect.

We can see this graphically from the graph (Fig. 5-11b) and mathematically from the equation (Eqn. 5-3). When we have a long TE, we enhance T_2^* contrast between tissues. Even though the signal to noise ratio is low (because there is greater signal decay for a longer TE), the tissue contrast is high.

Key Points

1.   Long TR: Reduces T_1 effect.

2.   Short TR: Enhances T_1 effect

3.   Short TE: Reduces T_2^* (T_2) effect

4.   Long TE: Enhances T_2^* (T_2) effect

Questions

5-1. In the graph in Figure P5-1, the T_1 and T_2 curves are plotted simultaneously for convenience. Assume the following values for T_1 and T_2:

$$\text{for WM: } T_1 = 500, T_2 = 100;$$
$$\text{for CSF: } T_1 = 2000, T_2 = 200 \text{ ms}$$

Also assume a spin density $N = 100$ for both WM and CSF.
(a) For a TR = 2000 ms, find the relative signal intensities for WM and CSF (i.e., points A and B on the graph).
(b) Calculate the crossover TE where WM and CSF have identical T_2 weighting (point C).
(c) Now, calculate the signal intensities of WM and CSF for TE = 25 (first echo) and TE = 100 (second echo), and the ratio CSF/WM
(d) Repeat (a)–(c) for TR = 3000, and observe how one gets more T2 weighting in the 2nd echo (higher ratio CSF/WM)
(e) Now, calculate the signal intensities for TR = 3000 and TE = 200. Notice that despite relative loss of signal for both WM and CSF, the ratio CSF/WM actually increases, indicating more T_2 weighting (i.e., CSF gets brighter on the images).

The following values may be helpful for those of you without a sophisticated calculator:

$$e = 2.72, e^{-1} = 1/e = .37,$$
$$e^{-2} = 1/e^2 = .14, e^{-3} = .05,$$

$$e^{-4} = .02, e^{-5} = .01, e^{-6} \cong 0,$$
$$e^{-.5} = .61, e^{-1.5} = 0.22, e^{-.13} = 0.88;$$
$$\ln .64 = \log_e .64 = -.45,$$
$$\ln .78 = -.25$$

5-2. Suppose that at 1.0 Tesla, the approximate T_1 and T_2 values for the following tissues are as follows:

Tissue	T_1 (ms)	T_2 (ms)
H_2O	2500	2500
fat	200	100
CSF	2000	300
gray matter	500	100

(a) Calculate the signal intensity *ratios* for:

1. H_2O/fat
2. CSF/gray matter

for the following pulse sequences:

1. T_1WI/SE with TR = 500 , TE = 25 ms
2. T_2WI/SE with TR = 2500, TE = 100 ms

Note: Assume similar spin densities for these tissues.
(b) Demonstrate the above graphically. *Hint:* $e^{-1} = .37$, $e^{-5} = .01$, $e^{-.04} = .96$, $e^{-1.25} = .29$, $e^{-12.5} \cong 0$ $e^{-2.5} = .08$, $e^{-.25} = .78$, $e^{-.2} = .82$, $e^{-.01} = .99$, $e^{-1/3} = .72$ $e^{-.25/300} = .92$.

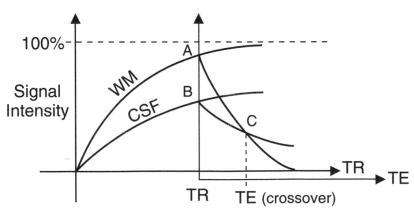

Figure P5-1

5-3. A longer TR
    (a) increases T1 weighting
    (b) reduces T2 weighting
    (c) reduces T1 weighting

5-4. A longer TE
    (a) increases T2 weighting
    (b) increases T1 weighting
    (c) reduces T2 weighting

5-5. Calculate the signal $N(H)(1 - e^{-TR/T1}) e^{-TE/T2}$ for the following theoretical situations
    (a) $TR = \infty$ (b) $TE = 0$
    (c) $TR = \infty$ and $TE = 0$

6 Tissue Contrast: Some Clinical Applications

INTRODUCTION

In the previous chapter, we talked about T_1 and T_2 weighting in terms of the time parameters TR and TE. Now let's discuss the T_1 and T_2 characteristics of the following tissues and see what physical properties affect them:

1. H_2O
2. Solids
3. Fat
4. Proteinaceous Material

T_2 CHARACTERISTICS

The T_2 characteristics of a tissue are determined by how fast the proton spins in that tissue dephase. If they dephase rapidly, we get a short T_2. If they dephase more slowly, we get a longer T_2.

H_2O

Because of the structure of the water molecule ($H-O-H$) and because of the sparsity of these molecules, spin-spin interaction among the hydrogen protons is minimal. Therefore, dephasing occurs at a much slower rate in water compared with other tissues. The T_2 relaxation time for H_2O is, therefore, long. Remember that T_2 decay is caused either by external magnetic field inhomogeneities or by spin-spin interactions within or between molecules. In H_2O, the effect of one hydrogen proton on another is relatively small. The distance between hydrogen protons both within each molecule and between adjacent molecules is relatively large, so there is little spin-spin interaction and, therefore, less dephasing.

Solids

The molecular structure of solids is opposite to that of pure water. It is a very compactly structured tissue, with many interactions between hydrogen protons. This large number of spin-spin interactions results in more dephasing. Thus, the T_2 for solids is short.

Fat and Proteinaceous Material

The structure of these materials is such that there is less dephasing than in solids, but more dephasing than in water. Therefore, T_2 for proteinaceous material or fat is intermediate.

T_1 CHARACTERISTICS

The T_1 of a tissue has to do with the way the protons are able to give off their energy to the surrounding lattice, or to absorb the energy from the lattice. It turns out that the most efficient energy transfer occurs when the **natural motional frequencies*** of the protons are at the **Larmor frequency** (ω_0). Recall that the Larmor frequency is proportional to the strength of the magnetic field:

$$\omega_0 = \gamma B_0$$

For Hydrogen, $\omega_0 = 42.6$ MHz/Tesla

In other words, the precessional frequency of a hydrogen proton is 42.6 MHz in a 1 Tesla magnetic field. However, the *natural motional frequency* of hydrogen protons depends on the physical states of the tissue. It is influenced by the atoms to which they are attached or are proximal to.

H_2O

Hydrogen protons in the small H_2O molecule have higher natural motional frequencies than, for example, hydrogen protons in a solid structure. The natural motional frequency of hydrogen protons in water is also much faster than the Larmor frequency for hydrogen.

$$\omega(H_2O) \gg \omega_0$$

Solids

Hydrogen protons in solids have lower natural motional frequencies than do water protons.

---

* translation, rotation, and vibration

The natural motional frequencies of hydrogen protons in solids is somewhat slower than Larmor frequency for hydrogen.

$$\omega(\text{Solids}) < \omega_0$$

Fat

Hydrogen protons in fat have natural motional frequencies that are almost equal to the Larmor frequencies used for MRI.

$$\omega(\text{fat}) \approx \omega_0$$

This result is caused by the rotational frequency of the carbons around the terminal C—C bond. Because this frequency is near the Larmor frequency, the *efficiency of energy transfer from the protons to the lattice or from the lattice to the protons* is increased, thus decreasing T_1.

Proteinaceous Solutions

The foregoing discussion on the T_1 and T_2 characteristics of fluids such as water applies only to *pure* water (or **bulk phase water**). However, most of the water in the body is not in the pure state but is **bound** to a **hydrophilic macromolecule** such as a protein.

Such water molecules form hydration layers around the macromolecule and are called **hydration layer water** (Fig. 6-1). These bound H_2O molecules lose some of the freedom in their motion. As a result, the natural motional frequencies of the H_2O molecules get closer to the Larmor frequency, thus yielding a more efficient energy transfer. The net result is a shortening in the T_1 relaxation. Therefore, proteinaceous fluids, i.e. hydration layer water, are brighter than pure water on T_1 weighted images.

If the protein content is high enough, hydration layer water can cause some T_2 shortening. This shortening is generally seen in gels and in **mucinous** fluids. Such proteinaceous fluids may be darker than pure fluids on T_2 weighted images.

For H_2O and solid tissue, the energy transfer is not efficient and the T_1 for H_2O and solid tissue is long. Also, the T_1 of H_2O is longer than the T_1 for solid tissue because the difference between the Larmor frequency and the natural motional frequencies of hydrogen protons in

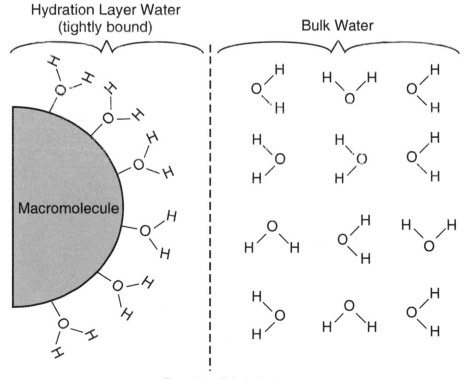

Figure 6-1. Hydration layer water.

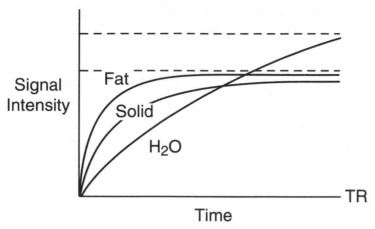

Figure 6-2.   T1 recovery curves of fat, water, and a solid tissue.

H_2O is much greater than the difference between the Larmor frequency and the motional frequencies of hydrogen protons in solid tissue.

Let's now draw the T_1 and T_2 curves for these different tissues (Fig. 6-2):

1. **Fat** has the shortest T_1, and will have the steepest T_1 recovery curve.
2. **Proteinaceous fluid** also has a short T_1.
3. **H_2O** has the longest T_1 and will have the slowest T_1 recovery curve.
4. **Solid** tissue has intermediate T_1.

For the sake of argument, we'll assume that they all have the same proton density. Actually, the proton density of H_2O is higher because there is more H_2O in the body than fat or solid tissue, and intensity is based not only on T_1 and T_2, but also on the proton density N(H):

$$I \propto N(H)(e^{-TE/T2})(1 - e^{-TR/T1})$$

At a time TR, we transmit another RF pulse. Let's superimpose the T_2 decay curve on the T_1 recovery curve (Fig. 6-3):

1. **H_2O** has a very long T_2, so it will have a very shallow T_2 decay curve.
2. **Solid** tissue has short T_2, and will thus decay fairly rapidly.
3. **Fat** has an intermediate T_2.
4. **Proteinaceous fluid** may have a short or intermediate T_2 depending on the protein content.

Therefore, we see that if we pick a long enough TE (TE_3) in Figure 6-3, the signals that we measure from each tissue show the following:

1. **H_2O** has the highest signal intensity (point a, Fig. 6-3).
2. **Solid** tissue has the lowest signal intensity.

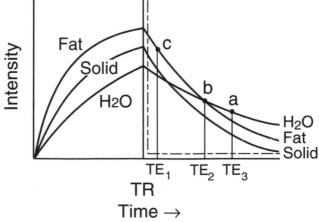

Figure 6-3.   T2 decay curves of fat, water, and a solid tissue.

3. **Fat** has an intermediate signal intensity.
4. **Proteinaceous fluid** has an intermediate or low signal intensity depending on its protein content.

If we take a shorter TE (TE_2), we might pick a point where fat and H_2O might have the same signal intensity. This is a crossover effect (point b, Fig. 6-3).

If the TE is really short (TE_1), we just get a T_1 or proton density effect, where

1. **Fat** has the highest intensity (point c, Fig. 6-3).
2. **Proteinaceous fluid** also has high intensity similar to fat.
3. **Solid** tissue has intermediate intensity.
4. **H_2O** has the lowest intensity.

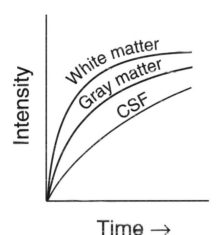

Figure 6-4. T1 recovery curves of CSF, white matter, and gray matter.

So, we can see from the curve that

1. If TR and TE are short, we get T_1 weighting.
2. If TR and TE are long, we get T_2 weighting.
3. If TR is long and TE is short, we get proton density weighting.

Let's now look at three different tissues in the brain: 1) gray matter, 2) white matter, and 3) CSF (Fig. 6-4). On a T_1 recovery curve:

1. **White matter** is white. The myelin sheath acts like fat; with more efficient energy exchange, it has a shorter longitudinal relaxation than does gray matter.
2. **Gray matter** is intermediate: without myelin, it acts more like a typical solid tissue.
3. **CSF** is dark: like water, it has inefficient energy exchange and thus the same long longitudinal relaxation, T_1.

Let's add the T_2 decay curves to the T_1 recovery curves (Fig. 6-5):

1. **CSF**, like H_2O, has the least dephasing, and thus the longest, T_2.
2. **White matter** has a slightly shorter T_2 than **gray matter**.

If we use a long TE (TE_3), then we'll get a typical T_2 weighted image. Therefore, at TE = TE_3, we have (Fig. 6-6)

$$@ \text{ TE} = TE_3 \begin{cases} \text{CSF is } \textbf{bright} \text{ (point a, Fig. 6-5)} \\ \text{Gray matter is intermediate (\textbf{gray})} \\ \text{White matter is } \textbf{dark} \end{cases}$$

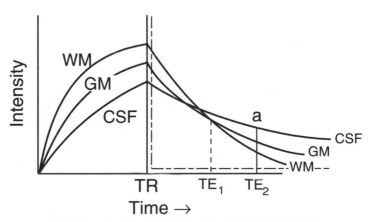

Figure 6-5. T2 decay curves of CSF, white matter, and gray matter.

Let's pick a shorter TE = TE_2 (Fig. 6-6). At this point, white matter and CSF are isointense (crossover point). We want to achieve this isointensity on a proton density image. We can see the advantages by considering what tumors and demyelinating plaques do on a T_1 recovery curve, or on a T_2 decay curve. Most pathological lesions have a slow T_1 recovery curve because of their **vasogenic edema** (which contains H_2O). However, their T_1 recovery curve is not as slow as pure water. Most pathologic lesions (e.g., tumor, edema, MS plaque) also have a long T_2 but not as long as that of CSF.

In Figure 6-6, we've included a T_1 recovery curve and a T_2 decay curve for a pathological lesion. If we are looking for MS plaques, let's first look at a T_2 weighted image (long TE = TE_3 in the graph):

1. White matter is dark.
2. CSF is bright.
3. MS plaque is also bright.

Even though brightness may be different between the CSF and MS plaque, the ratio is not great enough to discern a difference (e.g., the lesion is adjacent to a lateral ventricle).

If we now look at the intensities at a shorter TE (TE_2) corresponding to the CSF and white matter crossover point, then CSF and white matter will be isointense. The pathologic lesion (e.g., MS plaque) will be brighter than both CSF and white matter, and it can thus be detected more easily.

Remember also that if we chose a long TR and a very short TE (TE_1 on graph), the TE

Table 6-1. T_1, T_2, and Proton Density of Brain Tissues*

	T_1 (msec)	T_2 (msec)	N(H)
White matter	510	67	0.61
Gray matter	760	77	0.69
Edema	900	126	0.86
CSF	2650	180	1.00

* Stark and Bradley, p. 113

occurs before the crossover points of either CSF, gray matter, or white matter, resulting still in a proton density weighted image.

This is a good time to bring up the proton density factor: N(H). We've been, to a certain extent, ignoring it. We've talked about T_1 and T_2, and we've been assuming that all the tissues have almost the same proton density. However, in Table 6-1, we can see the differences in the proton densities of various tissues.

For instance, if the CSF has a proton density of 1 (or 100%), then white matter has a proton density of 0.61 (61% of CSF) and edema has a proton density of 0.86 (86% of CSF). How does this difference in proton density affect the graphs of T_1 and T_2? Let's talk about two different tissues (Fig. 6-7):

1. CSF
2. White matter

CSF has a higher proton density than white matter, so it has a higher maximum limit on the T_1 recovery curve. White matter has a lower proton density than CSF, but its T_1 is shorter. The two recovery curves cross at the point where white

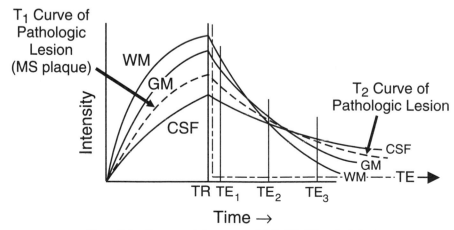

Figure 6-6. Recovery and decay curves of CSF, WM, GM, and a lesion.

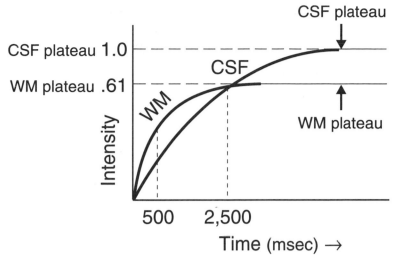

Figure 6-7. The plateau of the recovery curve of a tissue is determined by the proton density of that tissue N(H). For instance, N(CSF) is larger than N(WM).

matter and CSF have the same intensity (TR ≅ 2500 msec).

For the mathematically interested reader, this TR is the solution to the following equation:

$$1.0(1 - e^{-TR/2650}) = 0.61(1 - e^{-TR/510})$$

or

$$e^{-TR/2650} - 0.61\, e^{-TR/510} - 0.39 = 0$$

using the T_1 and N(H) values for WM and CSF from Table 6-1, resulting in a TR of approximately 2500 msec (2462 msec to be exact!).

Let's now consider two situations:

1. short TR
2. long TR

(1) First, draw the T_1 recovery curves for WM and CSF (Fig. 6-8). Now consider a **short TR** (say, 300 msec). White matter is initially brighter than CSF because of its shorter T_1. However, CSF has a longer T_2 than white matter. Therefore, after the T_2 crossover point, CSF will become brighter than white matter (e.g., at TE_2). Thus, at long TE, we get T2 contrast. If we pick a short TE (TE_1), we get T_1 contrast. Thus, with a short TR, which maximizes T_1 contrast, we want to

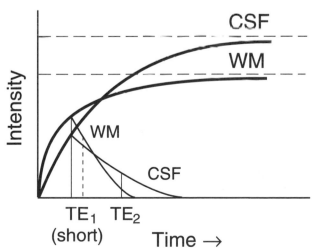

Figure 6-8. Recovery and decay curves for WM and CSF for a short TR.

choose as short a TE as possible to maximize the T_1 contrast.

T1W: Short TR/Short TE

(2) Now, draw the T_1 and T_2 curves again and this time pick a **long TR**. Remember that CSF has a greater proton density than white matter, so it will have a higher plateau value than white matter which is brought out by the long TR (Fig. 6-9). Then draw the T_2 decay curves, keeping in mind that CSF has a longer T_2 than white matter. If we now pick a very short TE (TE_1), the two signals are driven by their respective proton densities: CSF will have greater intensity than white matter (i.e., 39% from Table

6-1). At this point, the difference in intensity reflects their (*true*) proton density differences (assuming a *very* short TE).

PDW: Long TR/Short TE

If TE is long (TE_2), increase the signal intensity differences between white matter and CSF. This increased intensity difference reflects the T_2 difference:

T2W: Long TR/Long TE

Let's now introduce an abnormality—namely, edema—and incorporate it with CSF and white matter (Fig. 6-10). We know that the

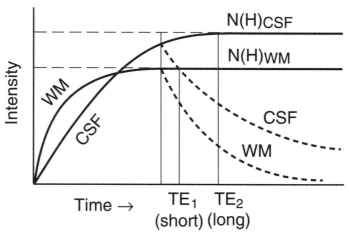

Figure 6-9.   Recovery and decay curves of WM and CSF for a long TR.

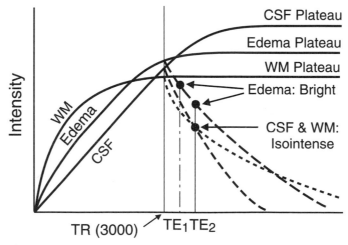

Figure 6-10.   Recovery and decay curves of WM, CSF, and edema for a long TR.

T_1 recovery curve for edema is in between CSF and white matter—it has a shorter T_1 than CSF and a longer T_1 than white matter. We also know that the plateau for edema is less than that for pure CSF, but more than that for white matter. Again, if we choose a TR that is long enough for white matter to reach its plateau, and then choose a TE that is short (either at or before the cross-over point for CSF and white matter T_2 decay), then edema has the highest signal intensity.

Therefore, for "proton density" images (long TR/short TE):

1. Edema is bright.
2. CSF and white matter are isointense.

Now, pick a TR at the point of intersection of the T_1 recovery curves for CSF and white matter—a point at which WM (white matter) has almost reached its peak intensity, but CSF has not (similar to the previous graphs, but TR is now longer in order to reach the crossover point) (Fig. 6-11). Now, apply the 90° pulse, and follow the T_2 decay curves. With a short TE, CSF is brighter than WM. With a long TE, CSF is still brighter than WM, but the difference in brightness gets magnified. On the long TR/short TE image, the difference in intensity reflects only the differences in proton densities between the two tissues, whereas the long TR/long TE image incorporates both proton

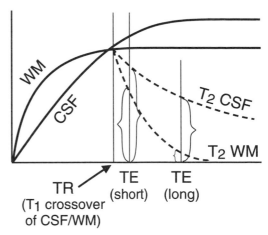

Figure 6-11. Recovery and decay curves of WM and CSF for a TR corresponding to the crossover point of CSF and WM.

densities *and* T_2 differences between the two tissues.

Parenthetically, in a **true** PD image (as in Fig. 6-9), CSF or H_2O has the highest signal (because water has more protons than any other tissue). Therefore, to minimize the T_1 and T_2 influences on what should be a **true** proton density weighted image, we need to make the TR long enough to allow the T_1 recovery curves to reach their plateaus, and then make the TE short enough to minimize T_2 decay. (Actually, this may not be a desirable image because lesions and normal fluid may be indistinguishable.)

Key Points

Table 6-2 summarizes the T_1 and T_2 properties of three tissues: water, solids, and fat/proteinaceous material. Table 6-3 contains the relative T_1 and T_2 values (short, intermediate, or long) for several tissues.

Table 6-2. T_1 and T_2 as a Function of Natural Motional Frequencies ω vs. the Larmor Frequency ω_0 for Different Tissues

	H_2O/Fluids	Solids	Fat and Proteinaceous Material
T_1	$\omega \gg \omega 0$ Non Efficient Energy Transfer **Very Long T_1**	$\omega < \omega 0$ Inefficient Energy Transfer **Long T_1**	$\omega \approx \omega 0$ Efficient Energy Transfer **Short T_1**
T_2	Less dephasing **Long T_2**	Most dephasing **Short T_2**	Intermediate dephasing **Intermediate T_2**

Table 6-3. Relative T$_1$ and T$_2$ Values for Several Tissues. a-d represent breakdown products of hemoglobin (a = oxyhemoglobin; b = deoxyhemoglobin; c = intracellular methemoglobin; d = extracellular methemoglobin; e = hemosiderin). GM = gray matter; WM = white matter; SI = signal intensity; Hgb = hemoglobin; IC = intracellular; EC = extracellular.

	long T$_1$ (low SI)	intermediate	short T$_1$ (high SI)
long T$_2$ (high SI)	water/CSF pathology edema		**d (EC metHgb)**
intermediate		muscle GM **a (oxyHgb)** WM	
short T$_2$ (low SI)	air cortical bone heavy Ca^{++} **b (deoxyHgb)** **e (hemosiderin)** fibrosis tendons		fat proteinaceous solutions **c (IC met Hgb)** paramagnetic materials (Gd, etc.)

Questions

6-1.   T/F   The most efficient energy transfer occurs at the Larmor frequency.

6-2.   Match
   (i)   air   (ii)   fat   (iii)   water
   (iv)   methemoglobin (intracellular)
   with
   (a)   short T1 and T2
   (b)   short T1, long T2
   (c)   long T1, short T2
   (d)   long T1, long T2

6-3.   T/F   Hydration layer water has a shorter T1 than bulk water.

7 Pulse Sequences

Part I (Saturation, Partial Saturation, Inversion Recovery)

INTRODUCTION

A **pulse sequence** is a *sequence* of RF *pulses* applied repeatedly during an MR study. Embedded in it are the TR and TE time parameters. It is related to a **timing diagram** or a **pulse sequence diagram** (PSD), which is discussed in Chapter 14. In this chapter, we'll discuss the concepts of "**saturation**" and consider pulse sequences partial saturation, saturation recovery, and inversion recovery. In the next chapter, we'll talk about the important spin-echo pulse sequence. Figure 7-1 illustrates the notations used for three types of RF pulses throughout this book.

SATURATION

Immediately after the longitudinal magnetization has been flipped into the x-y plane by a 90° pulse, the system is said to be **saturated**. Application of a second 90° pulse at this moment will elicit no signal (like beating a dead horse). A few moments later after some T_1 recovery, the system is "**partially saturated**." With complete T_1 recovery to the plateau value, the system is "**unsaturated**" or fully *magnetized*. Should the longitudinal magnetization only be partially flipped into the x-y plane (i.e., flip angles less than 90°), then there is still a component of magnetization along the z axis. The spins in this state are also **partially saturated**.

Partial Saturation Pulse Sequence

Start with a 90° pulse, wait for a short period TR, and then apply another 90° pulse. Keep repeating this sequence. The measurements are obtained immediately after the 90° RF pulse. Therefore, the signal received is an FID (free induction decay).

Let's see how this looks on the T_1 recovery curve (Fig. 7-2). At time t = 0, flip the longitudinal magnetization 90° into the x-y plane. Right after that, the longitudinal magnetization begins to recover. Wait a time t = TR, and repeat the 90° pulse. Initially, at time t = 0, the longitudinal magnetization is at a maximum. As soon as we flip it, the longitudinal magnetization goes to zero and then immediately thereafter begins to grow. At time t = TR, the longitudinal magnetization has grown but has not recovered its plateau before it is flipped into the x-y plane again. (Note that the length of the longitudinal magnetization vector before the second 90°RF pulse is less than the original longitudinal magnetization vector.)

Now, with a third 90° RF pulse, we again flip the longitudinal magnetization into the x-y plane. Again, the longitudinal magnetization goes to zero and immediately begins to recover. Again, at time 2TR, it is less than maximum, but is equal to the previous longitudinal magnetization (at time TR). Each subsequent recovery time

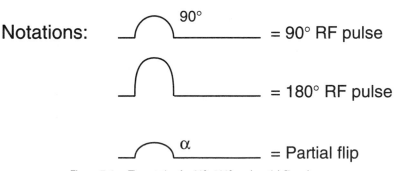

Notations:

= 90° RF pulse

= 180° RF pulse

= Partial flip

Figure 7-1. The notation for 90°, 180°, and partial flip pulses.

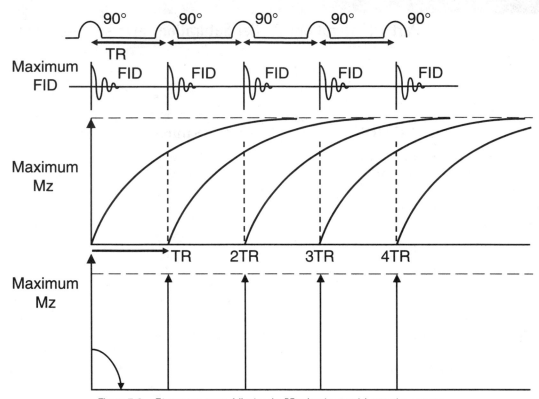

Figure 7-2.   T1 recovery curves following the RF pulses in a partial saturation sequence.

TR after each subsequent 90° pulse will also be the same. Thus, the maximum FID occurs at time t = 0 after the first 90° RF pulse, and all subsequent FIDs will have less magnitude but will have the same value.

> *Question:*   *Is there a residual transverse magnetization M_{xy} at time TR just before the next 90° RF pulse?*
> *Answer:*   *No! Because T_1 is several times larger than T_2, after a time TR has elapsed, the magnetization in the x-y plane has fully decayed to zero.*

In partial saturation, TE is minimal. The signal is measured immediately after the 90° RF pulse:

Partial saturation: TR is short, TE is minimal.

> *Question:*   *With short TR and minimal TE, what kind of an image would we be getting?*
> *Answer:*   *T_1 weighted image.*

A partial saturation pulse sequence generates a T_1 weighted image.

SATURATION RECOVERY PULSE SEQUENCE

The previous sequence is called partial saturation because at the time of the second 90° RF pulse (at time TR), we haven't yet completely recovered the longitudinal magnetization. Therefore, only a portion of the original longitudinal magnetization (M_0) is flipped at time TR (and subsequent TRs). Hence the name partial saturation.

In **saturation recovery**, we try to recover all the longitudinal magnetization before we apply another 90° RF pulse. We have to wait a long time before we apply a second RF pulse. Thus, TR will be long (Fig. 7-3).

After each 90° RF pulse, we measure it and an FID right away. Because we allow the longitudinal magnetization to completely recover before the next 90° pulse, the FID gives the maximum signal each time. In other words, we have recovered from the state of saturation.

In saturation recovery, TR is long and TE is minimal.

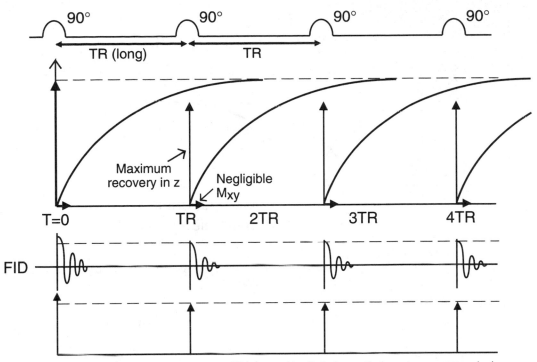

Figure 7-3. In a saturation recovery sequence, TR is long and longitudinal magnetization vectors are near maximal.

Question: With long TR and minimal TE, what kind of image do we get?

Answer: Proton density weighted (PDW).

The saturation recovery *pulse sequence results in a proton density weighted image.*

Neither of these sequences are really used any more, but they are so simple to understand that they are good springboards from which to learn about other, more complex pulse sequences. These pulse sequences are not used because it is very difficult to measure the FID without a delay period. Electronically we have to wait a certain period of time to make the measurements. Also, external magnetic inhomogeneity becomes a problem; that's why SE sequences (which we will discuss in the next chapter) are used to eliminate this problem.

INVERSION RECOVERY PULSE SEQUENCE

In inversion recovery, we first apply a 180° RF pulse. Next, we wait a period of time (the inversion time TI) and apply a 90° RF pulse. Then we wait a period of time TR (from the initial 180° pulse) and apply another 180° RF pulse (Fig. 7-4), beginning the sequence all over again.

Before we apply the 180° pulse, the magnetization vector points along the z axis. Immediately after we apply the 180° pulse, the magnetization vector is flipped 180°; it is now pointing south (−z), which is the opposite direction (Fig. 7-5).

We then allow the magnetization vector to recover along a T_1 growth curve. As it recovers, it gets smaller and smaller in the −z direction until it goes to zero, then starts growing in the +z

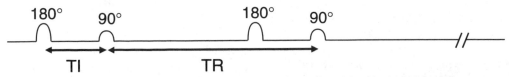

Figure 7-4. In inversion recovery, the time between the 180° pulse and the 90° pulse is denoted TI.

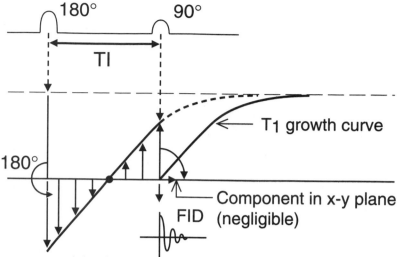

Figure 7-5. The recovery curves in inversion recovery. After the 180° pulse, the longitudinal magnetization vector is flipped 180° and starts to recover from a value that is the negative of its initial maximal value.

direction, ultimately recovering to the original longitudinal magnetization.

After a time TI, we apply a 90° pulse. This then flips the longitudinal magnetization into the x-y plane. The amount of magnetization flipped into the x-y plane will, of course, depends on the amount of longitudinal magnetization that has recovered during time TI after the original 180° RF pulse. We measure this flipped magnetization. Therefore, at this point we get an FID proportional to the longitudinal magnetization flipped into the x-y plane. Also, at this point, we begin the regrowth of the longitudinal magnetization. Recall that for a typical T_1 recovery curve, the formula for the exponential growth of the curve is

$$1 - e^{-t/T1}$$

However, when the magnetization starts to recover from $-M_0$ instead of zero (Fig. 7-6), the formula for recovery is

$$1 - 2e^{-t/T1}$$

EXERCISE:
Verify the above formula mathematically.

At time $t = 0$, signal intensity (SI) $= 1 - 2e^{-0/T1} = 1$
$- 2(1) = -1$
So at time $= 0$, magnitude of signal intensity $= -1$.
At $t = \infty$ (infinity), signal intensity $= 1 - 2e^{-\infty/T1}$
$= 1 - 2(0) = +1$
So at time $t = \infty$, the signal is maximal. These values correspond to the graph in Fig. 7-6.

Null Point

The point at which the signal crosses the zero line is called the **null point**. At this point, the signal intensity is zero. The time at this null point is denoted TI (null). We can solve the equation mathematically for TI(null) at which point the signal intensity is zero:

$$\text{Signal intensity} = 0 = 1 - 2e^{-TI/T1}$$

The solution to this equation is (see Problem 7-1):

$$TI(\text{null}) = (\log_e 2)T_1 = (\ln 2)T_1 \cong 0.693\ T_1$$

Let's go back and re-examine the recovery curves. Actually, there are two different exponentially growing curves occurring sequentially (Fig. 7-7):

1. recovery after the 180° RF pulse and
2. recovery after the 90° RF pulse

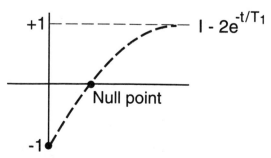

Figure 7-6. The recovery curve in IR is given by the formula $1 - 2\ e^{-t/T1}$.

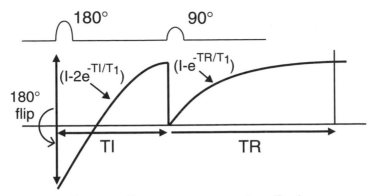

Figure 7-7. There are two recovery curves in one IR cycle.

(1) The T_1 recovery curve following the 180° pulse, starts at $-M_0$ and grows exponentially according to the formula:

$$M_0 (1 - 2e^{-TI/T1})$$

(2) The T_1 recovery curve following the 90° RF pulse, after the longitudinal magnetization flips into the x-y plane, starts at 0 and grows exponentially according to the formula:

$$M_0 (1 - e^{-TR/T1})$$

If we combine both of these T_1 recovery curves, we get a relationship that combines both T_1 and TR together. The result is the product of the above two formulas:

$$S \propto M_0 (1 - 2e^{-TI/T1})(1 - e^{-TR/T1})$$

Assuming that TI ≪ TR, the product of the terms within parentheses can be simplified to (see Problem 7-2)

$$(1 - 2e^{-TI/T1}) + (e^{-TR/T1})$$

Clinical Applications of Inversion Recovery

In an inversion recovery pulse sequence, we start out with a 180° RF pulse followed, after a time interval TI, by a 90° RF pulse. Next, after a certain time interval TR, the sequence is repeated with another 180° pulse.

TI = Inversion time, which represents the time interval between the 180° pulse and the 90° pulse.

TR = Time interval between successive 180° pulses (or, successive 90° pulses)

Consider graphically what happens to two tissues: edema and white matter (Fig. 7-8). In inversion recovery, we first flip the longitudinal

magnetization 180° with a 180° RF pulse. Subsequently, the magnetization vector still runs along the z axis but points in the negative (south) direction. Next, the longitudinal magnetization vectors begins to grow according to the T_1 growth curves of edema and white matter. Edema has a greater proton density than white matter, so its maximum magnetization along the z axis will be greater than the maximum for white matter. Likewise, after they have flipped 180°, the T_1 recovery curve for edema begins lower, i.e., is more negative along the z axis than is white matter.

From this initial position along the z axis, the longitudinal magnetization for edema grows along its T_1 recovery curve until it reaches its maximum. It starts decreasing in the negative z direction until it reaches zero (the null point) and then it continues increasing in the positive z direction until it reaches its maximum. The T_1 growth curve for white matter, because of its lower proton density, starts closer to zero on the negative z axis than edema after the 180° flip. Because of its shorter T_1, it recovers more rapidly along its T_1 curve than does edema to reach its maximum.

At time TI, a 90° excitation pulse is applied. Edema and white matter will have recovered their longitudinal magnetization at different rates depending on their individual T_1s. When both longitudinal magnetization vectors are flipped into the x-y plane by the 90° pulse, they generate FID signals. Immediately after the 90° pulse, each longitudinal magnetization vector goes to zero but begins recovering according to its T_1 recovery curve. Then, after a time interval TR, the process is repeated with another 180° inverting pulse.

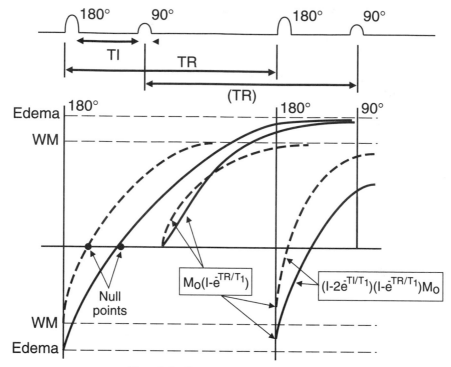

Figure 7-8. Recovery curves for WM and edema.

We saw earlier that the T_1 growth curve after the 180° pulse is given by the formula:

$$M_0(1 - e^{-TR/T1})(1 - 2e^{-TI/T1})$$

Magnitude Reconstruction

Magnitude reconstruction is another variable in inversion recovery. If we want to increase signal to noise by about 40% (more precisely, by a factor of $\sqrt{2}$), we can add the x and y channels of the coil together as the **root mean square (rms)**, i.e., $\sqrt{(S_x^2 + S_y^2)}$. This gives us a "**magnitude**" image, which is always positive. It appears like the mirror image of the negative growth curves, flipped about the time axis (Fig. 7-9) The dashed lines going from the positive z axis, down to the zero point, are actually the mirror image of the two T_1 growth curves of edema and white matter, "flipped" so that we only register their *magnitude*, not their positive or negative phase. This new method of displaying the inversion recovery process is called "**magnitude reconstruction**." Although it has $\sqrt{2}$ more signal to noise than the original "**phase construction**," its dynamic range is less than the original, i.e., 0 to M_0 vs. $-M_0$ to M_0. Thus,

magnitude reconstruction is used whenever S/N is limited, and phase reconstruction is used when greater contrast is needed.

In inversion recovery, TR is always long. By picking a long TR, we reach a steady state with maximum value on the T_1 growth curve of each tissue after the 90° pulse. What happens when TI is chosen to null white matter (Fig. 7-9)? If we consider just the *magnitude* of the signal, which is the distance of the T_1 recovery curve above or below the time line, then edema has a greater *magnitude* than white matter. Because edema has a longer T_2 than white matter, if we choose a long TE, then we will magnify the difference in intensity between the two tissues. In fact, the longer the TE, the greater the contrast difference will be between edema and white matter (Fig. 7-10).

FAT SUPPRESSION: STIR IMAGING

STIR stands for short TI (or Tau) inversion recovery. Let's draw two T_1 recovery curves, after the 180° RF pulse, for two tissues—fat and H_2O (Fig. 7-11). Pick the TI at the point where fat

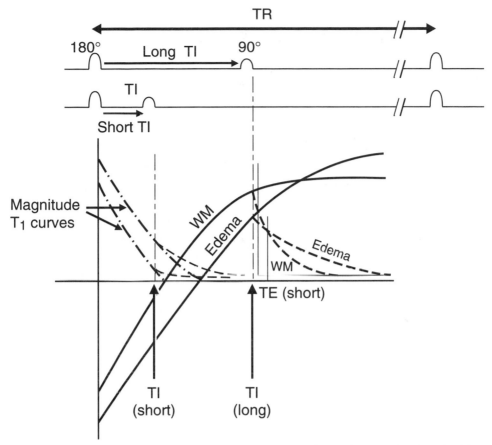

Figure 7-9. Recovery curves, magnitude recovery curves (mirror image curves to make everything positive), and associated decay curves for WM and edema.

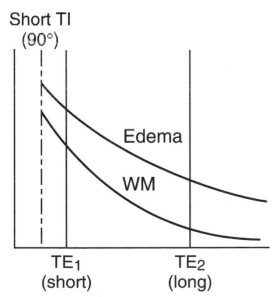

Figure 7-10. Tissue contrast for two different TEs.

crosses the zero point. (The null point is equal to *ln*2 [or 0.693] multiplied by the T_1 of fat [see Problem 7-1]).

At this null point for fat, if we draw the T_2 decay curves, fat starts at zero and will stay at zero. There will be no transverse magnetization from fat in the x-y plane, and water will have its usual T_2 decay curve. In effect, we have *suppressed* the fat signal. Therefore, after a 180° inverting pulse, we wait a time TI = 0.693 T_1 (fat) and we give the 90° pulse. All other tissues will have longitudinal magnetization that will flip into the x-y plane and give off a signal according to their T_2 curves. However, at its null point, fat will not have any longitudinal magnetization to flip into the x-y plane, and thus will not have any signal.

The term **STIR** is called "short TI inversion recovery" because fat has a very short T_1; therefore, a very short TI must be chosen to null it

Fat Supression:
Short TI Inversion Recovery (STIR) Imaging

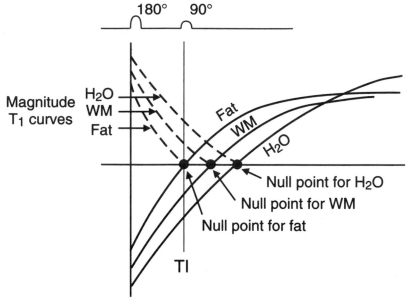

Figure 7-11. In the STIR fat suppression technique, TI is chosen so that the T1 recovery curve for fat crosses zero at the time of the 90° pulse.

(at high field [1.5 T] this TI is 140 msec, whereas at midfield [0.5 T] it is 100 msec). Fat will reach its null point before white matter, gray matter, H_2O, or edema (Fig. 7-11).

Key Points

We have discussed three types of pulse sequences: saturation recovery, partial saturation, and inversion recovery (IR). The latter one is very important because it allows suppression of any tissue by selecting TI to be 0.693 times the T_1 of that tissue:

$$TI \text{ (null)} = 0.693 \times T1$$

This subject is further elaborated upon in Chapter 24 on Tissue Suppression Techniques.

A partial saturation sequence results in T1 weighting (short TR and TE). A saturation recovery, however, renders PD weighting (long TR, short TE).

Questions

7-1. (a) Given an inversion recovery (IR) pulse sequence (Fig. 7-6), prove that TI that "nulls" or "suppresses" a certain tissue is equal to

$$0.693 \times T_1 \text{ (tissue), i.e.}$$
$$TI \text{ (null)} = 0.693 \times T_1$$

Hint: The IR curve is proportional to

$$S \propto 1 - 2e^{-t/T1}, \text{ where } t = TI$$

(b) Assuming a $T_1 = 180$ ms for fat, what TI would "suppress" the fat?

7-2. Consider the inversion recovery (IR) pulse sequence shown in Figure P7-1. Prove

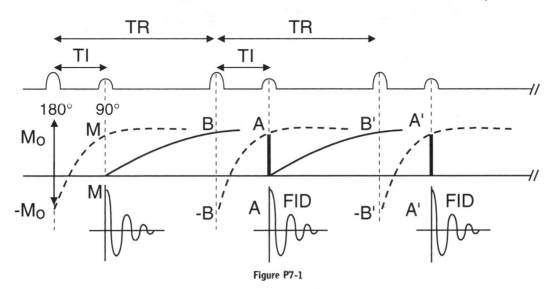

Figure P7-1

that the signal measured after each 90° pulse (i.e., at A, A') is given by

$$N(H)(1 - 2e^{-TI/T1} + e^{-TR/T1})$$

assuming that TI is much smaller than TR (i.e., TI ≪ TR).

7-3. Match
   (i)   partial saturation and
   (ii) saturation recovery
   with
   (a) T1 weighted
   (b) PD weighted

INTRODUCTION

This chapter focuses on the most frequently used pulse sequence—the spin echo (**SE**) pulse sequence. When the concept of **dephasing** was discussed in previous chapters, we brought up two main causes: 1) external magnetic inhomogeneity, and 2) inherent spin-spin interactions. The SE pulse sequence eliminates the former by an additional **refocussing** or **rephasing** 180° RF pulse. By using the spin-echo pulse sequence, we can eliminate dephasing caused by fixed **external magnetic field inhomogeneities**. (We can't eliminate **spin-spin interactions** because they are not fixed, i.e., they fluctuate randomly.)

SPIN-ECHO PULSE DIAGRAM

As a result of the 90° pulse, the magnetization vector M_z is flipped into the x-y plane. Consider the precession of three different magnetization vectors in the transverse plane, each in a slightly different magnetic environment (Fig. 8-1a). Initially, all of these vectors are *in phase* and they are all precessing at frequency ω_0.

In Figure 8-1a, say one group of spins is exposed to the magnetic field B_0, which causes them to precess at frequency ω_0. The adjacent group of spins sees a slightly higher field $B_0{}^+$ and precesses at a slightly higher frequency $\omega_0{}^+$, and another sees a slightly lower field $B_0{}^-$ with a precessional frequency of $\omega_0{}^-$. After the 90° pulse, the three spins will begin to get *out of phase* with each other (Fig. 8-1b). Eventually, the fast vector and the slow vector become 180° out of phase and cancel each other out (Fig. 8-1c).

ANALOGY

Let's consider the analogy of three runners running around the track (Fig. 8-2). Initially, they start out at the same point. After they run for a time τ, they are no longer together—one is running faster and gets ahead of the others, and one is running slower, falling behind the others.

At this time, if we make the runners turn around and run the opposite way, each one will still be running at the same speed (precessing at the same frequency in the case of the spins).

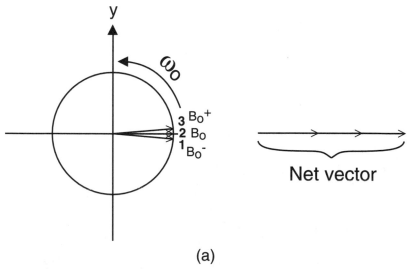

(a)

Figure 8-1. Three magnetization vectors in three slightly different magnetic environments. In **(a)** they are in phase and their vector sum is 3 times each individual vector. In **(b)** they are slightly out of phase, yielding a smaller net vector. In **(c)** vector 1 and 3 cancel each other out because they are 180° out of phase, leaving only vector 1.

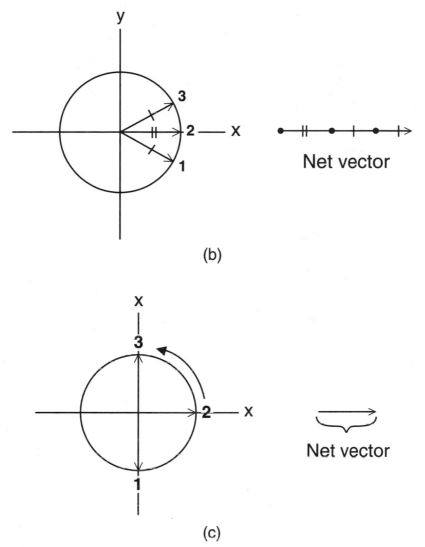

(b)

(c)

Figure 8-1. Continued.

They have just changed direction and are running back to where they started. Each one will then run the same distance if they run the same amount of time τ. Therefore, at time 2τ, they will all come back at the starting point *at the same time* and will be back together in phase. The action of making the runners change direction is done with the use of 180° refocusing pulse in the case of the spins.

Thus, at a certain time τ after the 90° pulse, when the spins have gotten out of phase, a 180° pulse is applied. Now all the spins flip 180° in the x-y plane and they continue precessing, but now in the opposite direction (Fig. 8-3). Let's look at the pulse sequence diagram (Fig. 8-4).

We start off with a 90° RF pulse to flip the spins into the x-y plane. We wait a time τ and apply a 180° RF pulse. Then we wait a long time, TR, and repeat the process.

If we draw the FID after the 90° pulse, we see that the FID dephases very rapidly, due to the T_2^* effect related to external magnetic field inhomogeneities and spin-spin interactions. The spins get out of phase. After time τ, we apply the 180° refocussing pulse. After an equal time τ, they will be completely in phase again, and the signal will reach a maximum.

1. Time τ is the time from 90° RF pulse to 180° RF pulse.

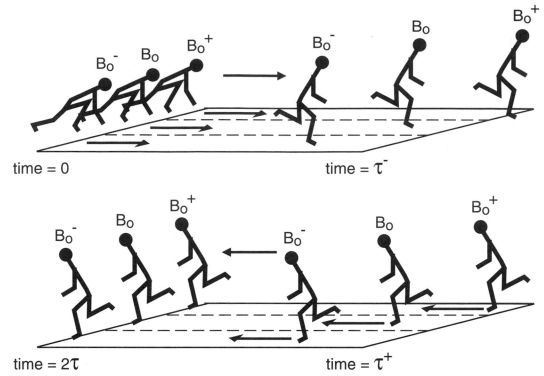

Figure 8-2. Analogy of three runners on a track. At time τ they are made to turn around and run back towards the starting point. Because the slowest runner is now in the lead, they will all reach the starting point at exactly the same time (at time 2τ).

2. Time τ is also the time from the 180° RF pulse to the point of maximum rephasing, i.e., the **echo**.
3. We call 2τ the **echo delay time** TE: the time after the 90° pulse when we get maximum signal again.
4. The 180° pulse is, therefore, called a **refocussing** or **rephasing** pulse.

We can apply a second 180° pulse. Now, instead of one 180° pulse following the 90° pulse, we have two 180° pulses in sequence after a 90° pulse (Fig. 8-5). After the first echo, the spins will begin to dephase again. A second 180° pulse applied at time τ_2 after the first echo will allow the spins to rephase again at time $2\tau_2$ after the first echo and a second echo is obtained. Each echo has its own TE.

1. The time from the 90° pulse to the first echo is TE_1.
2. The time from the 90° pulse to the second echo is TE_2.

Ideally, we would like to regain all the signal from the original FID. In practice, it can't happen. We are able to regain the signal lost due to fixed external magnetic field inhomogeneities by applying a refocussing 180° pulse, but dephasing caused by spin-spin interaction of the tissue cannot be regained. If we join the points of maximum signal due to rephasing as a result of the 180° pulses, we will get an *exponentially decaying curve* with a time constant given by T_2. Therefore, the decay of the original FID and the decay of each subsequent echo is given by $e^{-t/T2^*}$; whereas, the decay of the curve describing the maximum signal reached by each echo is given by $e^{-t/T2}$. This is the difference between T_2^* and T_2.

SYMMETRIC ECHOES

In Figure 8-5, if $\tau_1 = \tau_2$, then we get symmetric echoes.

EXAMPLE:

TR = 2000 and TE of 40 msec and 80 msec.

Here, $\tau_1 = 20$, so that TE1 = $2 \tau_1 = 40$, and $TE_2 = 80 = TE1 + 2 \tau_2 = 40 + 2 \tau_2$, then

$$2 \tau_2 = 40 \text{ and } \tau_2 = 20.$$

So $\tau_1 = \tau_2$ in symmetric echoes.

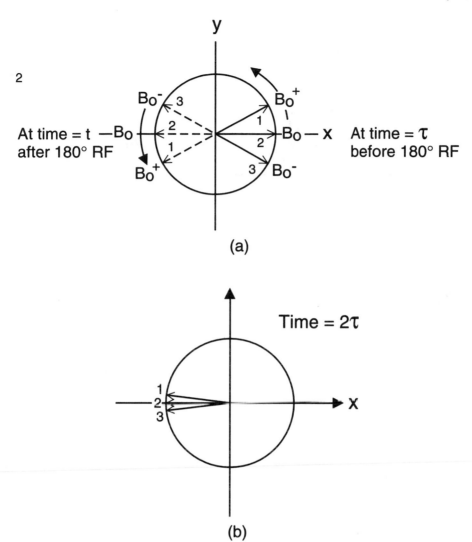

(a)

(b)

Figure 8-3.   The vectors in Figure 8-1 are reversed 180° in direction at time τ (a), so that at time 2τ they'll get in phase again (b).

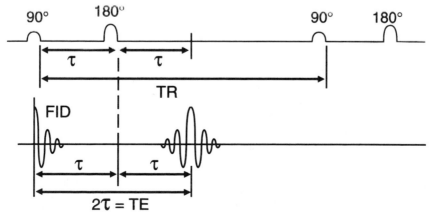

Figure 8-4.   In a spin echo pulse sequence, a 180° pulse is applied at time τ, causing the spins to get in phase at time 2τ. This leads to the formation of an echo from the FID.

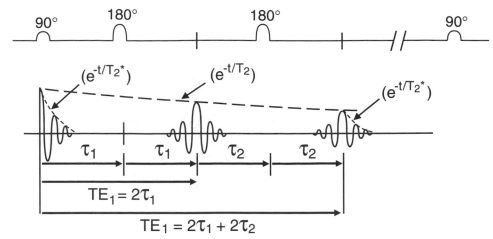

Figure 8-5.   An example of a dual echo, spine echo pulse sequence in which two echoes are formed via application of two 180° pulses.

ASYMMETRIC ECHOES

If $\tau_1 \neq \tau_2$, then we get **asymmetric echoes**.

EXAMPLE:
Take

$$TR = 2000, TE = 30 \text{ and } 80 \text{ msec.}$$
$$\text{Here } TE_1 = 2(\tau_1) = 30 \text{ msec, so } \tau_1 = 15 \text{ msec.}$$
$$TE_2 = 80 \text{ msec} = TE_1 + 2\ (\tau_2)$$
$$= 30 \text{ msec} + 2\ \tau_2 = 80 \text{ msec}$$
$$\text{then } 2\ \tau_2 = 50 \text{ and } \tau_2 = 25 \text{ msec}$$

So $\tau_1 \neq \tau_2$ in asymmetric echoes.

Question: What does the 180° pulse do to the longitudinal magnetization?
Answer: It inverts it. However, at time TE/2 (on the order of 10 msec), the recovered longitudinal magnetization is negligible and its inversion does not cause any significant signal loss. In fact, at t = TE/2, we have

$$M_z = M_0(1 - e^{-TE/2TR}) \cong 0$$

because TE/2 $\ll$ TR, so that $e^{-TE/2TR} \cong 1$.

TISSUE CONTRAST

As discussed in Chapter 6, tissue contrast in SE depends primarily on TR and TE. There are three types of tissue contrast:

1. T_1 weighted (T1W)
2. T_2 weighted (T2W)
3. Proton density weighted (PDW) (also called "balanced," "intermediate," and "spin density")

Let's see what TR and TE must be for these three imaging scenarios (Table 8-1):

1. For T_1 weighting, we want to eliminate the T_2 effect and enhance the T_1 effect.
    (a) to eliminate (reduce) the T_2 effect, we want a short TE
    (b) to enhance the T_1 effect, we want a short TR
    (c) the signal is then proportional to $N(1 - e^{-TR/T1})$
2. For T_2 weighting, we want to eliminate the T_1 effect and enhance the T_2 effect.
    (a) to eliminate (reduce) the T_1 effect, we want a long TR
    (b) to enhance the T_2 effect, we want a long TE
    (c) the signal is, therefore, proportional to $N(H)\ (e^{-TE/T2})$
3. For proton density weighting, we want to eliminate the T_1 and T_2 effects.
    (a) to eliminate (reduce) the T_1 effect, we want a long TR
    (b) to eliminate (reduce) the T_2 effect, we want a short TE
    (c) the signal is then proportional to $N\ (H)$

Table 8-1

	TR	TE	Signal (Theoretical)
T1W	short	short	$N(H)(1 - e^{-TR/T1})$
T2W	long	long	$N(H)(e^{-TE/T2})$
PDW	long	short	$N(H)$

Remember that in practice we never totally eliminate any of these factors. We would have to have an infinitely long TR to eliminate all T_1 effects, and we would need a TE of 0 to eliminate all T_2 effects. Therefore, all T_1-weighted images in practice have some T_2 influence; all T_2-weighted images have some T_1 influence; and proton density weighted images have some influence from both T_1 and T_2. This is why we use the terms T_1 *weighting*, T_2 *weighting*, and proton density *weighting*:

1. We put more *weight* on the differences in T_1 by shortening the TE and the TR.
2. We put more *weight* on the differences in T_2 by lengthening TR and the TE;
3. We put less *weight* on T_1 and T_2 by lengthening TR and shortening TE, thus giving more *weight* to proton density.

Key Points

1. The SE (spin echo) pulse sequence is composed of a 90° excitation pulse followed by one or more 180° rephasing pulses.

2. The purpose of the 180° pulse is to eliminate the dephasing effects caused by external magnetic field inhomogeneities by rephasing the spins at the time of echo (TE).

3. The resultant echo then depends on T_2 decay rather than T_2^* decay, as seen with the FID (free induction decay).

4. Table 8-2 summarizes the tissue contrast in SE with respect to TR and TE.

Table 8-2

	Short TE	Long TE
short TR	T1W	mixed
long TR	PDW	T2W

Questions

8-1. Consider a dual echo SE sequence as in Fig. 8-5:
(a) What are the received signals at Point A (first echo) and Point B (second echo)?
(b) What would the signal at Point A be without a 180° refocusing pulse?
(c) Calculate the ratio of the signals at Point A *without* a refocusing pulse to that with a refocusing pulse for TE1 = 25, TE2 = 50, T_2 = 50, and T_2^* = 25 m sec.

8-2. Match
(i) T1W (ii) T2W
(iii) PDW
with
(a) short T1 and T2
(b) long T1 and T2
(c) short T1, long T2
(d) long T1, short T2

8-3. T/F The 180° pulses totally eliminate the dephasing of spins in the transverse plane.

9 Fourier Transform

INTRODUCTION

Fourier was an eighteenth century French mathematician. His picture, along with the Fourier transform of his picture, are shown in Figure 9-1. The Fourier Transform (FT) is a mystery to most radiologists. Although the mathematics of FT is complex, its concept is easy to grasp. Basically, the FT provides a frequency spectrum of a signal. It is sometimes easier to work in the frequency domain and later convert back to the time domain.

Let's start by saying that we have a signal g(t), with a certain waveform (Fig. 9-2). This signal is basically a *time* function, i.e., a waveform that varies with time. Now, let's say we have a "black box" that converts the signal into its *frequency* components. The conversion that occurs in the "black box" is the **Fourier transform**. The FT converts the signal from the *time domain* to the

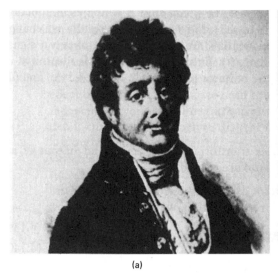

(a)

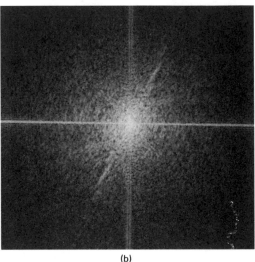

(b)

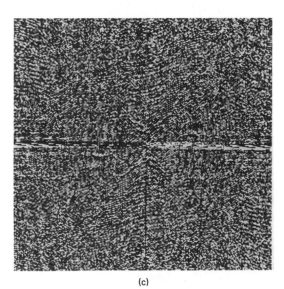

(c)

Figure 9-1. **(a)** The picture of French mathematician Fourier. **(b)** The magnitude of Fourier's 2-dimensional Fourier transform. **(c)** The phase of his Fourier transform. (Printed with permission from Oppenheim AV et al. Signals and Systems. Prentice Hall 1983).

g(t)   G(ω)

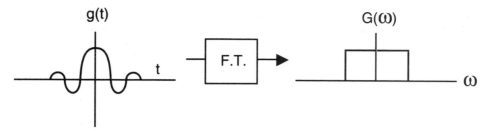

Figure 9-2. The Fourier transform of g(t), designated G(ω).

Example 1:

Cos function: cos ω₀t

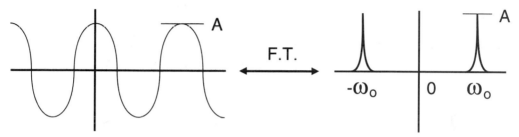

Figure 9-3. The FT of cos (ω₀t) consists of two spikes, one at ω_0 and on at $-\omega_0$.

frequency domain (Fig. 9-2). The FT of g(t) is denoted G(ω). (The frequency can be angular [ω] or linear [f].)

The FT is a mathematical equation (you don't have to memorize it). It is shown here to demonstrate that a relationship exists between the signal in the time domain g(t) and its Fourier transform G(ω) in the frequency domain:

$$G(\omega) = \int_{-\infty}^{+\infty} g(t)e^{-i\omega t}\, dt \qquad \text{(Eqn. 9-1a)}$$

$$G(f) = \int_{-\infty}^{+\infty} g(t)e^{-i2\pi f t}\, dt \qquad \text{(Eqn. 9-1b)}$$

where $\omega = 2\pi f$.

We are already familiar with the term $(e^{-i\omega t})$ from Chapter 1. This is the term for a vector spinning with angular frequency ω. The formula integrates the product of this periodic function and g(t) with respect to time. It also provides another function, G(ω), in the frequency domain (Fig. 9-2).

One interesting thing about the Fourier transform is that the Fourier transform of the Fourier transform provides the original signal. If the Fourier transform of g(t) is G(ω), then the Fourier

transform of G(ω) is g(t):

$$g(t) = 1/2\pi \int_{-\infty}^{+\infty} G(\omega)e^{+i\omega t}\, d\omega \qquad \text{(Eqn. 9-2)}$$

FT provides the *range of frequencies* that are in the signal. Here are some examples of functions and their Fourier transforms:

EXAMPLE 1:

The *cosine* function: $cos\ (\omega_0\ t)$

Obviously this signal (Fig. 9-3) has one single frequency. The frequency could be any number. The Fourier transform is a single spike representing the single frequency in the frequency domain (because of its symmetry, we also get a similar spike on the opposite side of zero[a]). The Fourier transform in this case tells us that there is only a single frequency because it shows only one frequency spike at ω_0 and is zero everywhere else on the line. We can, for simplicity, ignore the symmetric spike on the negative side of zero, and

---

[a] One can think of a negative frequency as oscillation in the opposite direction. For instance, if clockwise rotation is regarded as a positive frequency, then counterclockwise rotation would constitute a negative frequency. Also, see the discussion below regarding even and odd functions and their Fourier transforms.

just consider the single spike on the positive side to tell us that there is a single frequency (ω_0). The spike represents frequency and amplitude of the *cosine* function.

EXAMPLE 2:

The **sinc** wave: $sinc\,(\omega_0\,t) = sin\,(\omega_0\,t)/(\omega_0\,t)$

The Fourier transform of this signal (Fig. 9-4) has a rectangular shape and shows that the signal contains, not just a single frequency, but a *range* of frequencies from $-\omega_0$ to $+\omega_0$. The **bandwidth** of this range of frequencies is from $-\omega_0$ to $+\omega_0$.

$$Bandwidth = \pm\,\omega_0$$
$$= 2\omega_0$$

(We'll discuss bandwidth again later.) So the Fourier transform tells us the *range of frequencies*

that there are in a signal, as well as the amplitude of the signals at those frequencies. What's nice about the Fourier transform is that, if we have the range of frequencies and the amplitudes, we can reconstruct the original signal back.

EXAMPLE 3:

Let's consider two frequencies:

1.   cos ωt and
2.   cos $2\omega t$ (which is twice as fast as cos ωt)

The signal *cos(2ωt)* oscillates twice as fast as *cos(ωt)* (Fig. 9-5). If we add them up, we get a complex signal (Fig. 9-6). If we were just given the signal in Figure 9-6, we would have no idea that it is the sum of two *cosine* waves.

Question: *What is a good way to figure out what frequencies the signal is composed of?*

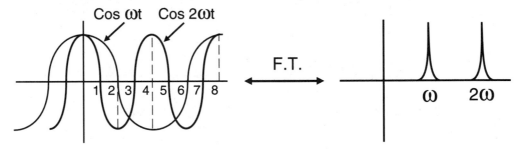

Figure 9-4.   The FT of a sinc function (sinc ω_0t = sin ω_0t/ω_0t) has a rectangular shape. The two ends of this rectangle are at ω_0 and $-\omega_0$ (where ω_0 is the frequency of the sinc function).

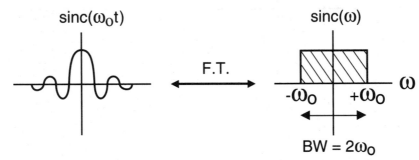

Figure 9-5.   The FT of cos 2ωt has two spikes: one at 2ω and one at -2ω (here, only the positive frequencies are shown).

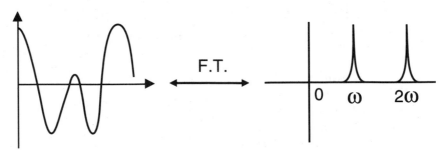

Figure 9-6.   The FT of cos ωt + cos 2ωt has two sets of spikes at $\pm\omega$ and $\pm2\omega$. By looking at the FT of this signal, it is easy to figure out its composition in the time domain.

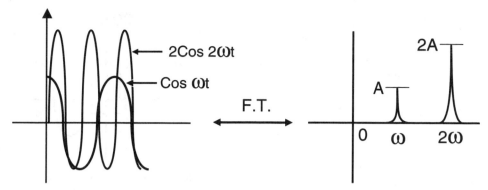

Figure 9-7. The signal cos ωt + 2 cos ωt and its FT. The FT has again two sets of spikes: one at ±ω and one at ±2ω (but with twice the magnitude).

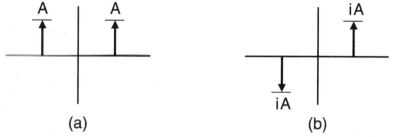

Figure 9-8. **(a)** FT of cos ωt. **(b)** FT of sin ωt. Here the spikes have opposite polarities and are also imaginary (i A as opposed to A).

Answer: The Fourier transform of this complex signal (which we know is the sum of 2 cosine waves, one twice as fast as the other) contains two spikes, one twice as far from the origin as the other (Fig. 9-6). This FT, then, demonstrates the composition of the signal in terms of its frequencies.

EXAMPLE 4:

Let's now have a complex signal with two *cosine* waves, with the second *cosine* wave not only twice as fast, but with twice the *amplitude* as well. Again, by looking at the signal in Figure 9-7, we have no idea what it is composed of, but by looking at the frequency spectrum (the Fourier transform of the signal), we can tell the composition of the signal: in this case, two separate *cosine* waves with differing frequencies and differing amplitudes. The Fourier transform provides the frequency spectrum of a signal with its amplitudes.

EXAMPLE 5:

Let's consider the Fourier transform of a *sine* wave: sin ωt. The Fourier transform of a *sine* wave is different than the Fourier transform of a *cosine* wave:

1. FT of a *cosine* wave is *symmetric* with two symmetric spikes on either side of zero (Fig. 9-8a).
2. FT of a *sine* wave is *anti-symmetric*. It has a positive

spike to right of zero, and a negative spike to left of zero[b] (Fig. 9-8b).

The reason for this is that a *sine* function is an **odd** function. In other words, if we take a time interval of *t* to the right of zero, the *sine* value is positive; whereas, if we take a similar interval in the other direction, the *sine* value is negative (Fig. 9-9). The *cosine* function, however, is an **even** function. If we go a certain interval to the right or left of zero, the *cosine* value is the same (Fig. 9-10). The FT of an even function is **real**, whereas the FT of an odd function is **imaginary**. Thus, *cosine* functions have Fourier transforms that are real (Fig. 9-8a). *Sine* functions have Fourier transforms that are imaginary (Fig. 9-8b).

FOURIER TRANSFORM VERSUS FOURIER SERIES

There is a difference between a **Fourier transform** and a **Fourier Series**. Admittedly this is

---

[b] Actually, the negative spike has an imaginary rather than a real amplitude (in the form of iA, where i is the imaginary unit $\sqrt{-1}$ and A is the amplitude of the spike). This concept is rather important in understanding the symmetry that exists in k-space, discussed in Chapters 13 and 16.

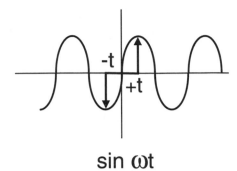

sin ωt

Figure 9-9.   sin ωt is an example of an *odd* function where the value of the signal at −t is the negative of its value at +t.

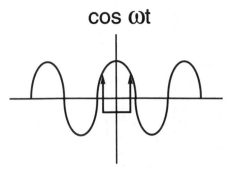

cos ωt

Figure 9-10.   cos ωt is an example of an *even* function where the values of the signal at ±t are the same.

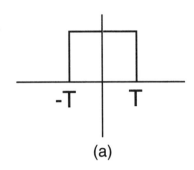

(a)

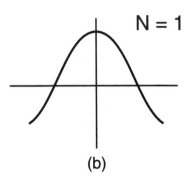

N = 1

(b)

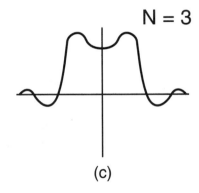

N = 3

(c)

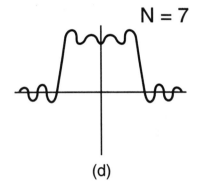

N = 7

(d)

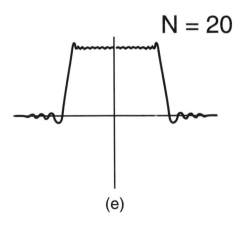

N = 20

(e)

Figure 9-11.   **(a)** A square or rectangular function can be approximated as the sum of a finite number (N) of sine and cosine functions. **(b)** N = 1. **(c)** N = 3. **(d)** N = 7. **(e)** N = 20. The signal in **(e)** more closely approximates a rectangle, except for the presence of a ring-down effect.

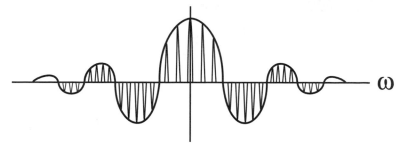

Figure 9-12. The FT of the signal in Eqn. 9-3 is a set of spikes whose envelope is a sinc function.

confusing. Let's talk about the original function g(t). This function can be represented by an infinite number of *sine* and *cosine* waves:

$$g(t) = a_0 + a_1 \cos(\omega_0 t) + a_2 \cos(2\omega_0 t) + \ldots + b_1 \sin(\omega_0 t) + b_2 \sin(2\omega_0 t) + \ldots$$

$$(\text{Eqn. 9-3})$$

What does this mean? Let's say that we have the rectangular function (Fig. 9-11a). We said that this is composed of an infinite number of *sine* and *cosine* waves:

1. If we start with a single *cosine* wave, the signal will be as in Figure 9-11b;
2. as we add *sine* and *cosine*, the signal will be as in Figure 9-11c;

3. as we continue to add *sine* and *cosine*, signal will be as in Figure 9-11d;
4. the more *cosine* and *sine* we add, the more the signal approximates a square wave (Fig. 9-11e);
5. it is impractical to go to infinity (∞). However, by eliminating the higher frequencies, we get a "ring-down" effect.

If we do a Fourier transform of the Fourier series of g(t) above, we get a series of spikes (Fig. 9-12). The **envelope** of this FT is the *sinc* wave.

In summary, the **Fourier series** tells us that a signal can be represented by a series of *sine* and *cosine* waves (in the time domain). The **Fourier transform**, however, gives the frequency spectrum of the function (in the frequency domain).

Key Points

The Fourier transform (FT), as intimidating as it may appear, represents a simple concept. Every signal (in the time domain) is composed of a series of frequencies. The FT is a way of representing that signal in terms of its frequencies. The FT also allows mathematical manipulations performed in the frequency domain, which are sometimes easier than in the time domain. The one-to-one relationship between a signal and its Fourier transform allows reconstruction of the original signal from its FT.

In other words, the FT represents a function in the frequency domain whose amplitude varies with the frequencies present in the signal. The bandwidth (BW) simply is a measure of the range of frequencies present in the signal (in Hz or in radians/sec).

Questions

9-1.   T/F   The Fourier transform represents the frequency spectrum of a signal, whereas the Fourier series decomposes the signal into a series of sine and cosine waves.

9-2.   T/F   (a)   It is always easier to perform calculations in the frequency domain.
(b)   It is always easier to perform calculations in the time domain.

10 Image Construction

Part I (Slice Selection)

INTRODUCTION

The signals received from a patient contain information about the entire part of the patient being imaged. They do not have any particular spatial information. That is, we cannot determine the specific origin point of each component of the signal. This is the function of the **gradients**. One gradient is required in each of the x, y, and z directions to obtain spatial information in that direction. Depending on their function, these gradients are called

1. the slice-select gradient;
2. the read-out or frequency-encoding gradient; and
3. the phase-encoding gradient.

Depending on their orientation axis they are called G_x, G_y, and G_z. Depending on the slice orientation (axial, sagittal, or coronal), G_x, G_y, and G_z can be used for slice select, readout, or phase encode.

A gradient is simply a magnetic field that changes from point to point—usually in a *linear* fashion. We temporarily create a magnetic field nonuniformity in a linear manner along all three axes to obtain information about position.

First, we'll consider the slice-select gradient, which is the easiest of all to understand. Once a slice has been selected, we worry about the problem of in-plane **spatial encoding**, i.e., discriminating position within the slice. As we'll see shortly, the principles behind slice selection and spatial encoding in MRI are different from the principles used in computerized tomography (CT).

HOW TO SELECT A SLICE

Suppose that we have a patient on the table and we want to select a slice at a certain level and of a certain thickness (Fig. 10-1). Remember that the patient is lying in the external magnetic field B_0 which is oriented along the z axis. If we transmit an RF pulse and get an FID or an echo back, the received signal would be from the entire patient. There is no spatial discrimination. All we get is a signal, and we have no idea yet from where exactly in the body the signal is coming.

The frequency of the RF pulse is given by the **Larmor frequency**:

$$\omega_0 = \gamma\, B_0$$

If we transmit an RF pulse that does not match the Larmor frequency (the frequency of oscillation at magnetic field B_0), we won't excite any of the protons in the patient.

However, if we make the magnetic field vary from point to point, then each position will have its own resonant frequency. We can make the magnetic field slightly weaker in strength at the feet and gradually increase in strength to a maximum at the head (Fig. 10-2). This effect is achieved by using a **gradient coil**.

Let's say the magnetic field strength is 1.5T at the center, 1.4T at the feet and 1.6T at the head. Then, the foot of the patient will experi-

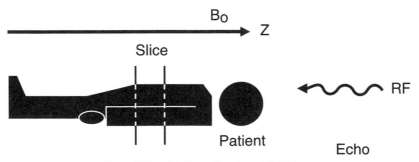

Figure 10-1. Selecting a slice of a certain thickness.

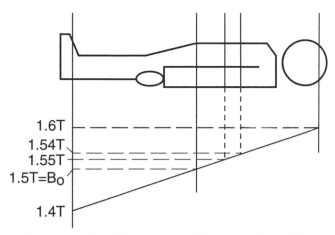

Figure 10-2. Slice thickness is determined by the slope of the gradient.

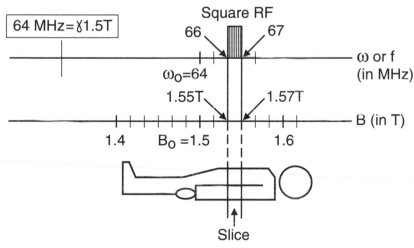

Figure 10-3. The relationship between field strength and Larmor frequency in determining slice thickness and position.

ence a weaker magnetic field than the head. Therefore, a *gradient* in any direction (x, y, or z) is a variation in the field along that axis in some fashion (the most common form of which is *linearly* increasing or decreasing). If we now transmit an RF pulse of a single frequency into the patient, we will receive signals corresponding to a line in the patient at the level of the magnetic field corresponding to that frequency (according to the Larmor frequency), but it will be an infinitely thin line. What we need to do is transmit an RF pulse with a **range** of frequencies—a **bandwidth** of frequencies.

What will the RF pulse look like in the frequency domain? First, note that for a 1.5T magnet, the Larmor frequency is 64 MHz for hydro-

gen protons:

64 MHz corresponds to B_0 of 1.5T magnet

To see how this is derived, recall that

$$\omega_0 = \gamma \, B_0, \text{ where } \gamma \cong 42.6 \text{ MHz/Tesla and} \\ B_0 = 1.5 \text{ Tesla}$$

This results in

$$\omega_0 = 42.6 \times 1.5 = 64 \text{ MHz}$$

The graph in Figure 10-3 shows the magnetic field strength and the corresponding Larmor frequency range. We are concerned here about a magnetic field strength ranging from 1.4T to 1.6T because, in our example, that is the magnetic field strength range to which we have exposed the patient. Let's excite one slice with an RF pulse. For example, let's excite a slice extending from 1.55T to 1.57T. This corresponds to a frequency range from 66 to 67 MHz.

If the RF has a square shape in the frequency domain with a range of frequencies that correspond to a range of magnetic field strengths, then we will excite only the protons that are in the slice containing that range of magnetic field strengths. The other protons in the rest of the body are not going to get excited because the range of frequencies from which we are transmitting the RF pulse does not match the Larmor frequencies of the other protons. The range of frequencies in the RF pulse will only match the Larmor frequency of a single slice.

So, we transmit an RF pulse with a range of frequencies that we know will correspond to a range of magnetic field strengths in a particular slice. This range of frequencies determines the slice thickness and is referred to as the **bandwidth**.

Bandwidth = Range of frequencies (determines the slice thickness)

We can measure the bandwidth (range of frequencies) by looking at the Fourier transform of the RF pulse. Let's now compare the RF signal to its Fourier transform. The RF pulse is generally a *sinc* wave and looks like Figure 10-4a with the Fourier transform that has a square shape.

If we have a narrower signal, we get a wider frequency bandwidth (Fig. 10-4b). The narrower signal reflects the fact that there are more oscillations in a given period of time so that the maximum frequency of the signal is greater. Because the Fourier transform depicts an infinite number of frequencies from zero to maximum, the bandwidth gets wider to depict a greater maximum frequency.

Let's apply this example to a *cosine* wave (Fig. 10-5a). The Fourier transform for this *cosine*

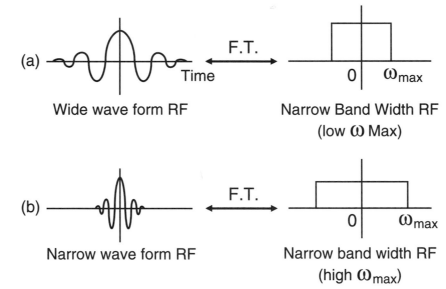

Figure 10-4. Comparison of wide and narrow waveforms and their FTs. The narrower the waveform in time domain, the wider its FT will be.

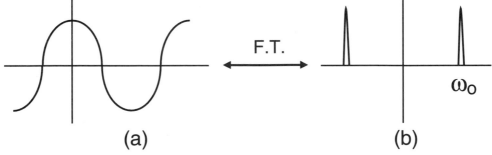

Figure 10-5. The FT **(b)** of **(a)** a cos signal ($\cos \omega_0 t$) has two spikes at $\pm \omega_0$.

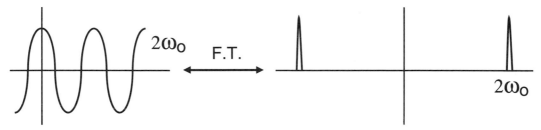

Figure 10-6. The FT of cos $2\omega_0 t$ has two spikes at $\pm 2\omega_0$.

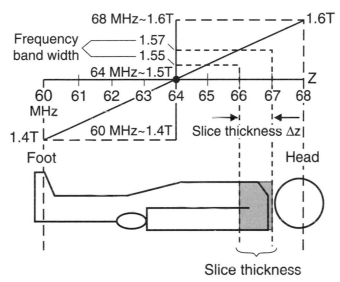

Figure 10-7. An example of the relationship between slice thickness and position, frequency and field strength.

wave contains two spikes, one on each side of zero (Figure 10-5b). If we then take a *cosine* wave with twice the oscillation frequency and look at its Fourier transform, we see that the spikes are farther apart (Fig. 10-6). Thus, as the *cosine* wave goes two times faster, the Fourier transform shows that the maximum frequency (in this case, the only frequency) is two times further away from the zero point. Furthermore, if we look at the diagram of the *cosine* waves, the faster *cosine* wave has a narrower oscillating wave form—the narrower the wave form, the faster the oscillation frequency. Again, the narrower the wave form of the RF signal, the wider its bandwidth (the greater the maximum frequency) (Fig. 10-6).

SLICE THICKNESS

Let's now talk about how we establish **slice thickness** (Fig. 10-7). The same principle would apply if we were to image from the base of the skull to the vertex rather than from the patient's head to toe. We establish a magnetic field strength **gradient** so that, at the midpoint of the field of study (in this instance, the entire body), the field strength is 1.5T; at the low end of the gradient (the foot), the field strength will be 1.4T; and at the high end of the gradient, the field strength will be maximum at 1.6T. These magnetic field strengths also correspond to different frequencies. Using the Larmor equation, we can calculate that approximately:

$$1.6T \sim 68\ MHz$$
$$1.5T \sim 64\ MHz$$
$$1.4T \sim 60\ MHz$$

If we pick a frequency bandwidth of a certain range, we would then get a slice of a certain thickness. Therefore, we transmit an RF pulse with a specific frequency bandwidth and no frequencies outside of this range (ideally). The frequency bandwidth will match the Larmor frequencies of the protons only in a section of the patient of a certain thickness, which corresponds to the range of magnetic field strengths corresponding to the Larmor frequencies. The magnetic field strength everywhere outside this slice is going to be either more or less than the mag-

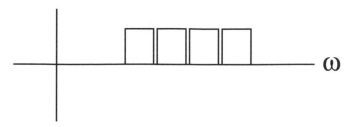

Figure 10-8. Ideal contiguous slices correspond to ideal rectangular shaped FTs that are positioned side by side.

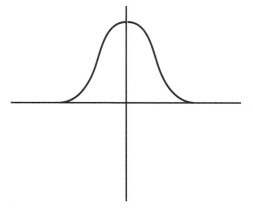

Figure 10-9. A more realistic FT has side lobes such as a Gaussian curve.

netic field strengths that correspond to the Larmor frequencies of the RF bandwidth.

> **Question:** *What happens if we put one slice right next to another?*
> **Answer:** *Ideally, the contiguous slices are right next to each other and the Fourier transform has a rectangular shape (Fig. 10-8). In other words, we want to have frequency ranges that are discrete and next to each other, so that each range of frequencies excites a different slice, and we can obtain contiguous slices.*

Cross Talk

In reality, the frequency spectrum of the RF pulse does not have a rectangular shape. Instead, it may have a bell shape or "Gaussian" curve

(Fig. 10-9). If we place these frequency spectrums close together, they will overlap; these areas of overlap cause "**cross-talk**" (Fig. 10-10).

Remember that cross talk is best explained in the **frequency domain**. It is more difficult to comprehend this in the time domain. To avoid this cross talk created by the overlap of adjacent frequency bandwidths, we create a **gap** between the consecutive bandwidths (in the frequency domain), thus creating a **gap** between consecutive slices in the actual image (Fig. 10-11). This will minimize or eliminate "cross-talk."

How to Change the Slice Thickness

There are two ways to change the slice thickness:

1. The first way to decrease the thickness is to use a *narrower bandwidth*. A narrower frequency bandwidth will excite protons in a narrower band of magnetic field strengths (Fig. 10-12a).
2. The second way to decrease slice thickness is to *increase the slope of the magnetic field gradient* (Fig. 10-12b), i.e., by increasing the gradient strength.

Slice Select Gradient

The change in the magnetic field strength along the z axis is called the **z gradient** (G_z). For an axial slice in a superconducting magnet, it is also called the **slice select gradient**. If we

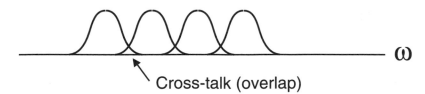

Cross-talk (overlap)

Figure 10-10. Crosstalk: in the absence of ideal rectangular shaped FTs, the side lobes of the FTs may overlap.

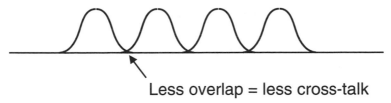

Less overlap = less cross-talk

Figure 10-11. To minimize cross-talk, the slices are set farther apart (by introducing gaps between successive slices).

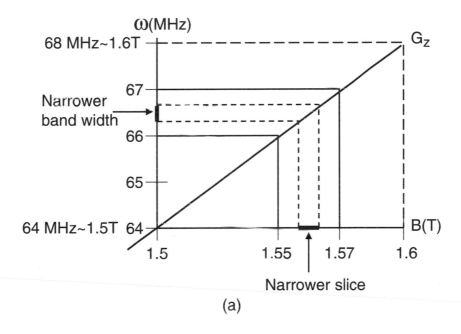

(a)

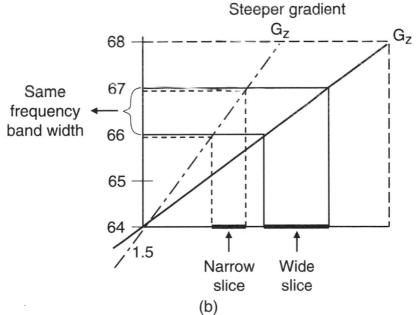

(b)

Figure 10-12. To decrease slice thickness, either a narrower BW **(a)** or a steeper gradient **(b)** is used.

increase the gradient and keep the frequency bandwidth the same, we get a thinner slice.

The slice thickness can be decreased by
1. *decreasing the bandwidth of the RF pulse, or*
2. *increasing the slice select gradient.*

There is an electronic limitation as to how much we can decrease the bandwidth. There is also a machine limitation as to how much we can increase the gradient. These factors set an absolute limit on how *thin* a slice can be.

By the foregoing procedure, we select a slice with a certain thickness. The slice is selected with a frequency range in the RF pulse that corresponds to the slice location and its thickness. The echo signal that we get back from the slice is from the entire slice. We have no way yet of discriminating points within the slice. This is where the **frequency encoding** and the **phase encoding** steps come into play.

REVIEW
RF Pulses

There are two types of RF pulses:

1. Nonselective
2. Selective

By **selective**, we mean an RF pulse that is slice selective—an RF pulse whose frequency bandwidth corresponds to a specific band of magnetic field strengths along a magnetic field gradient. Ideally, this RF pulse will select only a certain slice of the body that we are imaging (used in two-dimensional or 2D imaging).

A **non selective** RF pulse excites every part of the body that is in the coil (used in three dimensional or 3D imaging).

SINC RF PULSE

Earlier, we talked about one type of RF pulse in which we had a *sinc* wave in the time domain. The *sinc* function is mathematically expressed as

$$sinc(t) = sin(t)/t$$

This simply means that the oscillating function *sin t* is divided by *t*. Therefore, because *t* goes into an oscillating function (*sin t*), the result will be an oscillating function. As *t* goes from a large value to a small value, the result of (*sin t/t*) will get larger and will reach maximum when t approaches zero. The rectangular transform in the frequency domain has a positive maximum frequency (f_{max}) and a negative maximum frequency ($-f_{max}$) as shown in Figure 10-13. The bandwidth is thus 2 × (maximum frequency); i.e.,

$$BW = 2f_{max}$$

This is only one type of selective RF pulse. There are other types of selective RF pulses.

GAUSSIAN RF PULSE

The first generation of MR machines used an RF pulse that had a **Gaussian** shape (Fig. 10-14a). The Gaussian RF pulse has a bell shape in the time domain.

The Fourier transform of a Gaussian function is also a Gaussian curve (Fig. 10-14).

If we take another Gaussian curve in the narrower time domain, its Fourier transform will be wider (Fig. 10-15). An inverse relationship exists between the range of frequencies and the duration of the RF pulse, as we have discussed before.

A short pulse results in a wider bandwidth. The MR machine uses different types of RF pulses for different purposes, but for the sake

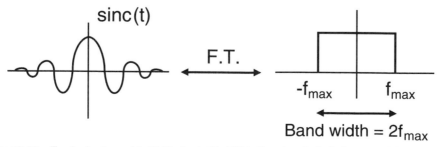

Figure 10-13.   The sinc function and its FT. The bandwidth (BW) is $2f_{max}$ where f_{max} is the frequency of the sinc function.

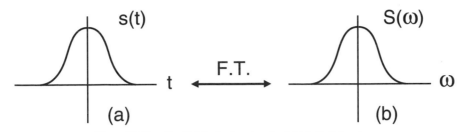

Figure 10-14.   The FT **(b)** of a Gaussian signal **(a)** is itself Gaussian.

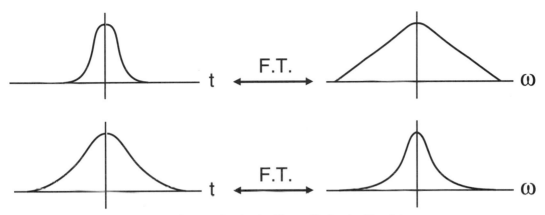

Figure 10-15.   A narrow Gaussian signal has a wide Gaussian FT, and vice versa.

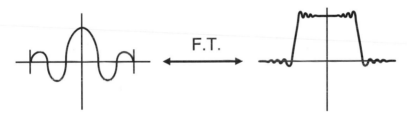

Figure 10-16.   The FT of a truncated sinc function has a rectangular-like profile containing rings or ripple effects.

of discussion, let's assume that we are dealing with an ideal *sinc* wave RF pulse that has an ideal square Fourier transform.

Remember that the RF pulse is an electromagnetic wave generated by an electric current through a coil. If we use the body coil to generate the RF pulse, we generate the RF throughout the body. If we use a surface coil, the RF pulse we generate is localized to the area of the surface coil. This is one reason why images are better with a surface coil. Most coils are transmit/receive—the coil transmits the RF pulse and also receives the signal from the body.

Going back to the *sinc* wave, in reality we can't go all the way to infinity in time when transmitting a signal. We have to **truncate** the

signal and deal with a certain finite time domain (Fig. 10-16). The Fourier transform of this truncated signal gives the "**ripples**" effect on the square wave as we saw in Chapter 9. The more we truncate the signal, the more "ripple" we get. Ripples are also called "overshoot" and "undershoot" artifacts.

Bandwidth

Bandwidth is a measure of the range of frequencies. We know that for a 1.5 T magnet, the Larmor frequency is about 64 MHz. The RF pulse that we generate is in the radio frequency range, but its bandwidth is in the **audible** frequency range.

This is analogous to a radio. When we tune into the FM station KOST 103.5 FM in L.A., are we really getting 103.5 MHz of soundwaves? If the signal you receive on your radio has this high a frequency, you can't hear it (we can't hear a MHz frequency signal [maybe dolphins can, but humans can't!]). However, the frequency that we receive is actually in the **audible** range. Each station has a certain frequency range that they deal with, and the bandwidth that they use is nearly the same for all radio stations in the audible frequency range; it is about 1–2 kHz (Fig. 10-17).

Now, the bandwidth of 1 kHz is 100,000 times smaller than the 103.5 MHz frequency. The audible frequency range gets **modulated** to the **center frequency** (e.g., FM 103.5 MHz). The modulated frequency is then transmitted. The antenna receives this modulated signal. The signal then goes into the radio and is **demodulated** (Fig. 10-18). Depending on which station we tune into (e.g., KOST FM at 103.5 MHz), we get that range of frequencies demodulated back to zero frequency.

Thus, the bandwidth of a signal transmitted by a radio station always stays at about 1 kHz,

but it is transmitted as a 1kHz bandwidth *modulated* to, say, 103.5 MHz. Then, in the radio, it is demodulated back to zero center frequency, still with a bandwidth of about 1 kHz. What we send and what we receive are in the same frequency range. In between, the frequency gets modulated from zero to 103.5 MHz. We are just changing *the center frequency*. Everything else stays the same.

The reason radio transmission does this is that each radio station is only allowed a narrow bandwidth (in the kHz range) for transmission. But we cannot transmit a kHz frequency. It just doesn't travel very far, and radio transmissions have to travel for miles. Besides, the signals from different stations will get all mixed up if they all work in a small frequency range on the order of a few kHz. Therefore, the kHz frequency bandwidth is modulated to the MHz range, still maintaining the same kHz bandwidth. Now with the MHz frequency as a **carrier**, the narrow 1 kHz bandwidth can be transmitted over long distances.

In MRI, the **center frequency** is the Larmor frequency. Thus, the RF pulse that we transmit into the patient is *centered* at the Larmor fre-

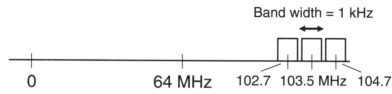

Figure 10-17.   An example of frequencies of FM radio stations.

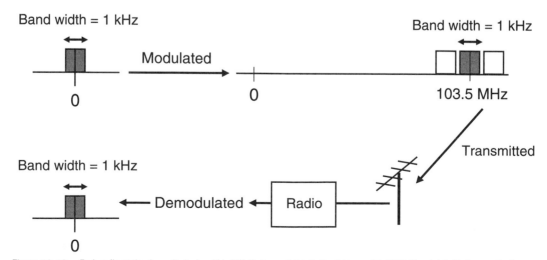

Figure 10-18.   Each radio station has a limited audible BW. To transmit this to the listeners, this BW is "modulated" via a carrier frequency (which is several orders of magnitude higher). In the radio, this frequency is demodulated back to the audible range.

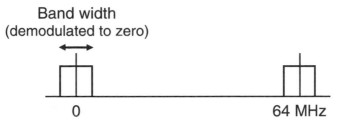

Figure 10-19. The process of demodulation in MRI.

quency of 64 MHz at 1.5 Tesla (Fig. 10-19). However, the bandwidth of frequencies in the RF pulse is *very narrow*. Again, for simplicity, we will assume that the bandwidth of the RF pulse has been demodulated to a center frequency of zero.

Slice-select Gradient

Let's go back to the slice select gradient. We purposely create a linear magnetic nonuniformity, so the foot will experience a weaker magnetic field than the head. The slope of magnetic field versus distance is called the **gradient**. A gradient is a measure of change of magnetic field with distance. We can have a **linear** gradient or a **nonlinear** gradient. The gradients that we use in MRI are usually linear. (In fact, nonlinearities may be present in the gradients that cause **geometric distortion artifacts** [see Chapter 10 on MR Artifacts].)

By creating this gradient, different magnetic fields are experienced from the foot to the head in an increasing order. The protons in the body will also experience a gradient in terms of their precessional frequency in that the protons in the foot are going to precess slower than the protons in the head.

We then transmit an RF pulse that matches the proton precessional frequency in a certain section of the body. Then, only the protons in this section will **resonate**; none of the other protons in any other portion of the body will resonate (i.e., flip into the transverse plane).

If we want to select a specific slice, then we transmit an RF pulse with a bandwidth that has the appropriate *center frequency*. This gradient is turned on only when we transmit the RF pulses. This makes sense because we only want the RF pulse to excite a thin slice of the body. When we transmit the 180° pulse for the same slice, we activate the same gradient.

When we study another slice, the gradient stays the same. We just alter the *center frequency* of the RF pulse. In this manner, we can excite different slices in any order desired.

Key Points

We have seen how one goes about selecting a slice in the body. This is done via a slice-select gradient. To vary the slice *thickness*, we can either vary the bandwidth of the transmitted RF pulse or the slope of the gradient. Thus, we can decrease the slice thickness by

1.   decreasing the bandwidth of the RF pulse, or
2.   increasing the slice select gradient.

Because the RF profiles are not ideal and may have side lobes or tails, if you try to have contiguous slices, you'll run into a problem called *crosstalk*. Basically, the transmitted signals in the frequency domain (i.e., their Fourier transforms)

will overlap and "cross talk." To avoid this, you must introduce *gaps* between the slices. This is done by excluding a certain range of frequencies (i.e., BW) in the transmitted RF pulses. The larger the gaps, the less cross you get, but the chance of missing a lesion within the gaps is greater.

The center frequency for each transmitted BW is like a *carrier* frequency around which the desired BW is centered, much like what goes on in radio-communication. Once a slice is selected, the question arises as to how to determine the pixels within that slice. This is the topic of the next chapter.

Questions

10-1. (a) The range of frequencies included in an RF pulse is referred to as its bandwidth (BW). Suppose that an RF pulse has frequencies ranging from -500 to 500 Hz (i.e., BW = 1000 Hz = 1 kHz). Now, to achieve a slice thickness of 5 mm, determine the amplitude of the slice-selection gradient.

(b) What is the minimum achievable slice thickness given a minimum RF BW = 426 Hz and a maximum gradient $G_z = 10$ mT/m?

Hint: $\omega = \gamma B$ so $\Delta\omega = BW = \gamma \Delta B$. Now, $B = G_z z$ so that $\Delta B = G_z \Delta z$.

Thus BW $= \gamma \Delta B = \gamma G_z \Delta z$ or $\Delta z = BW/(\gamma G_z)$, where Δz = slice thickness and $\gamma = 42.6$ MHz/T

10-2. Thinner slices can be achieved by
(a) decreasing the transmit (RF) bandwidth
(b) decreasing the receive (signal) BW
(c) increasing the slice select gradient strength
(d) all of the above
(e) only (a) and (b)
(f) only (a) and (c)

11 Image Construction

Part II (Spatial Encoding)

INTRODUCTION

In the last chapter, we learned how to select a slice and how to adjust its thickness. However, we did not address the question of from where within a particular slice each component of the signal comes. In other words, we still don't have spatial information regarding each slice. To create an image of a slice, we need to know how much signal comes from each **pixel** (picture element) or, more accurately, each **voxel** (volume element). This is the topic of spatial encoding, of which there are two parts: frequency encoding and phase encoding.

FREQUENCY ENCODING

After selecting a slice, how can we get information about individual pixels within that slice? As an example, consider a slice with three columns and three rows, for a total of nine pixels. This slice is selected using a selective 90° pulse (Fig. 11-1). We turn the Gz (slice-select gradient) on during the 90° pulse and turn it off after the 90° pulse.

We also send a selective 180° RF refocusing pulse, and we again turn the Gz gradient on during the 180° pulse. The **echo** is received after a time TE. The echo is a signal from the *entire* slice. To get spatial information in the x-direction of the slice, we apply another gradient Gx called the **frequency encoding gradient** (also called the **read-out gradient**) in the x-direction (Fig. 11-2). With this gradient in the x-direction, the center of this 3 × 3 matrix (the center volume) is not going to experience the gradient, i.e., it's not going to experience any change in magnetic field from that prior to turning on the Gx gradient. The column of pixels to the right of midline will experience a higher net magnetic field. The column of pixels on the left will have a lower net magnetic field.

The Gx gradient is applied during the time the echo is received, i.e., during read out.

Let's now assign some magnitude numbers to the pixels in the matrix (Fig. 11-3).

The numbers in each pixel and their specific location is what we ultimately want to discover because this corresponds to an image. We want to *recreate* this image using MRI.

Initially, all the protons in this section experience the same frequency of precession. Let's call that frequency ω_0. Now let's assign each pixel

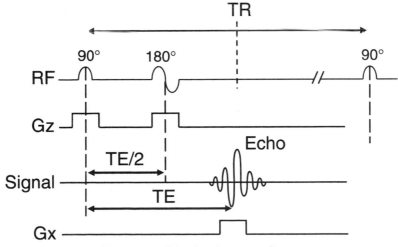

Figure 11-1. Spin-echo pulse sequence diagram.

its frequency at a specific point in time before turning on the Gx gradient, while they all still have the same frequency, and combine it with the magnitude we've assigned to each pixel (Fig. 11-4). For simplicity, we'll use a *cosine* wave as the received signal. In reality, the received signal is a more complicated one, such as a *sinc* wave.

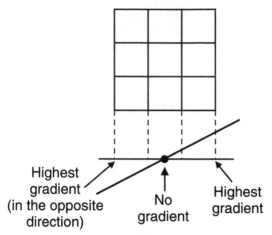

Figure 11-2. Frequency-encoding gradient along the x axis.

0	1	1
1	2	0
-2	0	1

Figure 11-3. In the previous example of a 3 × 3 matrix, each pixel is assigned a value (magnitude).

Each pixel has a designated magnitude (amplitude) and they all have the same precessional frequency ω_0 (except those pixels that have zero signal amplitude). Without any gradient in the x direction, this is the signal we're going to get. The signal will be the *sum* of all the signals from each pixel.

The sum of the amplitudes
$$= (0) + (1) + (-2) + (1) + (2) + (0) + (1) + (0) + (1) = 4$$

The frequency is the same for each pixel (i.e., ω_0), as is the shape of the signal (i.e., $\cos\omega_0 t$). So

sum of the pixels
$$= \text{signal from whole slice} = 4\cos\omega_0 t$$

We know that, in reality, the signal is more complex. For example, the signal is a decaying signal with time such as a *sinc* wave but, for simplicity, let's accept that we are dealing with a simple *cosine* wave as our signal with an amplitude of 4.

In summary, when we transmit an RF pulse with frequencies appropriate for a particular slice, all the protons in that slice will start to precess in phase at the Larmor frequency (ω_0). Each pixel contains a different number of protons designated by a number. For purposes of illustration, the number we have assigned to each pixel is proportional to the number of protons in each pixel. This number corresponds to the **amplitude** of the signal. The signal is designated as a *cosine* wave because it oscillates as a result of the precessing protons. However, we still do not have any spatial information; all we have at this point is a signal coming from

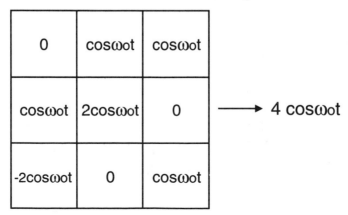

Figure 11-4. Each pixel is also assigned a frequency ω_0, and represented as A cos $\omega_0 t$, where A is the magnitude.

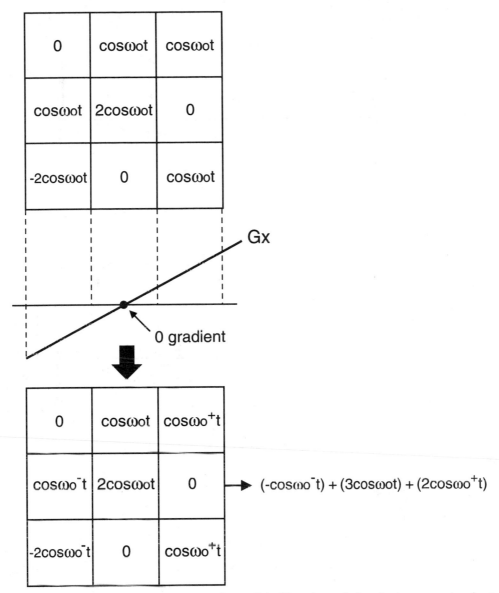

Figure 11-5. The matrix exposed to a frequency gradient results in different frequencies in each column; ω_0, ω_0^+, and ω_0^-.

the *entire slice* without spatial discrimination. What we want to be able to do is to separate the summed signal into its components and to tell, pixel by pixel, where each component of the received signal originated.

Let's now apply the frequency encoding gradient in the x-direction and see what happens to the pixels (Fig. 11-5). Let's look at the three columns in the matrix:

1. The pixels in the center column will not feel the gradient. Thus, they will remain

with the same frequency (ω_0). (And, of course, the amplitude of each pixel is constant because the number of protons doesn't change.)

2. The column of pixels to the right of midline is going to have slightly higher frequency. We'll call this (ω_0^+). This is because at a higher magnetic field strength, the protons in this column will oscillate at a higher frequency.

3. The column of pixels to the left of midline will experience a slightly lower field

Before Gx

Received Signal s(t) = (4cosω₀t)

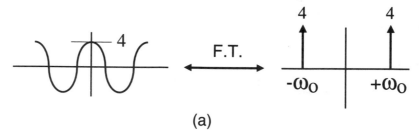

(a)

After Gx

Received Signal s(t) = (-cosω₀⁻t) + (3cosω₀t) + (2cosω₀⁺t)

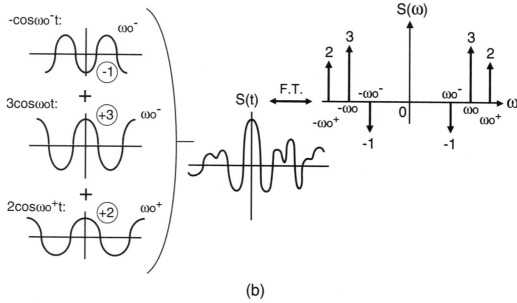

(b)

Figure 11-6. (a) The signal and its FT prior to the application of the gradient. The signal has a single frequency ω_0. **(b)** After application of the frequency gradient G_x, the resulting composite signal will be composed of 3 frequencies with a more complicated waveform and FT.

strength and thus have a precessional frequency a little lower than the other columns. We'll call this (ω_0-).

The signal that we get now is still the sum of all the individual signals; however, now each column of pixels has a different frequency, so we can *algebraically* only add up the ones that have the same frequency, as follows:

column #1:
$$0 + (cos\omega_0^-t) + (-2cos\omega_0^-t) = -cos\omega_0^-t$$
column #2:
$$(cos\omega_0t) + (2cos\omega_0t) + 0 = 3\,cos\omega_0t$$

column #3:
$$(cos\omega_0^+t) + 0 + (cos\omega_0^+t) = 2cos\omega_0^+t$$

---

sum of signals = $(-cos\omega_0^-t)$ + $(3cos\omega_0t)$ + $(2cos\omega_0^+t)$

Let's look at the Fourier transform of the signal *before* the Gx gradient is applied (Fig. 11-6a) and look at it again *after* the Gx gradient is applied (Fig. 11-6b). For a *cosine* wave, the Fourier transform is a symmetric pair of spikes at the *cosine* frequency, with an amplitude equal to the magnitude of the signal. (Remember that this is simplified. Usually, we deal with a band of frequencies, i.e., the *bandwidth*, as opposed to a single frequency. However, right now, for simplicity, we leave it as a single frequency, with its Fourier transform as a single spike.)

Now the computer can look at the Fourier transform and see that we are now dealing with three different frequencies:

1. The center frequency comes from the central column, and the amplitude of the frequency spike represents the sum of the amplitudes of the pixels in that column, i.e., ($3\,cos\omega_0 t$).
2. The higher frequency comes from the column to the right, and the amplitude of that frequency spike represents the sum of the amplitude of the pixels in that column, i.e., ($2cos\omega_0^+ t$).

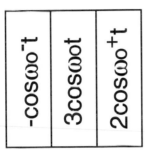

Figure 11-7. The sum of the signals in each column. Since the signals belonging to the same column have the same frequency, they are additive.

3. The lower frequency comes from the column to the left, and the amplitude of that frequency spike represents the sum of the amplitude of the pixels in that column, i.e., ($-cos\omega_0^- t$).

The way frequency encoding works is that frequency and position have a one-to-one relationship:

---

frequency ↔ *position*

So far we have done some spatial encoding and have extracted some information from the slice. We are now able to decompose the slice matrix into three different columns (Fig. 11-7). That is, we have three different shades of gray corresponding to the three columns.

So, now we've done our job in the x-direction. The next thing we want to do is to decompose the individual columns into their three individual pixels (i.e., work in the y direction). The two ways of doing this are as follows:

1. Back projection
2. 2 DFT (two-dimensional Fourier transform)

Back Projections

If we think in terms of CT imaging and apply gradients, we start out with an area we want to image and apply a gradient (Fig. 11-8a). Then

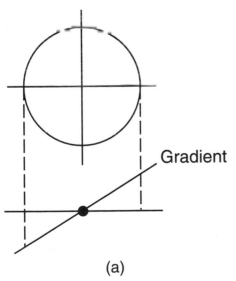
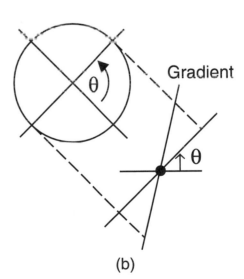

(a)　　　(b)

Figure 11-8. Back projection. By gradually rotating the gradient (from **a** to **b**), we get a set of equations the solution to which gives the pixel values.

we can rotate the gradient by an angle θ and reapply the gradient (Fig. 11-8b). We can continue this to complete 360°, and each time we do this we get different numbers. At the end, we end up with a set of equations, which can be solved for values of the pixels in the matrix. This is the **back projection** approach performed by rotating the frequency gradient.

Advantages
1. It is possible to pick a small FOV (field of view).

Disadvantages
1. This technique is very dependent on external magnetic field inhomogeneities (i.e., it is sensitive to ΔB_0).
2. This technique is also very sensitive to the magnetic field gradients. If the gradient is *not* perfect, you get artifacts.

Because of these disadvantages, this technique was given up.

2DFT: 2-dimensional Digital Fourier Transform

2DFT is the method currently used, and is the topic of the remainder of this chapter.

Advantages
1. Lack of sensitivity to external magnetic field inhomogeneities.
2. Lack of sensitivity to gradient field inhomogeneities.

PHASE ENCODING

In the 2DFT technique, in addition to using the Gz gradient for slice selection and the Gx gradient for encoding in the x-direction, we add another gradient Gy in the y-direction. This is called the **phase-encoding gradient** (Fig. 11-9).

We turn on the Gy gradient before we turn on the Gx (read out) gradient. It is usually applied right after the RF pulse or just before the Gx gradient or anywhere in between.

Gy is usually applied between the 90° and the 180° RF pulses or between the 180° pulse and the echo.

So now let's again look at the slice with its 9 pixels before either the Gx (frequency encoding) gradient or the Gy (phase encoding) gradient is applied (Fig. 11-10a). The designation of the pixels on the right in Figure 11-10a is a way of denoting phase and frequency. The arrow

Phase Encoding

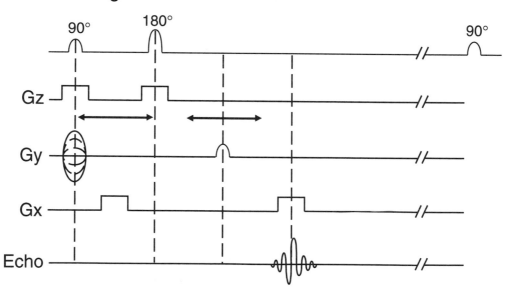

Figure 11-9. The phase-encode gradient G_y is applied along the y axis. It is usually applied between the 90° and the 180° pulse or between the 180° pulse and the echo.

Before Gx or Gy

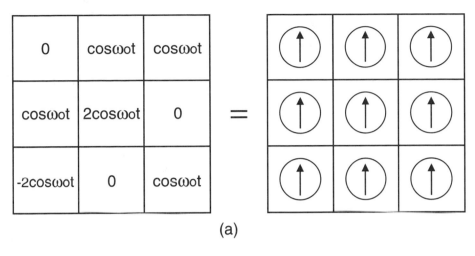

(a)

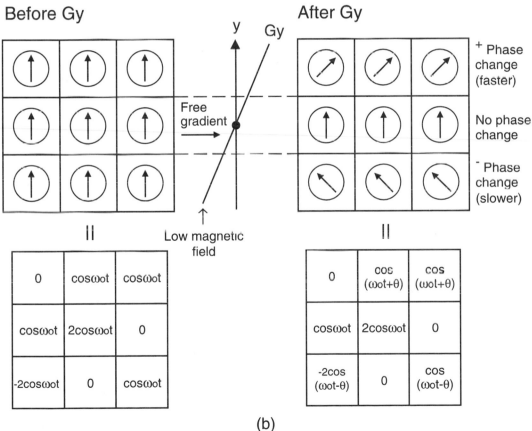

(b)

Figure 11-10. Analogy of clock handle: **(a)** Before application of G_x or G_y, the handles point north. **(b)** After application of Gy, the handles in different rows get out of phase. **(c)** After application of G_x, each pixel has a different frequency and phase (i.e., the handles rotate at different speeds and with different phase, keeping in mind that the speed is the same for all the elements belonging to the same column).

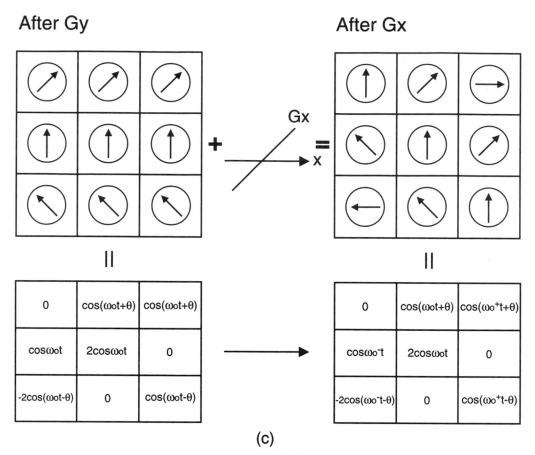

Figure 11-10. Continued.

represents the hand of a clock and denotes the position of precession (i.e., the phase) at a given point in time. After the 90° RF pulse, all the protons in the selected slice precess at the same frequency (ω_0). At any point in time *before* being exposed to a magnetic field gradient, the protons in all the pixels will all be pointing in the same direction (e.g., north) without any phase difference among them.

This is precisely what the clock diagram shows: prior to being exposed to a magnetic field gradient, all the protons in each pixel are in phase with each other, oscillating at the same frequency. (Note that we have eliminated magnitude from the clock diagram. All we are concerned about for now is the phase and frequency of the direction of the spins at a particular point in time.)

Now let's expose the slice to a Gy gradient—a magnetic field gradient in the y-direction (Fig. 11-10b). With the gradient now applied in the

y-direction, the pixels in the upper row will experience a higher net magnetic field, the pixels in the middle row will experience no change in the magnetic field, and the pixels in the lower row will experience a lower net magnetic field.

Consequently, the pixels in the middle row, because they experience no change in the magnetic field, will have no phase change after the gradient is turned on. They will continue to point in the same direction as they did before activation of the gradient.

Protons in the pixels on the top row will all start precessing faster because they are now experiencing a stronger magnetic field. Therefore, they will all remain in phase with one another but will be out-of-phase with the protons in the middle row.

The pixels in the bottom row will all start precessing more slowly because they are now experiencing a weaker magnetic field. They will all be in phase with one another but will be out of phase with the protons in the middle and upper rows.

Once the Gy gradient is turned off, all the protons will now be at the same magnetic field strength once again, so they will all again precess at the same frequency.

However, look at what has happened. A permanent **phase shift** has occurred in the protons of each row. True, they are now all spinning at the same frequency; however, those that were previously exposed to the higher magnetic field and were out of phase with the protons in the middle row will continue to be out of phase now that all protons are spinning at the same frequency again. Likewise, those protons previously exposed to the lower magnetic field that went out of phase with the protons in the middle now will continue to be out of phase now that all protons are spinning at the same frequency again.

Now we have caused a difference in the rows of pixels based on phase (designated by θ in Fig. 11-10b). Differences in spatial position up and down are reflected in that phase value. Hence the term **phase encoding**.

Remember that the Gy gradient is turned on before reading out the signal. So when we read the signal, we turn on the Gx gradient, which, as we learned from our earlier discussion, allows us to frequency encode in the Gx direction (Fig. 11-10c). With the Gx gradient on, the middle column protons won't experience any change in their precessional frequency, so their frequency is unchanged. However, as you can see, each pixel in the middle column already has a distinct *phase shift*, which had occurred when the Gy gradient was on, and this phase shift persists.

With the Gx gradient turned on, the protons in the columns to the right of midline will experience a greater magnetic field so that all the protons in this column will have a faster precessional frequency. However, we notice that each pixel in this column was already out of phase with the other pixels in the column due to the phase shift which had occurred when the Gy gradient was on. Therefore, protons in each pixel of the right column shift the same amount (because they all have the same increased frequency). But because they shift from a unique position, they will then each move to a phase shift that is different for each pixel.

Likewise, the protons in the column to the left of midline will experience a lower precessional frequency with the Gx gradient on. But, again, we notice that each pixel in this column is already out of phase with the other pixels in the column due to the phase shift that had occurred when the Gy gradient was on. So, again, after the Gx gradient is turned on, each pixel will move to a specific phase-shift distinct for each pixel. In summary, x position is represented by a unique *frequency* and y position by a unique *phase*.

The protons in each pixel have a distinct frequency and a distinct phase, which are unique and encode for the x and y coordinates for that pixel.

Question: How does one determine the phase shift between adjacent rows?
Answer: First, to figure out the phase shift, we divide 360° by the number of rows:

$$\Delta\theta = 360/\text{\# of rows}$$

Because we have three rows, the phase shift between rows is (see Figure 11-11)

$$\Delta\theta = 360/3 = 120° \ (or\ 2\pi/3)$$

Therefore, in the middle row, there will be no phase shift. In the upper row, the phase shift will be 120°. In the lower rows, the phase shift will be +240° (which is the same as −120°)

Each row has its own *unique phase shift* caused by the Gy gradient:

row 1: Phase shift of +120°.
row 2: No phase shift
row 3: Phase shift of −120°

Also, each *column* has its own *unique frequency* caused by the Gx gradient.

column 1: frequency of ω_0-
column 2: frequency of ω_0
column 3: frequency of ω_0+

When combined, as it is during the read-out of the signal, we see that each pixel has its own unique phase shift and frequency.

Question: Why does it take time to do phase encoding?

Received Signal After Gx & Gy

0	$\cos(\omega_0 t + 120°)$	$\cos(\omega_0^+ t + 120°)$
$\cos(\omega_0^- t)$	$2\cos(\omega_0 t)$	0
$-2\cos(\omega_0^- t - 120°)$	0	$\cos(\omega_0^+ t - 120°)$

Figure 11-11. The received signal after application of both G_x and G_y for the 3 × 3 matrix used in previous examples.

Answer: It takes time because we need to do a separate phase encode for each row of pixels that we need to discriminate in the slice. In this case, we have 3 rows of pixels, so we would do 3 phase-encoding steps. Each time we do a separate phase encode, it is a new spin echo taking time TR after a new 90° RF pulse. With each new phase-encoding step (taking time TR), we change the magnetic gradient Gy:

TR#1: No Gradient—no phase shift between rows.

TR#2: Gradient with 120° phase shift between rows.

TR#3: Gradient with 240° (or −120°) phase shift between rows.

We wouldn't need another TR because 240° + 120° = 360° phase shift, and this would give us the same information as a 0° phase shift. What would happen to the signals with the three different phase-encoding steps (Fig. 11-12)?

During TR#1, where we don't apply a gradient Gy in the y direction, we get no phase shift between the rows. Then, when we apply the frequency encoding gradient Gx in the x direction, we get the frequency difference between the columns.

During TR#2, we apply a Gy gradient so that there is a 120° phase shift between the rows. Then, when we apply the frequency encoding gradient Gx in the x-direction, we get the frequency difference in the columns on top of the 120° phase shift between the rows.

During TR#3, we apply a steeper Gy gradient so that now there is a 240° (or −120°) phase shift between the rows. Then, when we apply the frequency encoding gradient in the x direction, we get the frequency difference in the columns on top of the 240° phase shift between the rows.

Notice that in each case the middle row never experiences any phase shift, and the middle column never experiences any frequency change. Therefore, the center pixel never experiences any frequency or phase shift. Also notice that we need a separate TR for each phase encoding step. That is why phase encoding takes time. We need one TR time period to perform each phase encoding step. Hence, part of the formula describing the acquisition time for a sequence includes TR and the number of phase encoding steps (as well as the number of excitations).

As an example, if we need to discriminate 256 rows, then we need to perform 256 phase encoding steps, each with a different gradient Gy, taking time 256 × TR. The difference in

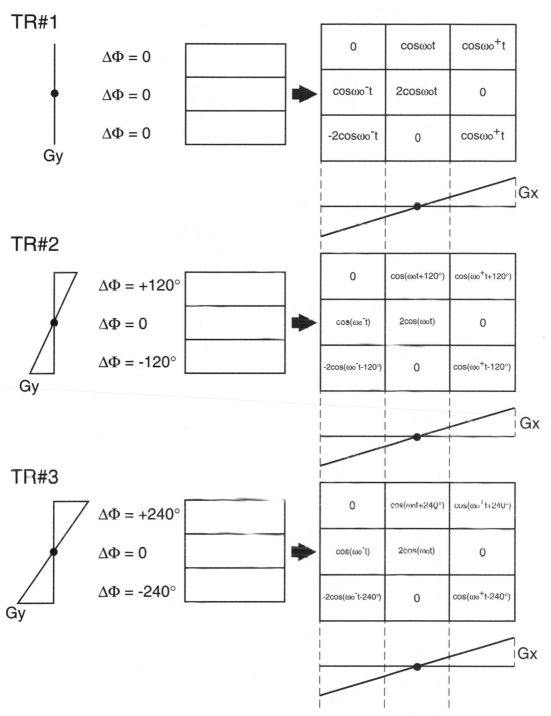

Figure 11-12.   The received signal during each cycle.

the phase shift between the rows in this case would be:

360°/256 phase encoding step ≅ 1.45°

1. TR#1 = No gradient ∴ no phase shift
2. TR#2 = gradient to allow a phase shift = 1.45° between rows
3. TR#3 = steeper gradient to allow a phase shift = 2 × (1.45°) between rows
4. TR#4 = steeper gradient to allow a phase shift = 3 × (1.45°) between rows

....

256. TR#256 = the steepest gradient to allow a phase shift = 255 × (1.45°) between rows

If we do these steps once more, we get the same information as the first phase encoding step, which is redundant. Each time we do a phase encoding step followed by frequency encoding, we get a *signal*. The first signal we get is without any phase shift (TR#1). Then we activate the phase encode gradient, add some phase shift and get another signal (TR#2), and so on. Each signal is different because it has a different phase shift.

Data Space

Each of these signals fills one line in a set of rows referred to as the **data space** (Fig. 11-13). **k-space** can be thought of as a digitized version of the data space (more on this in Chapter 13). Let's see how this is done within each TR period:

1. With TR#1, we have no phase shift. After the frequency encoding step, a signal is received and placed into one row of the data space. In the previous example, we happened to put it into the center row of the data space (this is arbitrary, though).
2. With TR#2, we add a phase shift and, after the frequency encoding step, a signal (which will be different than the signal from the first TR) is received and put into another row in the data space. In the previous example, we put it into the top row of the data space (again, this is arbitrary).
3. With the third TR, we add more phase shift. After the frequency encoding step, a third signal (which is different from the other two signals because of the increased phase shift) is received and put into another row of the data space. In

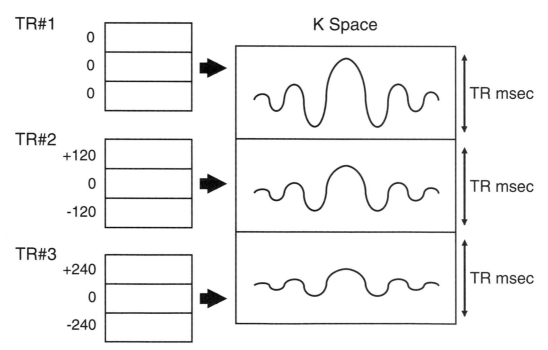

Figure 11-13. Each row in the Data Space (analog K space) contains the received signal corresponding to a particular phase-encode gradient.

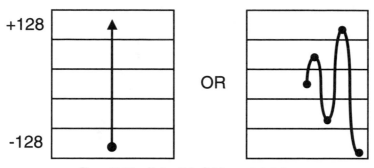

Figure 11-14. Various K (or Data) space trajectories.

the previous example, we put it into the bottom row of the data space.

The interval between the rows in the data space is given by TR msec, going through a cycle from one 90° pulse to the next 90° pulse.

SUMMARY

TR#1: place the signal into the center of the data space
TR#2: place it one above the center of the data space
TR#3: place it one below the center of the data space

If we had a TR#4, we would place it two above the center, and if we had a TR#5, we would place it two below the center. We could continue along filling the data space in this manner.

Remember that in our example, we start in the center of the data space with TR#1, which has no phase shift. In each subsequent row (as we go farther out in the data space) there is progressively greater and greater phase shift in each phase encoding step. Also remember that each phase encoding step has a different magnetic field gradient; thus, its phase shift will be different from each preceding and each subsequent phase encoding step.

However, also note that the selection of phase encoding steps, i.e., the order in which we perform them, is *arbitrary*. We can start with no phase shift and go progressively to maximum phase shift, or we can start with maximum phase shift and go down to no phase shift. Likewise, the position to which they are assigned in the data space is also *arbitrary*.

When we discuss fast spin echo in later chapters, we will see the arbitrariness of this phase encoding assignment. Even in conventional spin echo imaging, the placement of signals into the data space can vary. For example, two different patterns of the data space filling with 256 phase encoding steps are shown in Figure 11-14. We can put the first signal in the bottom of the data space and work up with successive phase encoding steps. Or, as in our example, we can start in the center and go alternately up and down. Usually, the center row of the data space corresponds to no phase gradient.

Note, however, that the center of the data space does not represent the center of your picture. Each signal has information in it about the entire picture. Remember that each signal

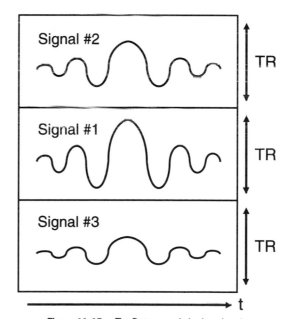

Figure 11-15. The Data space is in time domain.

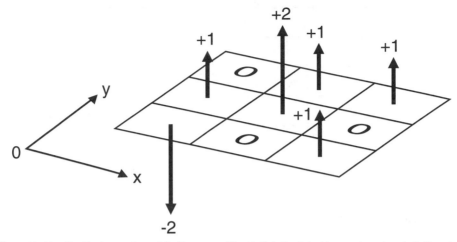

Figure 11-16. The Fourier transform of the Data space (Fig. 11-5) is the desired image, shown here in 3 dimensions.

that goes into each row of the data space is the *sum* of all the signals from individual pixels in the slice.

The information in the data space is in the **time domain** (so it is not as scary as it looks). In fact, it is in the time domain in both directions: the received signal is displayed over a period of time (t) and signals in two successive rows are obtained at every TR (Fig. 11-15).

The information in this data space has not yet been digitized. In fact, a digitized version of this information is the true **k-space**. We will see in a later chapter (Chapter 16) that the "digitized" k-space is in a **spatial frequency domain.** But let's not get confused now! Let's see how we can digitize this information in the data. This is accomplished via sampling.

SAMPLING

The signal that goes into the data space has been phase-encoded and frequency encoded. But it has not yet been **sampled** (more on this in the next chapter).

When we describe a matrix of, say, 256 × 192, what do we mean by it? If we only have 192 phase-encoding steps, why do we have 256 (instead of 192) frequency encodes if we only need one frequency encode for every encoding step?

Actually, the 256 number refers to the different number of frequencies we have for each phase encoding step. These two steps are thus independent from one another. For example, let's look at a 4 × 5 matrix. This means that we do 5 different frequencies for each phase encoding step, with the center column having no change in frequency and two different frequencies for the columns on either side; there will be four different phase encoding steps. Therefore, the result will be **asymmetric** pixels. Let's go back to our original 3 × 3 matrix, with its data space as in Figure 11-15.

How do we go from the data space (Fig. 11-9a) to the desired image Figure 11-3? The answer is via **Fourier transformation**. The Fourier transform of the signals in Figure 11-15 is a set of spikes, which in a 3-dimensional space looks like Figure 11-16. More on this in chapters to come.

Key Points

In the previous chapter, we learned how to select a slice using a slice-select gradient Gz. In this chapter, we saw how to determine the pixel values in a slice using two gradients: a frequency encoding (or readout) gradient Gx and a phase encoding gradient Gy.

Gx is applied during the readout (i.e., during reception of the echo). It is used to sample the echo. Therefore, each TR interval contains one readout (Gx) per slice.

Gy is applied in increments between the 90° RF pulse and each echo. Thus, for every slice, each TR interval contains one phase-encoding step (i.e., one gradient strength of Gy). This process completes one line in k-space corresponding to the selected Gy. This process is repeated Ny times to fill the entire k-space.

We have not yet discussed the mechanism of performing frequency and phase-encoding operations. This is the topic of the next chapter.

Questions

11-1.   Match
(i) Gx   (ii) Gy   (iii) Gz
with
(a)   applied during the echo
(b)   applied during the RF transmission
(c)   applied between the RF and the readout

11-2.   T/F   In conventional SE imaging, during each cycle (one TR period), only a *single* value of the phase encode gradient strength Gy is applied.

11-3.   What is the phase increment for 128 phase encode steps (i.e., Ny = 128)?

11-4.   Match:
(i)   position along x axis
(ii)   position along y axis
with
(a)   phase encode gradient G_y
(b)   frequency encode gradient G_x
(c)   absolute phase ϕ_y
(d)   absolute frequency f_x

12 Signal Processing

INTRODUCTION

Signal processing refers to analog and/or digital manipulation of a signal. The signal could be an electric current or voltage, as is the case in MR imaging. **Image processing** is a form of signal processing in which the manipulations are performed on a digitized image. **Analog-to-digital conversion** (ADC) is a process where a time-varying (analog) signal is converted to a digitized form (i.e., a series of 0s and 1s) that can be recognized by a computer. An understanding of signal processing requires a basic understanding of the concept of frequency domain and Fourier transform because the majority of the "processing" of a signal is accomplished in the frequency domain and, at the end, the results are converted back into the time domain.

One of signal processing's key concepts, as we shall see shortly, is the **Nyquist sampling** theorem. An understanding of the sampling procedure allows one to appreciate the relationship between the samples of a signal (in time domain) and its bandwidth (in frequency domain). Once

this concept is grasped, the issue of **aliasing (wraparound)** artifact can be explained very easily. A knowledge of signal processing will also help the reader understand the more complicated, newer fast scanning pulse sequences presented in later chapters.

SEQUENCE OF EVENTS

First, let's summarize what has been discussed so far. Figure 12-1 illustrates a summary of a spin echo pulse sequence. The following is a summary of the sequence of events:

1. We have 90° and 180° pulses separated by a time of (TE/2) msec;
2. After a time of TE msec after each 90° RF pulse, we get an **echo**;
3. We turn on the slice-selective gradient (Gz) during the two RF transmissions. This causes a linear gradient of magnetic field along the z axis. By choosing an RF pulse with an appropriate frequency and bandwidth, we can select a slice at a

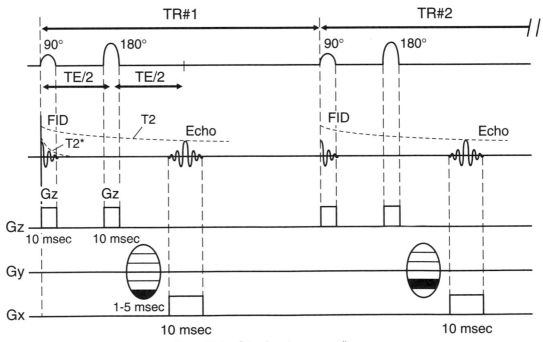

Figure 12-1.   Spin-echo pulse sequence diagram.

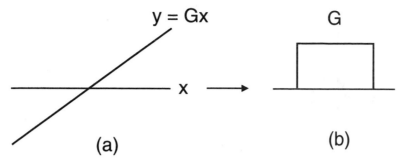

Figure 12-2. A linear gradient G represents a linear function G_x, which can either be represented as a linear line with slope G **(a)** or as a rectangle with height G **(b)**.

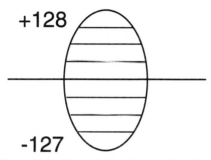

Figure 12-3. The symbol for phase-encode gradient.

particular position with a particular thickness.

As an aside, consider Figure 12-2. Plotting field strength versus position (Fig. 12-2), the gradient is represented as a sloped line. The slope of the line is a constant that we call G. The value y along this line with slope G at point x is y = G x. This is a simple linear equation. Figure 12-2b plots gradient strength versus time. Figures 12-2a and 12-2b are used interchangeably to illustrate a *linear* gradient with strength G.

4. Right before we receive the echo, we apply a phase encoding gradient (Gy). The symbol for the phase encoding grading is in Figure 12-3. This symbol denotes the *multiple* phase encoding steps that are necessary as we cycle through the acquisition.

5. The frequency encoding gradient (Gx) is turned on during the time period during which the echo is received.

6. *Time Requirements*

   (a) the frequency encoding step takes about 10 msec (4–8 msec at high field; 16–30 msec at lower fields);

   (b) the phase encoding step takes 1–5 msec;

   (c) each RF pulse (with a Gz gradient) takes 2–10 msec.

Then we repeat the whole sequence of events after time TR. The time spent from the center of the 90° pulse to the end of the echo read-out is

TE + 1/2 (sampling time) = (TE + Ts/2)

The **sampling time** Ts is the time it takes to sample the echo, which is the time that the Gx gradient (read-out or frequency encode gradient) is on. The Gx gradient is on throughout the echo readout—from beginning to end (Fig. 12-4). The time from the beginning of the 90° pulse to the midpoint of the echo is TE. Because half of the sampling time continues past the midpoint of the echo, we need to add half the sampling time to TE to account for the entire "active time" from the beginning of the RF pulse to the end of sampling time:

Active time = TE + Ts/2

There may also be time taken up by other events that occur before the RF pulse (such as presaturation pulses) that we include as **overhead time** (T_o). Thus,

Active time = TE + Ts/2 + T_o

Let's assume a TE of 40 msec, a sampling time Ts = 10 msec, and an overhead time T_o = 5 msec. Then,

Active time = 40 msec + 10 msec/2 + 5 msec
= 50 msec

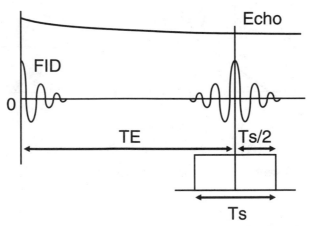

Figure 12-4. The frequency gradient is turned on during readout (i.e., during the echo).

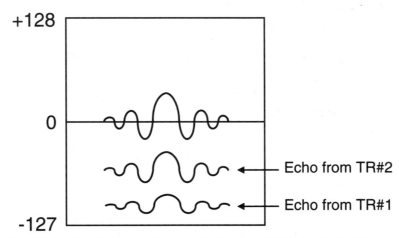

Figure 12-5. For each phase encoding step, a signal is obtained that is placed in the Data space.

Therefore, it takes 50 msec to read out the signal from one echo. We then place this signal into the data space (Fig. 12-5). We have designated 256 rows in the data space (from −127 to +128) and in this instance we've placed the first signal at position −127.

7. In the next TR cycle, we do exactly the same thing, except this time, the phase encoding step will be done with a slightly weaker magnetic gradient and will be one step higher in K (data) space.

Question: Why does the magnitude of the signal differ with each phase encoding step? For example, in the diagram above, the signal from the echo of TR#2 seems to have higher maximum amplitude than the signal from the echo of TR#1.

Answer: The strength of the phase encoding gradient affects the magnitude of the signal.

When the phase encode gradient is at a maximum (when we have the largest magnetic field gradient), we have the maximum dephasing of proton spins. Recall that we are dealing with proton spins that have been flipped into the transverse plane by a 90° pulse, and the signal is maximum as long as these proton spins stay *in phase*. By using a magnetic field gradient, we are introducing an artificial external means of dephasing. Also, remember that when we flip the protons into the transverse plane, they are initially in phase, and then rapidly go out of phase due to external magnetic inhomogeneities and spin-spin interactions (Fig. 12-6a). Next, the protons are flipped with a 180° pulse and, after a period of time = TE/2, they go back in phase (Fig. 12-6b).

On top of this, we introduce a magnetic inhomogeneity by way of a linear gradient where the inhomogeneity increases linearly, causing *additional dephasing* of proton spins. We realize that we have to accept this additional dephasing because this is the way we obtain *spatial* information along the axis of this gradient. This process is called **phase encoding**.

However, this explains why, when we use the magnetic field gradient for phase encoding, the additional dephasing caused by the gradient will necessarily decrease the overall signal we receive during that phase encoding step. It then allows us to conclude:

(a) The largest magnetic gradient we use for maximum phase encoding will give us the lowest magnitude signal.

(b) When the magnetic gradient in the phase-encode direction is zero, we will not introduce any additional dephasing, and we will get the largest magnitude signal.

Therefore, if we go back and examine the signal from TR#1 and TR#2 we see that:

(a) TR#1 at position (−127) in the data space has a lower amplitude signal than TR#2 at position (−126). This is because during TR#1 a larger phase-encoding gradient is used than during TR#2 (keep in mind, however, that assignments of gradients to different TR intervals in the data space is *arbitrary*).

k-space, as we mentioned in the last chapter (with more to come in Chapters 13 and 16) can be thought of as a digitized version of the data space. The signal in the center of k-space

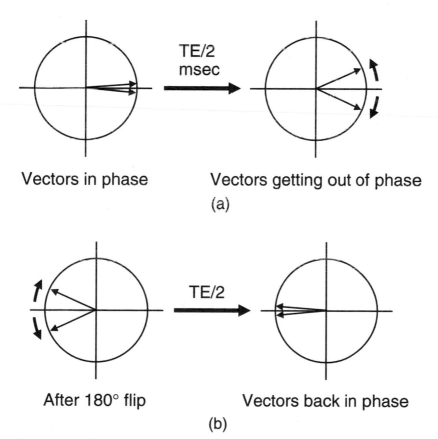

Vectors in phase   Vectors getting out of phase

(a)

After 180° flip   Vectors back in phase

(b)

Figure 12-6. The spins are initially in phase **(a)**, then get out of phase at time TE/2. At this point, a 180° pulse is applied, reversing the vectors **(b)** so that they come back in phase after another period TE/2 (i.e., at time TE).

(at position 0) has the maximum amplitude. This is because this signal is obtained at a phase-encoding step where no magnetic field gradient is used (i.e., no phase gradient and hence no extra dephasing due to phase encoding). In fact, the center line of k-space will always be occupied by the phase encoding step that uses no gradient.

The center line of k-space will always contain the phase encoding step with the **weakest gradient** *and thus with the* **most signal.**

The most peripheral lines of k-space will be occupied by the phase encoding steps that use the strongest gradients.

The periphery of k-space will contain those phase encoding steps with the **largest gradients** *and thus with the* **least signal.**

8.   Multi-slice Technique:

Remember that TR is much longer than the *active time* needed to perform all the functions necessary to select a slice, phase encode, and frequency encode. The TR might be, say, 1000 msec. The *active time* in our example was 50 msec. There is a lot of "**dead time**" in between the 50 msec of active time and the next 90° pulse. We can take advantage of this "dead time" in order to get information regarding other slices.

As an example, in Figure 12-7 we will have time for two additional slices to be studied during the dead time within one TR period. After we obtain the signal from slice #1, we can apply another 90° pulse of a different center frequency ω and transmit bandwidth to specify the next slice (Fig. 12-8). Here we are talking about the transmitted bandwidth (of the RF pulse) that determines slice thickness, not to be confused with the receiver bandwidth (of the echo) that determines noise. More on this later.

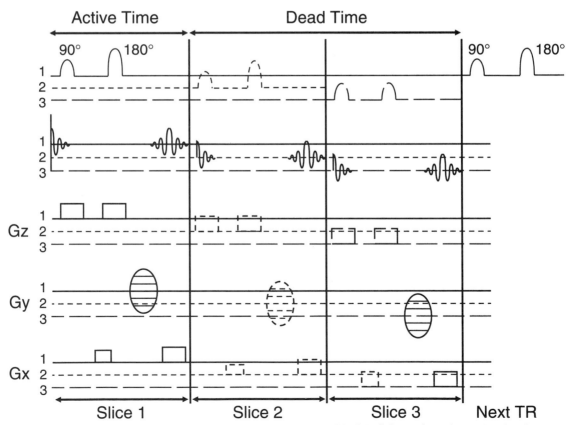

Figure 12-7.   Multislice acquisition. During each TR cycle, there is a certain "dead time" that can be used to acquire other slices.

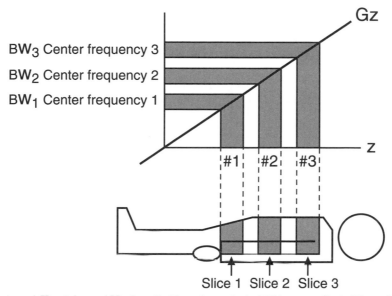

Figure 12-8. During each TR period, several RF pulses with different frequencies (and BWs) corresponding to different slices are transmitted.

To choose the next slice, we keep the same magnetic gradient Gz, but we choose a bandwidth at a higher or lower *center* (or Larmor) frequency to flip the protons 90° in a different slice. The *bandwidth is the same* as the first slice, but the *center frequency is different*.

We choose the same phase encoding gradient Gy so we get the same amount of dephasing in this next slice. We sample the echo with the same frequency encoding gradient as we did with the first slice. Because we still have time during the dead time to acquire a third slice, we repeat everything and again choose a 90° RF pulse of a different Larmor frequency so we can flip the protons of a different slice into the transverse plane. The signal from each slice will be placed in a different k-space.

Each slice has its own k-space.

Slice selection can be performed in several different ways. We can have *contiguous slices*; *sequential slices* with a *gap* between slices; and *interleaved slices*, where we do odd numbered slices (i.e., 1, 3, 5) and then go back and do even numbered slices (i.e., 2, 4, 6).

9. Number of Slices (Coverage)

The number of slices we can do within any TR is limited by the *dead time* after (TE + Ts/2 +

To). Furthermore, if we choose to have two echoes per TR (as in dual-echo spin-echo sequence), the number of slices we could have would be cut back more. The formula for the maximum number of slices one can obtain is

$$\text{\# slices} < \frac{TR}{TE + Ts/2 + To} = \frac{TR}{\text{active time}}$$

If we do multiple echoes (or just one long echo) the formula is governed by the *longest* TE.

EXAMPLES:

1. TR = 1000, TE = 35 msec, Ts = 10 msec, T_o = 10 msec (short TE)

$$\text{Max \# slices} = \frac{TR}{TE + Ts/2 + To}$$
$$= \frac{1000}{35 + 5 + 10}$$
$$= 1000/50 = 20 \text{ slices}$$

2. TR = 1000, TE = 75, Ts = 10 msec, T_o = 10 msec (long TE)

$$\text{Max \# slices} = \frac{1000}{95 + 5 + 10}$$
$$= 1000/90 \cong 11 \text{ slices}$$

We usually don't know what the sampling time (Ts) or overhead time (T_o) is; therefore, a rough approximation is

---

Max # slices < TR/TE

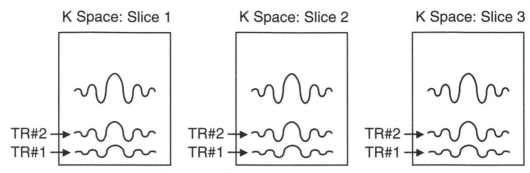

Figure 12-9. Each slice has its own K (Data) space.

It is said that in a double echo sequence, the first echo is "free." This means that the number of slices in a double echo sequence is determined only by the TE of the second echo

$$TR = 1000, TE_1 = 30, TE_2 = 80$$

$$\text{Max \# slices} = \frac{TR}{TE \text{ (second echo)} + Ts/2 + To}$$
$$= 1000/(80 + 15) = 1000/95 \cong 10.5$$

In actual fact, the maximum number of slices is determined by TR, and the time it takes to get one line in the data space as follows:

Max number of slices $<$ TR/time to get one line
of signal into the data space
$$= TR/(TE + Ts/2 + To)$$

Also remember that each slice has its own data space (and, thus, its own k-space), and if we are doing a double echo sequence, *each echo has its own data space (k-space)*. The signal obtained from each slice during the same TR will be obtained with the same phase-encoding step. Thus, the equivalent line in each data space of the slices for a given TR will be subject to the same dephasing effects of the phase-encoding gradient (Fig. 12-9).

10.   Center Frequency:

A few more words about the *center frequency* and *transmit bandwidth*. As we go from slice to slice, the RF center frequency, (i.e., the Larmor frequency) changes, but the bandwidth remains the same. In Figure 12-10, the bandwidth (the range of frequencies) remains the same. The *center frequency* of the bandwidth changes: it increases as we go higher on the magnetic field gradient and it decreases as we go lower on the magnetic gradient.

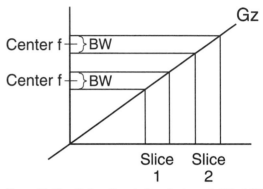

Figure 12-10. During slice selection, the transmit BW of RF pulses remains the same but their center frequencies vary.

The bandwidth (range of frequencies) should be constant because we want each slice to be of the same thickness. At the low end of the magnetic gradient the frequencies are lower, and at the top end of the gradient the frequencies are higher. Thus, as we go up the gradient, we approach higher center frequencies for the RF pulse; however, the bandwidth won't change.

If the duration of the RF pulse is short, then its bandwidth will be wide and vice versa (Fig. 12-11). In our pulse sequence, we use the same RF bandwidth (i.e., the same RF duration) each time, but the center frequency is changed. Think of the center frequency as a **carrier** frequency. We are sending the same signal, but we are carrying it at a different center frequency, and the bandwidth around it is the original signal (Fig. 12-12).

If we use a *wider* bandwidth with the same center frequency, then we get a *thicker* slice; a *narrower* RF pulse whose Fourier transform has a wider bandwidth gives us a thicker slice. A *carrier* is a signal that determines the center frequency. For more details, refer to the discussion on bandwidth in Chapter 10.

Figure 12-13a displays a typical signal from the echo. After the signal is received at the receiver coil, it is digitized (through signal sampling) because the computer analyzing the signal can only work with digitized numbers. The vertical bars in Figure 12-13a demonstrate the sampling procedure. Instead of having a continuum of signal amplitudes, **samples** of the signal at certain time intervals (usually equidistant intervals) are taken.

The computer now only has these **discrete** (as opposed to analog) values. Each value is represented in the computer as a **binary number** (0s and 1s) so the computer doesn't deal with the whole signal—just discrete samples of the signal. A computer **bit** is either a 0 or a 1. A **byte** consists of 8 bits and represents the basic building block of computer characters. Each sample of an analog signal is encoded into a series of bytes, which is recognized by every computer. This process is the basis for **ADC** (**analog-to-digital conversion**).

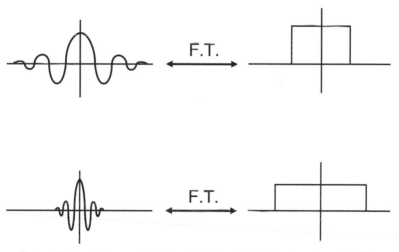

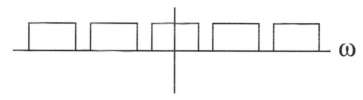

Figure 12-11. An inverse relationship exists between the duration of a pulse and its BW.

Figure 12-12. The FT of RF pulses—the BWs are the same but the center frequencies are different.

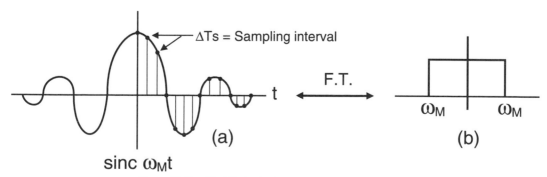

Figure 12-13. The FT of a sinc function contains a single rectangle.

The idea behind ADC is to just use the samples of a signal and be able to reconstruct the original signal from its samples.

Let's consider a *sinc* signal with frequency ω. As we have seen in previous chapters, this signal has a rectangular-shaped Fourier transform (Fig. 12-13b). The time between successive sampling points is called the sampling interval ΔTs.

$$\Delta Ts = \text{sampling interval}$$

After it is sampled, the aforementioned signal will look like Figure 12-14a. The **envelope** of this function is a curve connecting the sample points (which resembles the original *sinc* function). The Fourier transform of this sampled signal is given in Figure 12-14b. This Fourier transform looks like a *periodic* version of the original Fourier transform (Fig. 12-13b) because the Fourier transform of a discrete and periodic function is also periodic (see later text). If ΔTs is the sampling interval, the first center frequency is give by the following formula (Fig. 12-14b).

$$\text{center frequency} = 1/\Delta Ts$$

If we make the sampling interval very short, we will spread out the square waves in the Fourier transform; i.e., if we take several samples/cycle, the square waves spread out (Fig. 12-15). If we make the sampling interval very wide, the square waves of the Fourier transform are going to get closer; i.e., if we take few samples/cycle, the square waves get closer (Fig. 12-16).

ALIASING

We don't want to take too few samples/cycle; i.e., we don't want the sampling interval to be too wide because then the square waves will **overlap** and **aliasing** will result (Fig. 12-17).

Why is the Fourier transform of a continuous *sinc* function a single wave, whereas that of its sampled version shows repetitive square waves? (Fig. 12-18). The reason for this is *mathematical*. We will try to give an explanation that doesn't involve the complicated mathematics behind it.

To sample the signal, we have to multiply the signal by a sequence of spikes (each spike is called a "Delta" function). Each spike is separated from the next by the sampling interval (ΔTs) (Fig. 12-19).

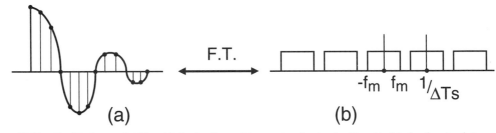

Figure 12-14. The FT of a sampled (discrete) sinc function contains a series of rectangles. The midpoint of each rectangle is a multiple of $1/\Delta Ts$.

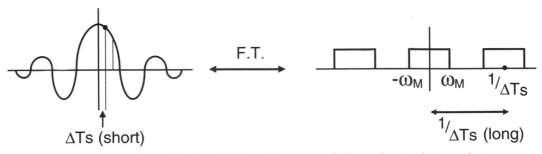

Figure 12-15. A short sampling interval ΔTs (i.e., taking more samples) causes the rectangles to spread out.

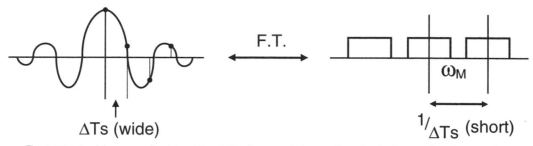

Figure 12-16. A longer sampling interval (i.e., taking fewer samples) causes the rectangles to move closer to one another.

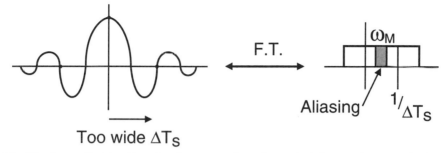

Figure 12-17. When the sampling interval is too long (i.e., not enough samples are taken), the rectangles may overlap (causing aliasing).

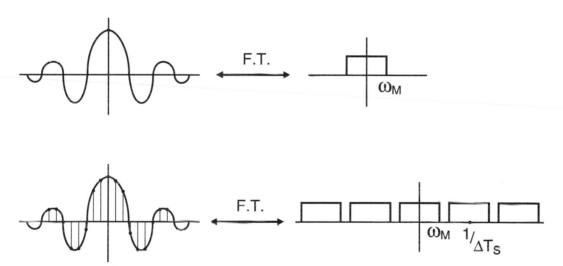

Figure 12-18. The FT of a sinc function is a rectangle, but that of its sampled variant is a series of rectangles.

Because the value of the series of spikes is zero everywhere between the spikes and is positive where the spikes are located, then multiplying the signal by the spikes will result in a value of 0 throughout the signal except where the spikes are located (Fig. 12-20).

Now, the Fourier transform of a series of spikes is also a series of spikes (Fig. 12-21). Whereas the spikes are separated by ΔTs, the Fourier transform of the spikes are in the frequency domain and are separated by 1/ΔTs (Fig. 12-21). The Fourier transform of the signal multiplied by the spikes is the Fourier transform of the signal "**convolved**" with the Fourier transfer of the spikes. (This has to do with a mathematical operation called "**convolution**"). Convolution basically means that we take the Fourier transform of the signal and center it around each spike (Fig. 12-22).

Eventually, we want to get back our original signal. If we take these repetitive Fourier trans-

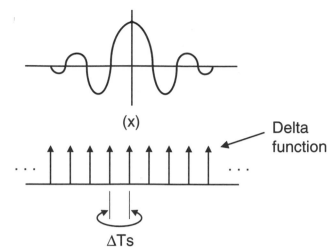

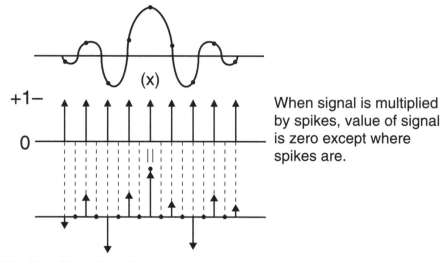

Figure 12-19. To sample a continuous, analog signal, a series of spikes (called Delta functions) is multiplied by the signal.

When signal is multiplied by spikes, value of signal is zero except where spikes are.

Figure 12-20. After multiplying the signal by a series of spikes, the result is zero except at the points of the spikes. The value of each resulting spike is equal to the value of the signal at that point.

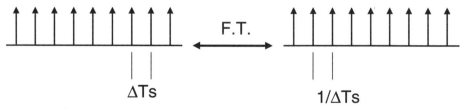

Figure 12-21. The FT of a series of spikes (separated by ΔTs) is also a series of spikes (separated by 1/ΔTs).

forms and pass them through a **low pass filter** (LPF) we will ultimately retrieve our original signal (Fig. 12-23). But remember, we really don't need to know the above mathematics to understand the principles of sampling.

Let's consider an easier signal: a *cosine* function $cos\omega_0 t$ and its Fourier transform (Fig. 12-24). The sampled version of this signal (with 4 samples/interval) is shown in Figure 12-25a with its Fourier transform in Figure 12-25b. Notice how the Fourier transform of this digi-

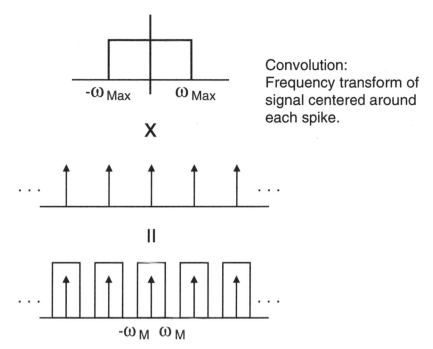

Convolution:
Frequency transform of
signal centered around
each spike.

Figure 12-22.   The FT of the product of a signal and a series of spikes is the FT of that signal (e.g., a rectangle) "convolved" with a series of spikes. The result is the FT of that signal replicated an infinite number of times.

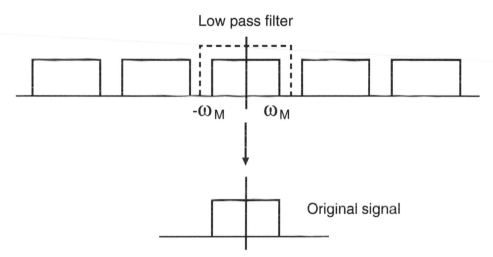

Figure 12-23.   When the previous FT is passed through a low pass filter, the result is the desired FT.

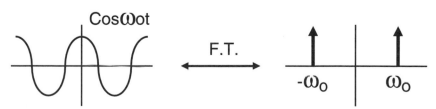

Figure 12-24.   FT of cos $\omega_0 t$.

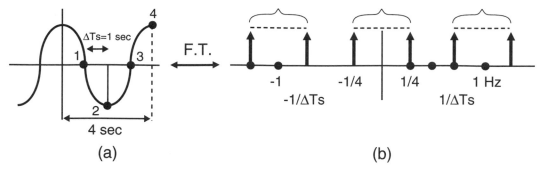

Figure 12-25. The FT of a sampled cosine signal.

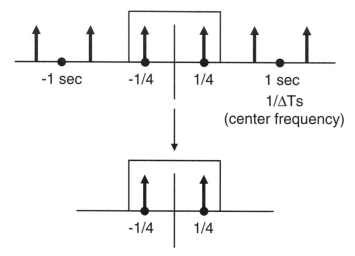

Figure 12-26. The previous FT passed through a LPF gives the FT of the original cosine function.

tized cosine function has multiple replicas. Briefly,

1. the cycle is 4 seconds long;
2. ΔTs is 1 second;
3. frequency = number of cycles/second = 1/4 cycle/second = 1/4 Hz;
4. $1/\Delta$Ts = 1/1 sec = 1 Hz.

On the Fourier transform (Fig. 12-25b), we have the center frequency 1/4 Hz corresponding to one replica, and the center frequency $1/\Delta$Ts (= 1 Hz) corresponding to the second replica. If we now pass this Fourier transform through a *low pass filter* (LPF) as in Figure 12-26 to eliminate all the high frequencies, we will recover our original pair of frequency spikes, which is the Fourier transform of the original *cosine* wave.

Visually, if we had the 4 sampling points in Figure 12-25a, we could still see quite easily what the original signal should look like (Fig. 12-27) by connecting the dots. It would be easier

if we had more samples because the more samples we use, the easier it is to see the shape of the original signal (Fig. 12-27b).

Let's now take another example in which we have fewer than 4 samples. Let's try two samples/cycle (Fig. 12-28a). In this case,

1. The period is still 4 seconds;
2. ΔTs = sampling interval is 2 seconds;
3. $1/\Delta$Ts = 1/2 = 0.5 Hz.

Let's see the Fourier transform of this example (Fig. 12-28b). Frequency is still 1/4. The sampling internal is now 2 seconds, so $1/\Delta$Ts = 1/2 Hz. We show two spikes on either side of 1/2 seconds, which is the frequency range around the center frequency of ½ second.

We see now that the pair of spikes centered at 1/2 Hz come right next to the original pair of spikes of 1/4 Hz. They practically overlap. If we pass this Fourier transform through a low pass filter to eliminate the higher frequencies, we still recover the two frequency spikes, which are the Fourier transformer of the original *cosine* signal; however, they will be increased in amplitude because of the overlap (Fig. 12-29).

Now let's see what happens if we take even fewer samples (Fig. 12-30a). Here,

1. the period is still 4 seconds;
2. but $\Delta Ts = 3$ seconds;
3. $1/\Delta Ts = 1/3$ Hz;
4. the frequency is still 1/4 cycles/second.

So, let's look at the Fourier transform (Fig. 12-30b). If we put this Fourier transform through a *low pass filter*, the spikes associated with the center frequency ($1/\Delta Ts$) will *interfere* with the original signal (Fig. 12-31). We will not only have the original spikes but we will have two extra spikes that are closer to the center. Now we have the *sum of two cosine waves* rather than the spikes of the single original *cosine* wave. We have the spikes of another *cosine* wave which are closer together, meaning that its transform is a *cosine* wave of *lower frequency*. This is called **aliasing**.

What we wanted to approximate by sampling

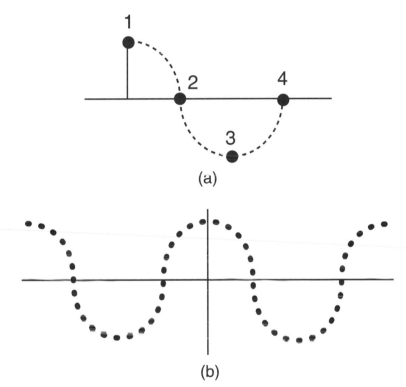

(a)

(b)

Figure 12-27. If enough samples are taken, the original signal can be visually reconstructed by connecting the dots. The more samples taken, the easier it is to visualize the original signal.

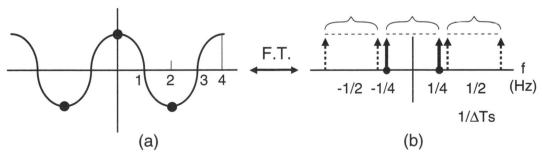

Figure 12-28. If exactly two samples are taken per cycle of a cosine function, the spikes will overlap exactly and the original signal is still decipherable.

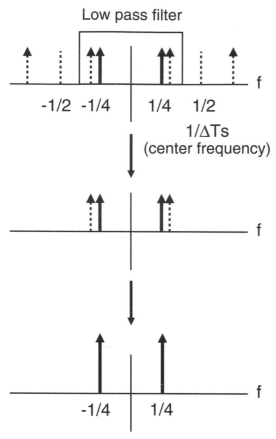

Figure 12-29.   An LPF applied to the previous FT allows recreation of the original signal (although the height of the spikes is doubled).

was the original signal, having a frequency of 1/4 Hz. But as a result of undersampling, we also obtain an undesired signal with a much lower frequency (Fig. 12-32).

Aliasing—An Analogy

As an analogy, let's consider a stage-coach wheel in a Western movie. Sometimes, it appears as if the wheel is turning in the reverse direction. Let's see how this happens. When we take a motion picture, we are actually taking *samples* in time. Let's take one point on the wheel and take a sample at time = 0 (Fig. 12-33). At a later time (t_1), we take another frame. The point rotates a certain distance forward as the wheel turns. When we watch this in a motion picture we see this point rotating in a *clockwise* direction.

Now let's see what happens when we **under-sample** (Fig. 12-34). Let's say the first frame

starts at the same point as before at t = 0. But on the next frame, we wait longer (t_2) to sample and don't sample until the point almost comes around to its original spot. We wait a similar time for the next sample and the point again comes around almost to the spot on the second frame. If we take a motion picture of this, the wheel will appear as if it's turning *counterclockwise*. This is because we are *undersampling*. This is an example of *aliasing*. The wheel is actually turning in a forward direction, but because of undersampling, it *appears* to be doing something else.

Undersampling causes aliasing.

Aliasing comes from the term **alias**: a *fake name*. We have a real frequency, but because of undersampling, we appear to have a *fake* frequency. In the previous example in which the *cosine* wave was undersampled, the real signal was a *cosine* wave with a frequency of 1/4 Hz, but the "alias" *cosine* wave had a *lower frequency* (Fig. 12-31). In the example of the wagon wheel, the real rotation was in a clockwise direction, but the alias was in a counterclockwise direction, probably with a slower rotation.

SAMPLING THEOREM (NYQUIST LAW)

Consider Figure 12-35. The sampling theorem states:

Nyquist Law: If ω_{max} is the maximum frequency in the signal, then the sampling rate must be at least twice the maximum signal frequency to avoid aliasing, i.e., $\omega_{sampling} = 1/\Delta Ts \geq 2 \, \omega_{max}$.

This is easy to see in the diagram (Fig. 12-35). We want the sampling rate to be at least equal to the sum of the maximum frequencies of adjacent boxes (to keep the boxes from overlapping). In other words, the sampling rate should be at least twice ω_{max}. In terms of sampling interval (ΔTs), it should be less than half of the period of the signal (remember that $\Delta Ts = 1/\omega_{max}$):

$$\Delta Ts < 1/2 \text{ (Period)}$$

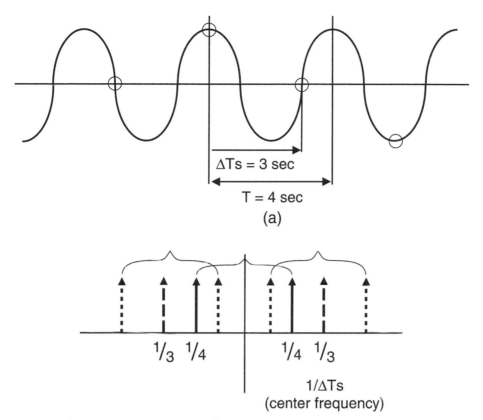

ΔTs = 3 sec

T = 4 sec

(a)

1/3 1/4   1/4 1/3

1/ΔTs
(center frequency)

Figure 12-30.   When too few samples are taken **(a)**, the spikes will get mixed up **(b)**.

Low pass filter

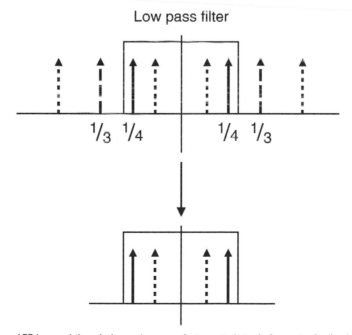

1/3 1/4   1/4 1/3

Figure 12-31.   When an LPF is passed through the previous example, two sets, instead of one set, of spikes is produced, which would yield a different signal than the original cosine function. This is called aliasing.

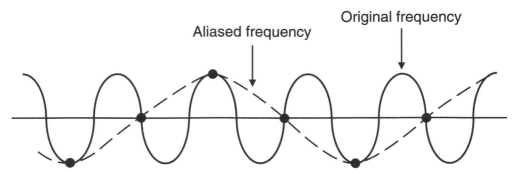

Figure 12-32.   When too few samples are taken, the perceived (aliased) frequency is different from the actual (original) frequency.

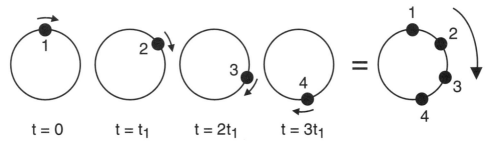

Figure 12-33.   Analogy of aliasing. If the motion picture frames of a stage-coach wheel are taken fast enough, the wheel appears to rotate correctly in the clockwise direction.

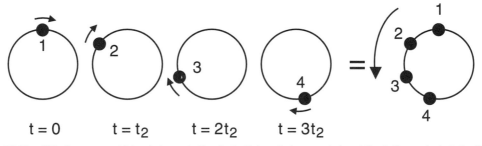

Figure 12-34.   If the frames are not taken fast enough, the wheel will deceptively appear to be rotating in the counterclockwise direction.

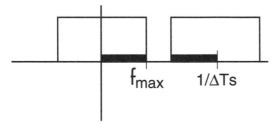

Figure 12-35. Nyquist Law: To avoid aliasing, the maximum frequency in the signal (f_{max}) should be less than half the sampling frequency ($1/\Delta Ts$). In other words, the sampling interval (ΔTs) should be at least twice the minimum period ($1/f_{max}$). That is, at least two samples per cycle (corresponding to the highest frequency in the signal) are required to avoid aliasing.

This is the **Nyquist Theorem**. Basically, it means that if we want to recover a signal from its samples, we need to take *at least two samples/cycle*. We can take as many samples as we like, but sampling takes time, so we want to *take the minimum number of samples necessary* to accurately recover the signal from its Fourier transform. We saw diagrammatically how, with a minimum of two samples per cycle, we could accurately approximate the original *cosine* signal (Fig. 12-36).

Nyquist Theorem Says:

The maximum frequency we can recover is one-half of the sampling rate.

$$\text{Max frequency} = 1/2 \ (\Delta Ts)$$

or

$$1/\Delta Ts = 2 \ (\text{Nyquist frequency})$$

Question: *What is the difference between sampling interval and sampling time?*
Answer: *Sampling internal (ΔTs) is the time between sampling points (Fig. 12-37). When we sample a signal, we can't possibly take an infinite number of samples. So we take (N) samples and then we stop. This gives the sampling time (Ts), the time it takes to sample the entire signal.*

$$Ts = N \times (\Delta Ts)$$

The sampling time (Ts) is the sampling interval (ΔTs) multiplied by the number of samples taken (N). The MR machine samples at a certain interval (say, about $\Delta Ts = 50 \ \mu s$). Let's say we have 256 frequency encoding steps (N = 256). Then, sampling time = $256 \times 50 \ \mu sec \cong 13$ msec.

Let's prove the following:

$$\text{Bandwidth} = 1/\text{sampling interval}$$
$$BW = 1/\Delta Ts$$

If the samples are close together, we get a higher bandwidth. If the samples are further apart, we get a lower bandwidth. Earlier, we were dealing with the bandwidth of an RF pulse. Now we are talking about the bandwidth of the received signal, i.e., the bandwidth of the echo. The Nyquist Theorem says that we should do a minimum of two samples per cycle to reconstruct the original signal. Is there any benefit in doing more samples/cycle?

The RF bandwidth is the **"transmission" bandwidth**. However, the bandwidth associated with the sampled signal is the **"receiver" bandwidth**. To prove the above relationship between BW and ΔTs, recall that frequency (which is

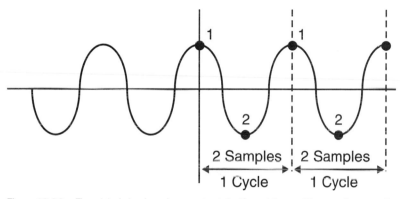

Figure 12-36. The original signal can be reconstructed with a minimum of two samples per cycle.

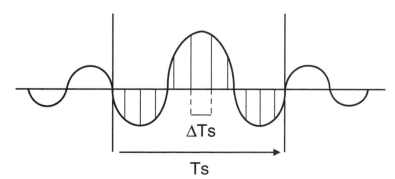

Figure 12-37. The sampling interval ΔTs is the time interval between two successive samples. The sampling interval Ts is the total sampling time, which is the product of ΔTs and the number of samples N, i.e., $Ts = N \cdot \Delta Ts$.

number of cycles/seconds) is the reciprocal of time (1/time):

ΔTs is the sampling interval
(in the time domain),
$1/\Delta Ts$ = frequency,

and if we're operating at the Nyquist frequency,

$1/\Delta Ts$ = frequency bandwidth (Fig. 12-38).

From the diagram, we see that if we operate at the Nyquist frequency, then the bandwidth is equal to 2 × (maximum frequency ω_{max}). Thus,

$$\text{Bandwidth} = 2(\omega_{max}) = 1/\Delta Ts$$

We generally do not want to take more than the minimum number of samples to recreate the signal because more samples requires more time. We want to operate as efficiently as possible, i.e., take as few samples as possible, without causing *aliasing*.

We can, under certain circumstances, take more samples than two samples per cycle. For example, when we activate the feature on the scanner to avoid wraparound along the frequency-encode direction, the scanner automatically performs **oversampling** to prevent aliasing. This is done to play it safe by doubling the number of samples taken.

DIGITIZED k-SPACE

We've already shown how we fill lines of the data space with our signal, with each line performed using a different phase encoding step. What we actually put into each line of the data space are the *sampled* data from each signal. Once we put these samples into each line of data space, then we complete the data space.

All MRI machines operate under the same principle when it comes to sampling the signal. A minimum of two samples/cycle is taken and put into the data space (Fig. 12-39a). If more than two samples/cycle are taken, then the bandwidth is wider, but it won't give us a better approximation of the signal (Fig. 12-39b). If we take less than two samples per cycle, the adjacent bandwidths may overlap and cause aliasing (Fig. 12-39c).

SIGNAL-TO-NOISE RATIO (SNR OR S/N)

When the bandwidth is narrowed, the SNR is increased. (This topic is discussed at length in a later chapter). SNR is inversely proportional to the square root of the bandwidth. SNR is also proportional to the volume of the pixel and to the square root of the number of phase encoding steps (Ny) and the number of excitations (NEX):

$$\text{SNR} \propto (\text{Pixel Volume}) \sqrt{\frac{\text{Ny.NEX}}{\text{BW}}}$$

Therefore, when we activate the feature on the scanner to lower the bandwidth on the second echo of a dual-echo T_2-weighted spin-echo image, we increase the SNR on the second echo. Remember that when we decrease the bandwidth, we are increasing the sampling interval (ΔTs). By increasing the sampling interval, we necessarily increase the sampling time (Ts) because Ts = N(ΔTs). We do this only on the second echo because the magnitude of the signal is always weaker on the second echo, so we want to increase the SNR on the second echo.

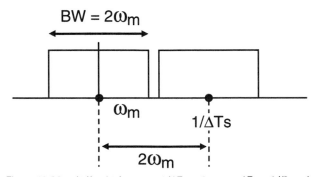

Figure 12-38.   At Nyquist frequency, $1/\Delta Ts = 2\ \omega_{max}$ or $\Delta Ts = 1/(2\ \omega_{max})$.

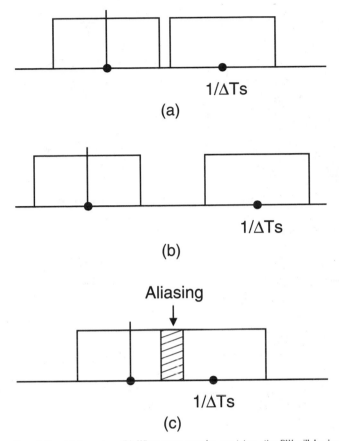

Figure 12-39. **(a)** Operating at Nyquist frequency. **(b)** When more samples are taken, the BW will be increased. **(c)** When too few samples are taken, aliasing may occur.

However, as we decrease the bandwidth to improve SNR, we are necessarily decreasing the number of samples per cycle; thus, we are increasing the possibility of aliasing. This is the reason behind why there is a limit on how much the bandwidth can be decreased. If we sample too fast, the bandwidth is wider and SNR goes down. If we sample too slowly, the bandwidth is narrow and we may get aliasing.

If we increase the sampling time (Ts), we then decrease the number of slices we can take per TR because of the following formula:

$$\text{number of slices} = \frac{TR}{TE + \tfrac{1}{2}Ts + To}.$$

$\downarrow BW \rightarrow \uparrow \Delta Ts$ *and* $\uparrow \Delta Ts \rightarrow \uparrow Ts$
since Ts = N (ΔTs).
Also $\downarrow BW \rightarrow \downarrow$ *#slices*
since $\uparrow Ts \rightarrow \downarrow$ *#slices.*

SAMPLING OF COMPOSITE SIGNALS

Let's discuss the sampling theorem in the case of a more complicated signal such as in Figure 12-40. When we have a *composite* signal (i.e., a signal composed of two or more frequencies), we need to take a minimum of two samples per cycle of the highest frequency present in the signal.

Presume that the complex signal above is a combination of three different *cosine* waves, each of a different frequency (Fig. 12-41). We have three different signals that are added up to give us a certain signal. The sampling theorem refers to the component of the signal that has the highest frequency. Therefore, we want to take two samples per cycle of the highest frequency component of the signal; this obviously means more than two samples per cycle for the other lower frequencies of the signal.

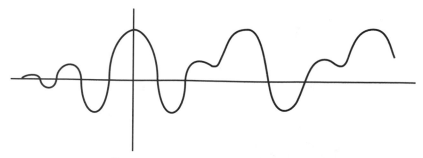

Figure 12-40.   An example of a composite signal.

2 Samples/cycle of highest frequency component of signal

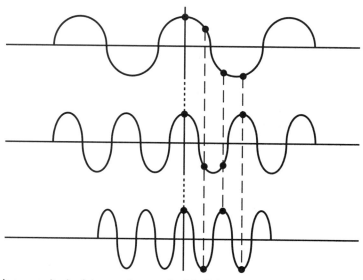

Figure 12-41.   In a composite signal, two samples per cycle of the highest frequency component is required to avoid aliasing.

We are taking samples of the composite signal. Therefore, even though we take a minimum of two samples per cycle of the highest frequency component of the signal, we will necessarily be taking more than two samples per cycle of all the lower frequency components of the signal.

Nyquist Sampling Theorem: A minimum of two samples/cycle (corresponding to the highest frequency present in the signal) are required to accurately reconstruct the original signal from its samples.

Example 1:
(a) At 1.5 Tesla, it typically takes 8 msec to perform one read-out: Ts = 8 msec.
(b) We have a matrix of, say, 256 × 256 pixels.

By convention, the first number refers to the number of frequency encoding steps. The second number refers to the number of phase-encoding steps. What is the bandwidth? We know that

$$BW = 1/\Delta Ts.$$

What is ΔTs?

$$\Delta Ts = \text{Sampling Time/Number of samples we test.}$$
$$= 8 \text{ msec/256 samples.}$$
$$BW = 1/\Delta Ts = 1/(8 \text{ msec/256})$$
$$= 256/8 \text{ msec} = 256/.008 \text{ sec}$$
$$= 32,000 \text{ Hz} = 32 \text{ kHz} = \pm 16 \text{ kHz}$$

This is a typical bandwidth for a typical read-out with 256 frequency encoding steps and a sampling time of 8 msec. Therefore, a frequency bandwidth of 32 kHz (±16 kHz) is a fairly typical frequency bandwidth that we deal with in routine imaging. This means that the bandwidth extends to $+16$ kHz on the right and -16 kHz on the left side of the center frequency.

EXAMPLE 2:
What would happen if we go to a 512 $\times$ 512 matrix, i.e., with 512 frequency encoding steps?

(a) We could either have a larger frequency bandwidth:

$$BW = \frac{1}{\Delta Ts} = \frac{1}{Ts/N}$$
$$= \frac{1}{.008 \text{ sec}/512}$$
$$= 512/.008 \text{ sec} = 64 \text{ kHz} = \pm 32 \text{ kHz}$$

(b) Or we could double the sampling time and keep the sampling interval (and the bandwidth) the same.

(We'll get into the relationship between the field of view and bandwidth later.)

Key Points

In this chapter, we have presented the basic concepts of signal processing, of which image processing is a subset. As mentioned in the introduction, the understanding of these concepts is crucial in understanding the intricacies of image optimization, which is one of the goals of every imagist. Again, memorizing the formulas is not as important as understanding the concepts behind them. Let's summarize:

1. ADC (Analog-to-Digital Conversion) is the process in which an analog (time-varying) signal is *encoded* to a digital signal (containing a series of binary numbers 0s and 1s) represented as *bytes* (8 *bits*) in the computer.

2. This is done by *sampling* the signal.

3. To be able to reconstruct the original signal from its discrete samples, the *Nyquist Law* must be satisfied. Otherwise, *aliasing* will occur.

4. The Nyquist Theorem states that the sampling frequency must be at least twice the highest frequency present in the signal.

5. Stated differently, if you take the waveform of the component signal with highest frequency (remember that each signal is a *composite* of many different signals with varying frequencies), then at least *two samples per cycle* are required to avoid aliasing.

6. Therefore, aliasing occurs because of *undersampling*. To assure that aliasing will not

happen, MR scanners may automatically perform *oversampling*.

7. The bandwidth (BW) is defined as the range of frequencies in the signal.

8. $BW = 1/\Delta Ts$, where ΔTs is the sampling interval (interval between two samples).

9. At Nyquist frequency, $BW = 2\,\omega_{max}$, where ω_{max} is the highest frequency in the signal, so that $\Delta Ts = 1/BW = 1/(2\,\omega_{max})$.

10. Total sampling time $Ts = Nx \cdot \Delta Ts$, where Nx is the number of frequency encodes.

11. SNR is given by

$$SNR \propto \text{volume} \cdot \sqrt{(Nx \cdot NEX/BW)}$$

12. So,

$$SNR \text{ is } \uparrow \text{ if BW } \downarrow$$

13. A narrower BW is used when a higher SNR is desired (e.g., on the second echo of a dual-echo SE image).

14. BW is $\downarrow$ if ΔTs is $\uparrow$ (i.e., less samples are taken), which may cause aliasing!

15. Now, if ΔTs is $\uparrow$ then $Ts = Nx \cdot \Delta Ts$ is $\uparrow$ which causes TE to $\uparrow$. Because

$$\text{\# slices} \cong TR/TE$$
then a narrower BW will reduce the *coverage*.

Questions

12-1. According to the Nyquist theorem, to avoid aliasing:
(a) At most, two samples per cycle corresponding to the highest frequency is required.
(b) At least two samples per cycle corresponding to the highest frequency is required.
(c) At most, two samples per cycle corresponding to the lowest frequency is required.
(d) At least two samples per cycle corresponding to the lowest frequency is required.

12-2. According to the Nyquist theorem, to avoid aliasing:
(a) The sampling frequency must be at least half the highest frequency in the signal.

(b) The sampling frequency must be at least twice the lowest frequency in the signal.
(c) The sampling frequency must be at least twice the highest frequency in the signal.
(d) The sampling frequency must be at least half the lowest frequency in the signal.

12-3. T/F Aliasing occurs because of oversampling.

12-4. T/F SNR is directly proportional to 1/BW

12-5. A narrower BW (all other things remaining unchanged) will result in:
(a) more SNR   (b) less coverage
(c) longer sampling time
(d) all of the above
(e) only (a) and (b)

13   Data Space

INTRODUCTION

Before we can understand k-space, we need to discuss the data space, which is a matrix of the processed image data. To most radiologists, k-space is in the twilight zone! We have already seen some of the basic concepts of the data space and k-space in the previous chapters. In this chapter, we will learn some of the properties of k-space in greater detail. The understanding of k-space is crucial to the understanding of some of the newer MRI fast scanning techniques, such as fast spin echo (FSE) and echo planar imaging (EPI).

WHERE DOES k-SPACE COME FROM?

k-space is derived from the data space, so it's really not as intimidating as it initially appears.

Figure 13-1 demonstrates a typical representation of the data space with a 256×256 matrix.

1. Figure 13-1 is an "**analog**" version of k-space. The true k-space, as we'll see later, is a **digitized** version of this figure, with axes referred to as "**spatial frequencies**."
2. In Figure 13-1, we have 256 phase encoding steps. We keep the zero-step (i.e., no phase-encoding) in the middle of k-space, so we go from -127 phase encode to $+128$ phase encode (bottom to top).
3. We also have 256 frequencies.
4. The y axis, then, is the phase encoding direction.
5. In the center, we put the signal acquired with no phase encoding gradient.

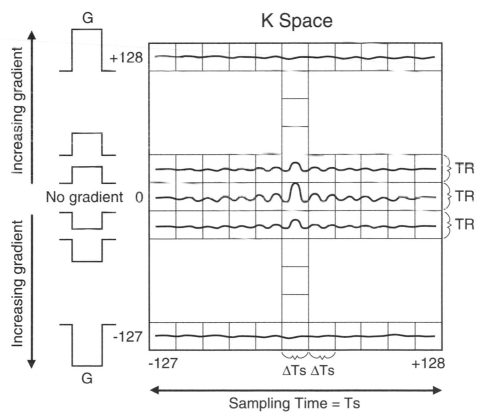

Figure 13-1. The Data space (with both axes as time variables) is an "analog" version of k-space.

6. As one advances on the y axis, each set has signal acquired with an increasing phase encoding gradient with maximum gradient at +128 phase encode step. Likewise, as one goes down from zero gradient in the y axis, each step has signal acquired with an increasing phase encoding gradient in the opposite direction with maximum gradient at −127 phase according step.

Let's now go back and review the spin echo pulse sequence (Fig. 13-2).

1. We apply the 90° pulse using an appropriate slice select gradient, Gz.
2. Next, we apply a 180° pulse and, after a time, TE receive an echo.
3. During this time, we apply the read-out gradient, Gy.
4. Then we place a *sampled version* of this echo in one of the rows in k-space. Let's say that this echo was obtained without using a phase encoding gradient in the y-direction. We *sample* the signal and then put it into the zero line in the data space.
5. With, say, a 256 × 256 matrix, we take 256 samples. Each of the 256 points in a row of the data space is a *sample* of the echo. (It's hard to draw discrete samples, so we'll draw continuous signals in the data space rows, realizing that each point in a row is a **digitized sample** of the signal).

6. For the second row in the data space, we do the exact same thing, except in this step the signal is obtained using a small phase encoding gradient in the y-axis.

Remember that the phase encoding gradient causes **dephasing** of the signal. Therefore, the signal for the second line of the data space will be similar in shape to the first signal (because both are signals from the same slice of tissue, just obtained at a different time) but smaller in **magnitude** than the first signal (because it undergoes additional dephasing due to phase-encoding gradient). Thus, when we draw this signal into the second line in the data space, we see that it is similar in shape to the first signal, but slightly *weaker*—because it's been *dephased*.

The signal that goes into the last line of the data space (+128) will be almost flat because it has undergone maximum dephasing; likewise, as we alternate to the signals placed below the zero-line (i.e., −1, −2 . . . −127), a certain symmetry results. For instance, line (−1) is similar in strength to line (+1) in that while line (+1) experiences mild dephasing due to slight increase in magnetic field strength, line (−1) experiences similar mild dephasing due to slight decrease in magnetic field strength. Likewise, the signal that goes into the first line in the data space (−127) will be almost flat due to maximum dephasing in the opposite direction of line (+128).

Remember that each line in the data space contains the signal obtained from the entire im-

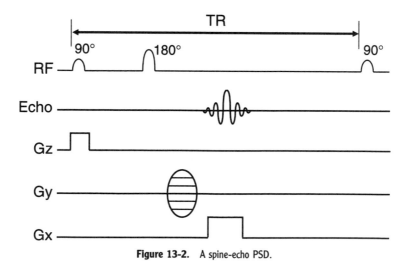

Figure 13-2. A spine-echo PSD.

age slice during a single TR. Each TR is obtained using a different phase encoding step in the y-axis.

Question 1: *How long does it take to go from one row in the data space to another?*
Answer: *It takes the time of one TR.*

Question 2: *How long does it take to go from one point (sample) in a row to the next point (sample) in the same row of the data space?*
Answer: *It takes the time spent between samples, i.e., the sampling interval (ΔTs).*

Question 3: *How long does it take to fill one row of the data space?*
Answer: *Let's say that $\Delta Ts \cong 50\ \mu sec$ and that there are 256 (N) samples along the readout axis. The sampling time is*

$$Ts = (\Delta Ts)(N)$$
$$\cong (50\ msec)(256)$$
$$= 8.12\ msec$$

Therefore, it takes about 8.12 milliseconds to fill one line of the data space. In general, it takes

$$Ts = Nx \cdot \Delta Ts$$

to fill one line of the data space.

Question 4: *How long does it take to fill one column of the data space?*
Answer: *It is the acquisition time $N_p \times TR$, where Np is the number of phase encoding steps.*

Let's say TR = 3000 msec and Np = 256.

Acquisition time = (3000 msec)(256)
= 12.5 minutes

If TR = 500 msec, then

Acquisition time = (500) (256) $\cong$ 2 minutes.

It takes several milliseconds to fill one row of the data space. But it takes several minutes to fill the columns of the data space.

MOTION ARTIFACTS

The preceding concept is one of the reasons why motion artifacts manifest themselves mainly in the phase encoding direction. In other words, it takes much longer to gather the signal in the phase encoding direction than in the frequency encoding direction, leaving more time for motion to affect the image in the phase direction. Another reason, as we shall see later, is that motion in any direction results in a phase change; thus, motion artifact propagates along the phase-encode direction.

PROPERTIES OF k-SPACE
Center of k-Space

The center of the data space contains maximum signal. This finding is caused by two factors:

1. Each of the signals has its maximum signal amplitude in the center column (Fig. 13-3). Recall that when we apply the 180° refocusing pulse, the dephased signal begins to rephase and reaches maximum amplitude when the protons are completely rephased. It then decreases in amplitude as the protons dephase once more.

   The middle column in the data space corresponds to the center of each individual echo, and the more peripheral columns refer to the more peripheral segments of the echoes: columns to the left of center depict rephasing of the echoes toward maximal amplitude in the data space; columns to the right of center depict dephasing of the echoes away from maximal amplitude in the data space.

   Therefore, as we go further out to the more peripheral columns, the signal weakens. The most peripheral points in the signal to the left is the weakest point of the signal as the signal just begins to rephase (Fig. 13-3). Likewise, the most peripheral point in the signal to the right is the weakest point after the signal has been refocused and then has regained maximum dephasing.

2. The maximum amplitude occurs in the center row because this line is obtained without additional dephasing due to phase encoding gradients; subsequent rows with progressively larger phase en-

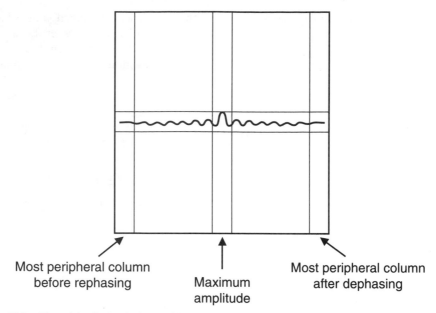

Most peripheral column
before rephasing

Maximum
amplitude

Most peripheral column
after dephasing

Figure 13-3. The peripheral points in the signal have the weakest amplitude; the center point has the maximal amplitude.

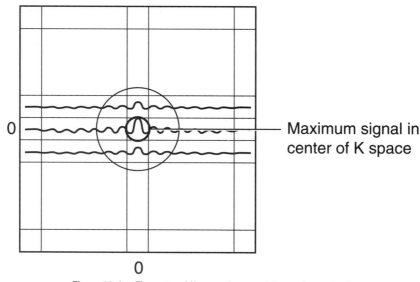

0

Maximum signal in
center of K space

0

Figure 13-4. The center of K space always contains maximum signal.

coding gradients have weaker signal amplitude.

Therefore, because the middle row has the strongest of all echoes and the middle column contains all the peaks of the echoes, the center point of the data space contains maximum amplitude, i.e., maximum signal-to-noise ratio (Fig. 13-4).

As we go farther out to the periphery in both directions, the signal weakens:

1. in the y direction because of progressively larger phase encoding steps;
2. in the x direction because the echo signal has either not yet reached maximum amplitude or is losing maximum aptitude due to dephasing.

Image of k-Space

Because of the *oscillating* nature of the signals, the image of the data space (and, thus, k-space) will appear as a series of concentric rings of signal intensity with alternating bands of high and low intensity as the signal oscillates from maximum to minimum, but an overall decrease in intensity as one goes from the center to periphery (Fig. 13-5a). So, the white and dark rings in k-space correspond to the peaks and valleys of the echoes, respectively. The original raw data (k-space) and the original image are shown in Figure 13-5.

Edges of k-Space

You might wonder that if the center of k-space contains the maximum signal, why not eliminate the periphery of the signal and just make an image from the central high signal intensity data (Figs. 13-4 and 13-6a)? We can actually make an image with this data, but the edges of the structures imaged will be very coarse (Fig. 13-6b). The periphery of k-space contributes to the

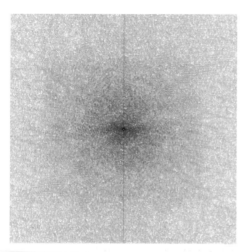

Orignal raw data
(a)

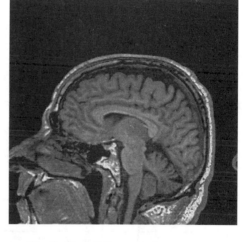

Original base image
(b)

Figure 13-5. **(a)** The original raw data (k-space) of **(b)** the original image (midline sagittal T_1- weighted image of the brain).

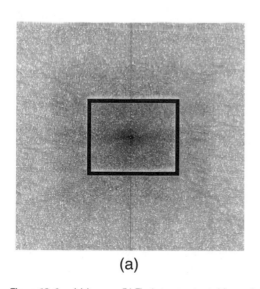

(a)

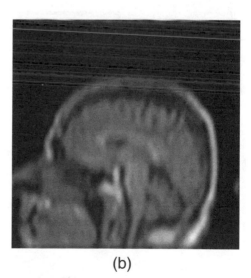

(b)

Figure 13-6. **(a)** k-space. **(b)** The image constructed from only the center of k-space. The details are reduced due to exclusion of peripheral points in k-space.

fine detail of the image. Let's see how this happens.

> **Question:**   *What type of information is available in the periphery of k-space?*
> **Answer:**   *The periphery of k-space provides information regarding "fineness" of the image and clarity at sharp interfaces.*

Recall the following Fourier transforms of a *sinc* wave and its truncated version from an earlier chapter (Fig. 13-7). As you can see, by truncating the signal (echo), ring artifacts are introduced in the Fourier transform. Therefore, by eliminating the samples in the periphery of the data space, the sharp interfaces in the image are degraded and the image gets coarser. In other words, the *fine detail* of the image is compromised when the edges of k-space are excluded. Figure 13-8b is the image corresponding to the periphery of k-space (Fig. 13-8a).

Image Construction

We can take a single line in k-space and make a whole image. It wouldn't be a very pretty image, but it would still contain all the information necessary to construct an image of the slice.

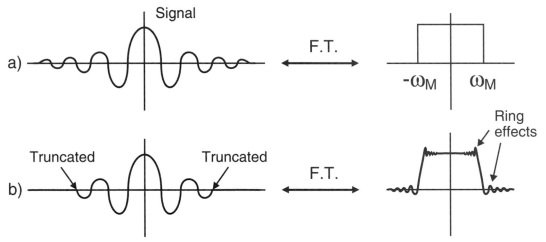

Figure 13-7.   **(a)** The FT of an ideal sinc function is a rectangle. **(b)** The FT of a truncated sinc function has ring down effects.

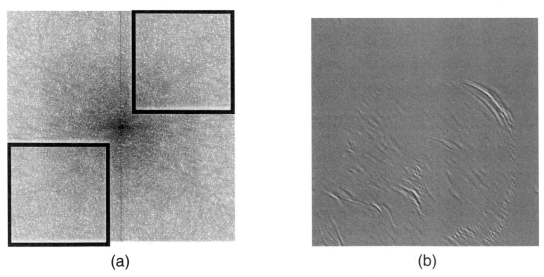

(a)   (b)

Figure 13-8.   **(a)** k-space. **(b)** The image constructed from only the periphery of k-space. This image has minimal signal but contains details about the interfaces in the original image.

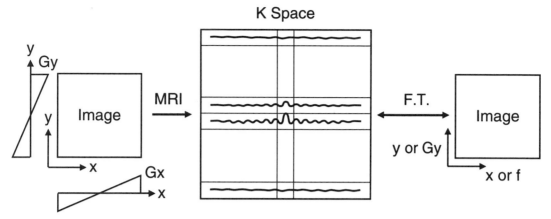

Figure 13-9. There is a one-to-one relationship between frequency and position along x axis and between phase-encode gradient increment and position along y direction.

There is absolutely no direct relationship between the center of k-space and the center of the image. Likewise, there is no direct relationship between the edges of k-space and the edges of the image.

A point at the very edge of k-space contributes to the entire image. It doesn't contribute as much to the image in terms of signal-to-noise as does a point in the center of k-space because the center of k-space has maximum signal, but the peripheral points still contribute to the clarity and fineness of the image.

Once we have all the data in k-space, we take the Fourier transform of k-space to get the image.

Question: *Why is the Fourier transform of k-space the desired image?*
Answer: *Because there is a one-to-one relationship between frequency and position in the x direction and between phase-encoding gradient strength[a] and position in the y direction.*

Question: *Why is there a one-to-one relationship between frequency and position?*
Answer: *Because, in our method of spatial encoding, we picked a linear gradient in the x direction that correlated sequential frequency increments with position; likewise, we picked a*

linear gradient in the y direction that correlated sequential phase gradient increments with position in the y direction (Fig. 13-9).

Thus, the center of the field of view of the image experiences no frequency gradient and no phase gradient, and the points in the periphery of the image experience the highest frequency and phase gradients. In other words, there is a $1:1$ relationship between frequency and position in the image.

In summary, the frequency and phase encoding gradients provide the position of a signal in space. They tell us which pixels each component of the signal goes into in the slice under study.

Question: *How are the shades of gray determined?*
Answer: *The shades of gray are determined by the **magnitude** or **amplitude** of the signal (actually its Fourier transform) at each pixel.*

Recall that the image of k-space looks like a series of concentric circles of alternating intensity on a two-dimensional surface. If we now incorporate *amplitude* as a third dimension, we would have the areas of greater amplitude coming off the surface of k-space towards us like a "warped" image (Fig. 13-10).

k-Space Symmetry

One step needs to be completed after receiving the signal and before placing it in k-space

---

[a] The one-to-oneness in the y direction is related to the phase-encoding gradient strength—and not just the phase. This is because the rows in the Data Space are differentiated by different phase-encoding gradient strengths Gy.

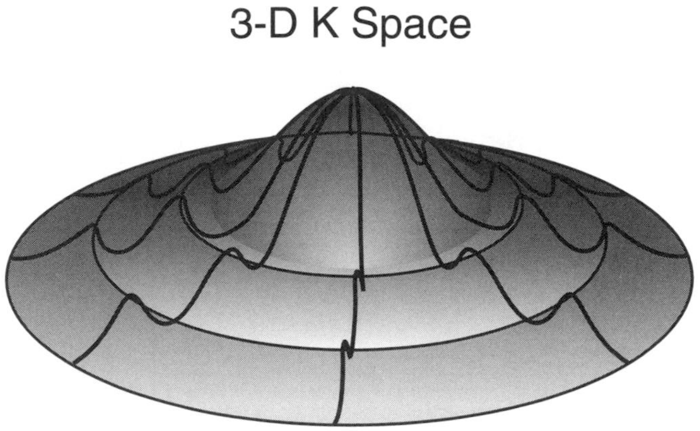

3-D K Space

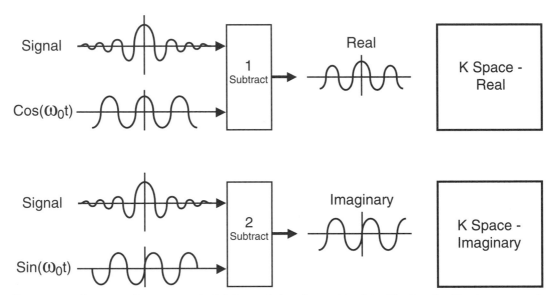

Figure 13-10. A three-dimensional line drawing of k-space.

Figure 13-11. The process of image construction includes a preliminary decomposition of signal into its real and imaginary components. This in turn yields a real and an imaginary k-space, i.e., a real and an imaginary image.

that we have so far ignored. This step is called **Phase-Sensitive Detection**. We want to take the echo signal, which is on a **carrier frequency**, shift it to zero frequency, and divide the signal into its real (*cosine*) and imaginary (*sine*) components.

First, we start off with the signal that is being frequency- and phase-shifted around a carrier frequency of 64 MHz for a 1.5T magnet. However, it's hard to tell if a signal has been frequency- or phase-shifted unless we "ground" the signal back to "zero."

Therefore, we first subtract the carrier frequency of 64 MHz from the signal (Fig. 13-11). We first take the signal and subtract a *cosine*

wave of center frequency ω_0 from the signal. Then we take the signal and, in a separate computation, subtract the *sine* wave of center frequency ω_0 from the signal.

If we subtract ω_0 from the signal, we center the signal at zero (in the frequency domain). We then have a resultant signal whose center frequency is 0. Perform this step twice to separate the signal into its real component (*cosine*) and its imaginary component (*sine*).

Each data space has two components:

1. The data space with "real" (*cosine*) data: the signal that has (cos ω_0t) subtracted from it and brought back to 0 frequency.

2. The data space with "imaginary" (*sine*) data: the signal that has (*sin* ω_0t) subtracted from it and brought back to 0 frequency.

We now have two data spaces (Fig. 13-12): one with *cosine* data (real); one with *sine* data (imaginary). Both have data centered at 0 frequency . In the data space with *cosine* data, we know that a great deal of symmetry exists. A cosine function is an example of an **even** function. If we look at a *cosine* function, we see that there is symmetry to the right and left of zero. In addition, there is symmetry above and below zero. Thus, if we put a pixel in a line of the data space to the right of the 0 column, and above the 0 line (point *a*), the symmetry of the *cosine* function would make us unable to discriminate between the other (*a*) positions. The computer couldn't tell the difference between any of the four pixel positions. This is why we use the *sine* version of the data space.

Now look at the data space with the *sine* data (Fig. 13-12b). Again, the pixel is in the same place as the *cosine* data space; it is in a line of the data space above the 0 line and to the right of the 0 column. However, (unlike the *cosine* data space) here we can distinguish it from the pixel below the 0 line ($-b$). We can also differentiate it from the pixel to the left of the 0 column ($-b$).

Why are these pixels different in the *sine* data space? Let's review the *sine* function ($sin\omega_0$t) of the two pixels to the right of the 0 frequency (Fig. 13-13a). The *sine* function is an example of an **odd** function because of its inherent antisymmetry. The *sine* function changes polarity above and below the 0 line. This allows us to differentiate the two pixels.

Now, let's examine the *sine* function ($sin\omega_0$t) above the zero line of the data space (Fig. 13-13b). Again, because of inherent antisymmetry of the *sine* function on either side of the 0 frequency, the pixels will have opposite polarity.

COMPLEX NUMBERS

We said in Chapter 1 that a complex number can be divided into its real (*cosine*) and imaginary (*sine*) parts. If we consider the (*cosine*) function as the real component and the (*sine*) function as the imaginary component, then we can add the (*sine*) and (*cosine*) together to get the **magnitude** of the signal as well as its **direction**.

So now let's add up the data of the 4 pixels (Fig. 13-14). Because of the changing polarity of the *sine* function, when we add the *sine* function to the *cosine* function, we can distinguish the *direction* of the four pixels (whereas with *cosine* function alone, we couldn't tell the direction).

Spatial direction of K space Information:

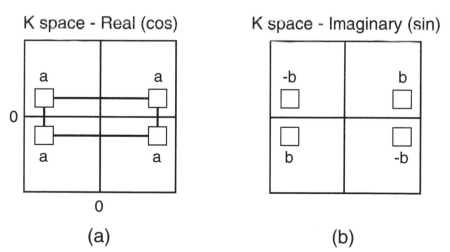

Figure 13-12. Spatial direction in k-space. The imaginary k-space provides a sense of left-right or up-down direction.

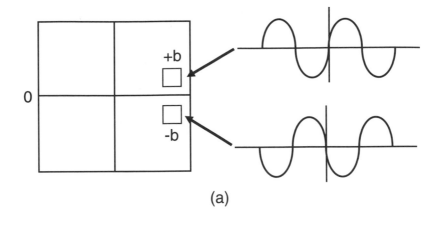

(a)

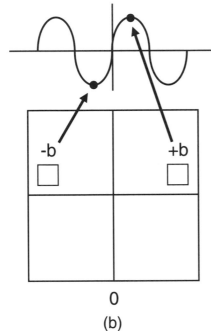

0

(b)

Figure 13-13. **(a)** Because the phase gradients corresponding to the top and bottom half of k-space generally have opposite polarities, the values in the corresponding imaginary k-space also will have opposite polarities. **(b)** Because the sine function is an odd function, the left half of the signal is the reverse of the right half, thus the corresponding points in the imaginary k-space also will have opposite signs.

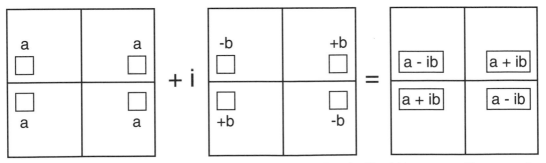

Figure 13-14. K-space conjugate (Hermitian) symmetry can be seen by adding the real and imaginary components of four corresponding data points. Notice the conjugate symmetry between left and right and between top and bottom.

In the lines above 0 phase encoding:

pixel $a - ib$ is to the left of the 0 frequency.
pixel $a + ib$ is to the right of the 0 frequency.

In the lines below 0 phase encoding:

pixel $a + ib$ is to the left of the 0 frequency.
pixel $a - ib$ is to the right of the 0 frequency.

Conjugate (Hermitian) Symmetry

The **conjugate** of a complex number $a + ib$ is the complex number $a - ib$ (i.e., with the same real component but a negative imaginary component). From this and from Figure 13-14 it is clear that **k-space possesses conjugate symmetry**, also known as **Hermitian symmetry.**

Half NEX (½ NEX)

In a "**½ NEX**[b]" technique (half-Fourier in phase), we acquire the data from the upper half of k-space and construct the lower part mathematically (Fig. 13-15), thus reducing the scan time. The trade-off is a reduced signal to-noise ratio (SNR) by a factor of $\sqrt{2}$, to be exact (see Chapter 17). Due to the presence of phase errors in the data, the symmetry previously discussed may not be perfect. This is why when employing such techniques, a few extra rows in the center of k-space—which contains maximum signal—are always added to allow for such phase corrections. That is, slightly more than 50% of k-space must be sampled to maintain phase information.

Fractional Echo

In "**fractional echo**," only the right half of the echo is sampled and the left half is constructed based on the right half (Fig. 13-16). (This allows TE to be shorter for fast scanning techniques like turbo FLASH and Fast SPGR—see Chapter 21.)

1/4 NEX

Because of the *conjugate symmetry* discussed previously, *theoretically* you should be able to create an image using only one *quadrant* of the combined real and imaginary data spaces (Fig. 13-17). That is, you should be able to construct

---

[b] ½ NEX is a misnomer because we are really halving the number of phase-encode steps—not the NEX.

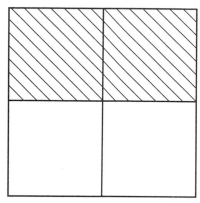

Figure 13-15.   In Half (or fractional) NEX, only half (or a fraction of) the rows in K space (plus a few extra central rows) are used, and the rest is constructed by symmetry.

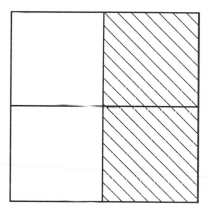

Figure 13-16.   In fractional echo, only a fraction of the echo is sampled.

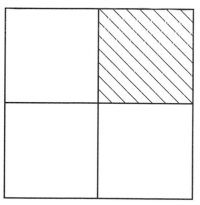

Figure 13-17.   Due to conjugate symmetry of k-space, *theoretically* you should be able to reconstruct the entire k-space from just one of its quadrants. In reality, however, this may create excessive phase errors due to actual imperfections in data symmetry.

the entire k-space data from only one quadrant. In reality, however, due to the presence of data acquisition errors, perfect symmetry does not exist and doing so may lead to phase errors and image distortion, which is probably why this technique is not being used.

Real and Imaginary Images

We discussed two components of the data space; namely, the real and imaginary components. Their respective Fourier transforms provide the real and imaginary components of the image (Fig. 13-18).

Magnitude (Modulus) and Phase Image

Recall that given a complex number $c = a + ib$, with a being the real and b the imaginary component, the phase (angle) is given by $tan\ \theta = b/a$ and the magnitude by $\sqrt{(a^2 + b^2)}$. This concept can be applied to the real and imaginary components of the image (Fig. 13-18) to generate the **magnitude and phase images** (Fig. 13-19).

The **magnitude image (modulus)** is what we deal with most of the time in MR imaging. The **phase image** is used in cases in which the *direction* is important. An example is phase contrast MR angiography, in which the phase indicates the direction of flow, i.e., up versus down, anterior versus posterior, or left versus right. In summary,

tangent (Phase angle) = (Imaginary/Real), or phase angle = arctan (Imaginary/Real), and modulus = $\sqrt{(\text{real})^2 + (\text{imaginary})^2}$

In actuality, when we do ½ NEX, we sample half of the phase encoding steps plus a few lines above or below the 0 line. We can then compensate for phase errors and determine the actual phase. This is referred to as **overscanning**.

Ideally, we want to have a *real* image with the *imaginary* part being *zero*, and thus a zero phase. In reality, however, we have all sorts of motion artifacts and gradient errors that create phase artifacts. Therefore, in reality, phase is never zero. Sometimes, when service engineers try to debug a system, they will sometimes look at the phase image to figure out the problem.

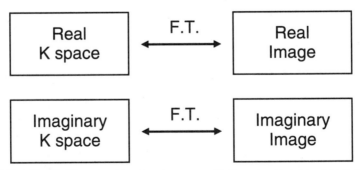

Figure 13-18.   The FT of the real and imaginary k-spaces provide the real and imaginary images, respectively.

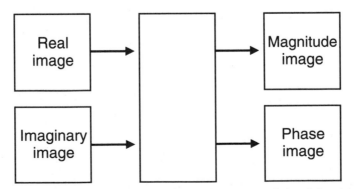

Figure 13-19.   The real and imaginary images **(a)** are used to create magnitude and phase images **(b)**.

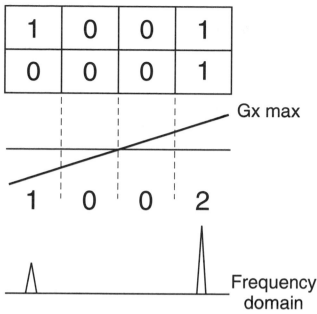

Figure 13-20. An example of a 2 × 4 matrix exposed to a frequency gradient and no phase gradient.

We too can look at the phase image. In flow imaging, the phase image is a *velocity image* and indicates magnitude and direction. For example, in imaging the CSF flow through the aqueduct, flow in the *antegrade* direction could be *black*, and flow in the *retrograde* direction could be *white* on the phase images. Thus, phase images in phase-contrast studies display the *direction* of flow.

Because the phase is never zero, we can combine the "real" image and the "imaginary" image to get a composite image, which is the image that we look at when we read an MR study. The **modulus** is the image we look at; it combines the data corresponding to the Fourier transform of the real and imaginary data spaces:

Image = Modulus
$$= \sqrt{(\text{Real Image})^2 + (\text{Imaginary Image})^2}$$

k-Space: An Example

The following is an example of a 2 × 4 matrix:

1	0	0	1
0	0	0	1

The number of frequency encoding steps = N_x = 4.

The number of phase encoding steps = N_y = 2.

We will give magnitudes of either 1 or 0 to each pixel, so that:

A pixel with a magnitude = 1 will be White.
A pixel with a magnitude = 0 will be Black.

In the first phase encoding step, with no gradient in the y direction, we apply a frequency encoding gradient in the x direction, which allows us to distinguish the rows. What we get then is a sum of pixels in each column, without knowing from which row the components of the sum originated (Fig. 13-20).

Remember that the Fourier transform can differentiate between different columns because each column has a different frequency. The Fourier transform of the signal will have two frequency spikes, with column 1 having an amplitude of 1 + 0 = 1, and column 4 having an amplitude of 1 + 1 = 2. Thus, applying the readout gradient allows us to differentiate between different columns. However, we still haven't differentiated between different rows. For instance, the amplitude = 2 in column 4 could be:

1 + 1 or 0 + 2 or 2 + 0

With the single phase encoding step, we have no idea how the sum of the amplitudes is decomposed to provide the amplitude of individual elements in each column. Remember that this first set of data was obtained with no gradient in the phase encoding (y) direction.

The first phase encoding step was at zero value of the phase-encode gradient. For the next phase encoding step, let's apply a gradient. The gradient will be 360° divided by 2, or 180°. This means that the first row will experience no gradient, and the second row will experience a gradient such that the spins will be 180° out of phase with the first row. This will result in no change in the numbers of the first row. But the numbers in the second row will be 180° phase shifted (i.e., they will be the negative of the original numbers).

1	0	0	1
0	0	0	-1

If we use the clock analogy to evaluate phase shift, the spins in the top row, experiencing no phase shift, will all point upward. The spins in the second row (which is experiencing a 180° phase shift) will all be pointing downward (Fig. 13-21).

Thus, whereas the values in the first row will remain unchanged, the values in the second row will be 180° reversed from what they were with no phase shift.

Row 1

1	0	0	1

Row 2 before 180° phase shift

0	0	0	1

Row 2 after 180° phase shift

0	0	0	-1

ASIDE: If we were to have four rows with four phase encoding steps, the steps would be: 0, 90°, 180° and 270° phase difference between rows, experiencing a steeper gradient with every successive TR (Fig. 13-22). In our study, with only two rows, we can only have two phase encoding steps:

1. zero phase difference (no gradient) between rows.
2. 180° phase difference, where one row experiences no phase difference and the second row experiences a 180° phase shift from the first row.

This division of phase encoding steps into equal divisions of 360° all relates to the cosine wave (Fig. 13-23). Therefore, for a phase difference of 180°, we get the negative value of the original number because $\cos 180° = -1$. For a different phase angle, we would get a fraction of the original value (from 0 to 1, or from 0 to -1, whatever $\cos \theta$ is).

With this phase-encoding step, let's see what the Fourier transform would be in the frequency-encoding direction (Fig. 13-24). The amplitude in columns 1, 2 and 3 remain unchanged from the 0 phase readings. However, there is a change in the amplitude of column 4.

With zero phase, column 4 adds up
to +2 (because $1 + 1 = 2$)
With 180° phase, column 4 adds up
to 0 (because $1 - 1 = 0$)

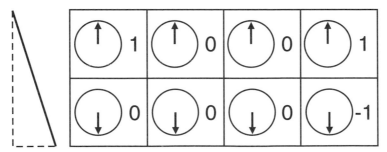

Figure 13-21. The same example exposed to phase encoding. The first row has no phase shift. The second row has a 180° phase shift (thus changing the sign of the pixel values).

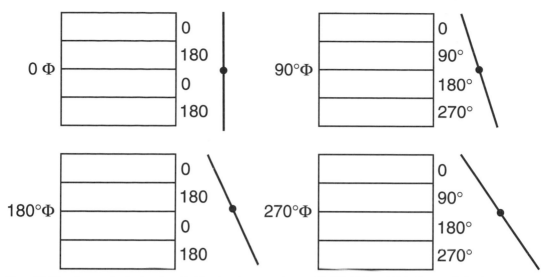

Figure 13-22. An example of a 4 × 4 matrix. The phase increments here are 0°, 90°, 180°, and 270°. (In general, the phase increment is 360°/Ny, where Ny is the number of phase-encode steps.)

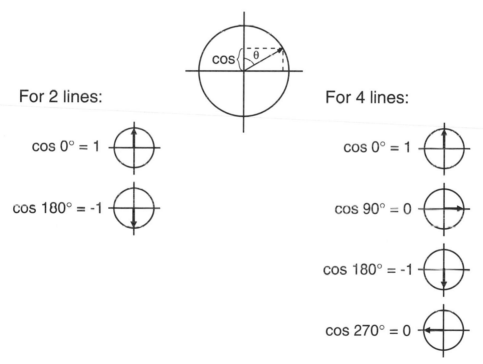

Figure 13-23. The effect of phase shifts on pixel values for two and for four rows.

With the change in phase, the second column is the sum of (+1) and (−1), which is equal to 0. We still don't know what the original value of each pixel was, but we do have a different total value in the Fourier transform of this second line in k-space when we compare it to the first line.

Now, let's do a little mathematics. The following is like solving two equations with two unknowns; solve for a, b, c, and d below:

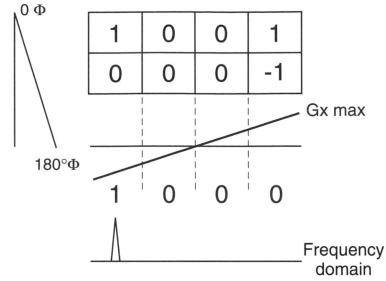

Figure 13-24.   The previous 2 × 4 example now exposed to a frequency gradient and a phase gradient (i.e., 180° phase shift).

1	0	0	1
0	0	0	1

0° phase

1	0	0	1
0	0	0	−1

180° phase

a	0	0	c
b	0	0	d

a	0	0	c
−b	0	0	−d

Let's look back at the pixel values in the phase = 0 line and:

1. designate the pixels in the first column (a and b)
2. designate the pixels in the fourth column (c and d)

Now look at the pixel values in the 180° phase line, and:

1. designate the pixels in the first column (a and −b)

   Note that pixel (a) remains the same as 0 phase line because neither experiences any phase change but pixel (−b) is negative because it experiences a 180° phase shift compared to pixel (b) in 0 phase line.
2. designate the pixels in column four as (c and −d)

Again note that pixel (c) remains the same as 0 phase line because neither experiences any phase change. However, pixel (−d) is negative because it experiences a 180° phase shift compared with pixel (d) in phase = 0 line.

first equations:

$$a + b = 1$$
$$a - b = 1$$

add $\overline{2a = 2}$

$$a = 1$$
$$b = 0$$

second equations:

$$c + d = 2$$
$$c - d = 0$$

add $\overline{2c = 2}$

$$c = 1$$
$$d = 1$$

By using the Fourier transforms of the two lines in k-space, we can determine the amplitude values of each pixel in each column. This is the concept of the **(digital) Fourier transform (DFT)**.

What is k-space in this example? Let's go back to Figure 13-20. The first line in the data space corresponds to the sum of all the signals obtained with 0 phase. With the gradient in the x-direction (Gx) causing different phase angles between the columns, the signal will consist of:

1. (cos of column 1 frequency) with (magnitude = 1), e.g., 1 cos t
2. (cos of column 4 frequency) with (magnitude = 2), e.g., 2 cos 4t

The sum of these signals will be the signal in the first line of the data space (in this case, $\cos t + 2 \cos 4t$) in time domain. Then the signal is sampled (four times in our example).

The second time around, the second line in the data space corresponding to the 180° phase shift will give us:

1. (cos of column 1 frequency) with (magnitude = 1), e.g., 1 cost
2. (cos of column 4 frequency) with (magnitude = 0), e.g., 0 cos 4t which is 0

Thus, we get a different signal in the time domain for the second line in the data space. Then this signal is sampled. Remember that no direct relationship exists between a point in the data space and the same point on the image.

The Fourier transform of the data space contains the four frequencies corresponding to the four samples taken during signal readout using the Gx gradient for frequency encoding. The *magnitude* (amplitude) of the frequencies correlates with the *brightness* on the image. In the x direction, a 1:1 relationship exists between frequency and position on the image. The amplitude at a certain frequency corresponds to the brightness at the corresponding pixel position. In the y direction, a 1:1 relationship exists between the position y and the *phase increment* $\Delta\phi$ (which is related to the gradient strength Gy).

To create the image, we perform a second Fourier transform on the data space. This step is just an additional mathematical step.

Question: How many calculations are necessary to solve the set of equations derived from k-space to create the image (i.e., the number of calculations to solve the DFT)?

Answer: In our example of two rows of k-space with four samples in each row, we had two equations per sample and four samples. So:

$$2 \times 4 = number\ of\ calculations$$

In general, with an $N \times N$ matrix, the number of calculations $= N \times N = N^2$.

EXAMPLE:
In a 256 × 256 matrix:

$$256^2 = 2^{16}\ calculations\ needed\ for\ DFT$$

FAST FOURIER TRANSFORM (FFT)

Fast Fourier Transform (FFT) is a signal processing transformation, similar to Fourier transform, that solves a DFT in a faster way. The number of calculations for FFT is:

$$Number\ of\ calculations = (N)(\log_2 N)$$

EXAMPLE:
For a 256 × 256 matrix:

$$256 \times \log_2 256 = (256)(8)$$

Because 8 is 1/32 of 256, we have cut down the number of calculations by a factor of 32. For $(\log_2 N)$ to be a whole number, the number of frequency encoding steps has to be a power of 2. This is why *frequency* encoding steps are always a power of 2 (i.e., 2^N such as 2, 4, 8, 16, 32, 64, 128, 256, 512), usually 128, 256, or 512, whenever FFT is used.

Key Points

We have introduced the often intimidating topic of k-space. k-space can initially be thought of as the "data space" (which can be thought of as an "analog" k-space), with each line in it representing a sampled version of the received signal (the echo). In the Data space, the coordinates are in time (horizontal scale is on the order of the sampling interval and the vertical scale is on the order of TR). The Fourier transform of k-space is the desired image. There is, however, one more step that comes after obtaining the data space and before construction of the true k-space, having to do with the concept of "spatial frequencies," which we shall discuss in a later chapter (Chapter 16).

Questions

13-1. T/F   Each row of Data space contains one of the received signals (echoes).

13-2. T/F   Each row of Data space corresponds to one frequency encode gradient strength.

13-3. T/F   The number of rows in the Data space equals the number of phase encode steps.

13-4. T/F   The center of Data space contains maximum signal.

13-5. T/F   The axes of the Data space are in the frequency domain.

13-6. T/F   The center of the Data space is directly related to the center of the image.

13-7. T/F   The right half of the Data (or k) space is the mirror image of the left half.

14 Pulse Sequence Diagram

"A pulse sequence diagram is to an MR scientist as sheet music is to a musician."

INTRODUCTION

A pulse sequence diagram (PSD) illustrates the sequence of events that occur during MR imaging. It is a timing diagram showing the RF pulses, gradients, and echoes. Having a good knowledge of the PSD will help the reader follow complicated pulse sequences (PS) with more ease and understand the interplay among various scan parameters.

PSD OF A SE SEQUENCE

Having been exposed to the concept of gradients, we are now able to illustrate a complete

pulse sequence diagram for, say, a spin-echo (SE) sequence (Fig. 14-1). Everything in the figure looks like what we have discussed before except for a few adjustments in:

1. slice-select gradient (Gz)
2. frequency-encoding gradient (Gx)

1a. Once the slice-select gradient (Gz) is applied, then a gradient in the negative direction is introduced in order to *refocus* the spins (Fig. 14-2). Basically, every time we apply a gradient, we dephase the spins. In the case of the Gz gradient, we dephase the spins in order to select a slice. But after

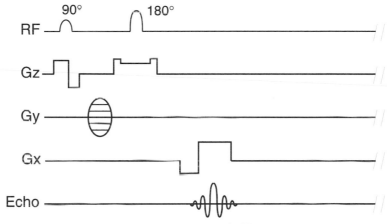

Figure 14-1. A spin-echo PSD.

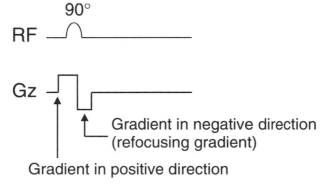

Gradient in negative direction (refocusing gradient)

Gradient in positive direction

Figure 14-2. The slice select gradient Gz is followed by a negative lobe to refocus the spins.

the slice is selected, we need to reverse the effect. The purpose of the *refocusing* gradient is to rephase the spins in the slice-select direction. (Alternatively, we can defocus the spins *prior* to slice selection so that they come back into phase with the *second* gradient pulse.)

1b. When the 180° pulse is applied, a slice-select gradient may or may not be applied. This is *optional* and depends on whether a single slice or multiple slices are being acquired. But before and after the 180° pulse, we apply a so-called "**crusher**" gradient so that the 180° pulse has a tri-lobed shape (Fig. 14-3). This is just a triviality. When the 180° pulse is applied, it may not be exactly 180°. It may not refocus everything at time TE as we would expect. So these "crusher" gradients are applied to *offset* that error. (The first lobe is used to balance the third; the second is slice selective; the third destroys the FID.)

2. There is an important adjustment in the read-out gradient (Gx). If we just apply a gradient while we're reading out the echo, we end up dephasing everything (Fig. 14-4). By the time we get to the middle of the signal, the signal intensity will be decreased because of the dephasing caused by the gradient, and by the time we get to the end of the signal,

there will be maximum dephasing and so much signal loss that there may not be any signal to read!

So we apply a gradient in the negative direction that has an area equal to 1/2 of that of the readout gradient (Fig. 14-5). The length of the read out gradient is the sampling time (Ts). For *stationary spins*, application of a gradient will make the spins go faster and faster and, as they go faster, they'll get out of phase. With the negative gradient, the stationary spins will have a maximum phase difference at the end of the negative gradient. As the gradient is reversed and a gradient in the positive direction is applied, the spins will *rephase* once again. This occurs right at the mid point of the read- out, i.e. at time TE. Subsequently, they'll go out of phase again. We can see that at time TE everything is refocused (Fig. 14-5).

If we didn't have the negative gradient lobe, the spins would begin to dephase when the gradient is turned on, and at time TE there would be an undesirable *phase difference*. Phase difference means a smaller signal (Fig. 14-6).

Sometimes, we'll see the notation for the extra Gx gradient illustrated differently (Fig. 14-7). It will be shown as a positive gradient rather than a negative gradient (as we just discussed). You might wonder that if the pre-read out Gx gradi-

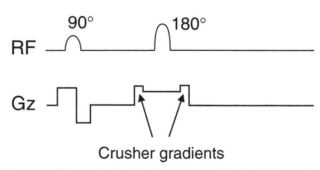

Figure 14-3.   Crusher gradients are applied at each side of the slice-selective gradient (applied during the 180° pulse) to achieve more accurate refocussing at time TE.

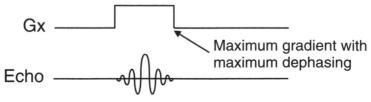

Figure 14-4.   If only a constant gradient Gx is applied during readout, we end up dephasing all the spins.

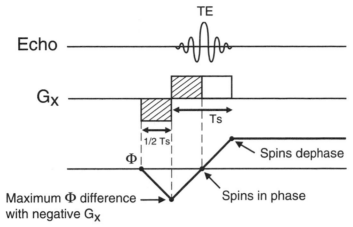

Figure 14-5. Prior to the application of the readout gradient, a negative gradient is applied resulting in a tri-lobed gradient. The negative lobe causes the spins to get out of phase. Then the spins get back in phase in the center of the echo.

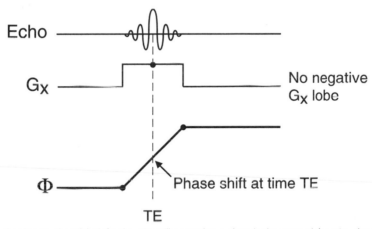

Figure 14-6. In the absence of a trilobed Gx, the spins will accumulate a phase in the center of the echo, thus yielding less signal.

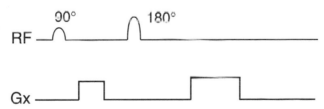

Figure 14-7. The first lobe of Gx can either be applied after the 180° as a negative lobe (as in previous figures) or as a positive lobe prior to the 180° pulse.

ent is positive, aren't we going to create *more* phase difference with an additional positive lobe?

The answer lies in the fact that in Figure 14-7 the positive pre-read out Gx gradient comes *before* the 180° refocusing pulse. After the Gx pre-read out gradient, we'll have a positive phase difference. This phase difference will stay constant until the 180° pulse is applied (Fig. 14-8).

After the 180° RF pulse is applied, the phase difference will be reversed. Then it will remain constant until the Gx gradient is applied. Then, the spins will begin going back in phase, reaching a zero phase difference at time TE, and going out of phase afterwards. So, we get the same thing with both the positive and negative pre-read out Gx gradients, depending on where in the pulse sequence the gradient is applied.

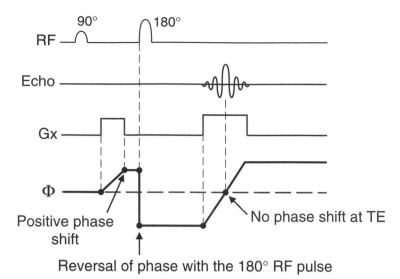

Figure 14-8. This diagram demonstrates how the spins get back in phase at the center of the echo when an additional refocussing positive gradient is applied prior to the 180° pulse.

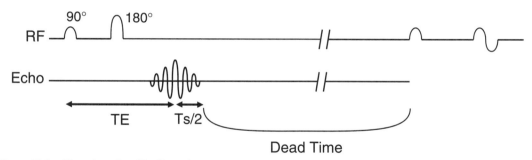

Figure 14-9. There always is a "dead" time between the completion of readout and the next 90° pulse. This dead time can be taken advantage of to acquire other slices.

ACQUISITION TIME

In previous chapters, we talked about multi-slice imaging and we said that there was a lot of "dead" time between the end of the echo and the next 90° RF pulse (Fig. 14-9). We can use this "dead" time to our advantage to process other slices.

Question 1:   *If we manage to fit in all the slices we want within the dead time, what will the acquisition time for the study be?*
Answer: *It takes TR seconds to fill one line in the data space. Thus, the acquisition time, which is the time it takes to fill the entire data space, is TR times the number of lines in the data space.*

Question 2:   *How many lines (rows) do we have in the data (or K) space?*

Answer: *The number of lines in k-space equals the number of phase encoding steps Np or Ny.*

Question 3:   *Does it help to repeat the sequence all over again?*
Answer: *We can repeat the whole sequence over again (or repeat each phase encoding step over again) to average out the noise and increase the signal to noise ratio (SNR).*

Each cycle is called an **excitation**. The term **NEX** stands for the **N**umber of **EX**citations. So the acquisition time depends on:

1.   TR (the time to do one line of the data space)
2.   Ny (the number of phase encoding steps)
3.   NEX (the number of times we repeat the whole sequence)

Acquisition time = (TR) (Ny) (NEX)

This formula is for a conventional spin-echo sequence. Notice that the number of slices doesn't even enter the equation. This is somewhat counter-intuitive if one is used to the principles of scan time in CT because, in CT, the more slices we obtain, the longer the sequence will be. This is not necessarily true in MR because of the fact that we can do multiple slices within the time of one TR. Obviously, though, if we decrease the TR, we decrease the number of slices we're able to obtain. So the number of slices is *indirectly* determined by the TR parameter.

Let's say that we want to do a T1-weighted study with a fairly wide coverage. Increasing the TR to allow more slices per TR might be counter productive because T1 weighting will be reduced. Thus, there is a *trade-off* between increasing coverage and achieving more T1 weighting.

EXAMPLE 1:

TR = 1000 msec, Ny = 256, NEX = 1

$$\begin{aligned} \text{Acquisition Time} &= (TR)\,(Ny)\,(NEX) \\ &= (1000\text{ msec})\,(256)\,(1) \\ &= 256\text{ sec} \cong 4.27\text{ min.} \end{aligned}$$

Let's say that we fit 10 slices in the TR. Then we could obtain the 10 slices in 4.27 min.

EXAMPLE 2:

If, on the other hand, we were to only obtain one slice per TR at a time, we would have to repeat the sequence 10 times to obtain 10 slices, then the scan time would instead be

$$(10)\,(1000\text{ msec})\,(256)\,(1\text{ NEX}) \cong 10 \times 4.27\text{ min}$$
$$= 42.7\text{ min}$$

which is, obviously, impractical.

Key Points

We have discussed the topic of PSD (pulse sequence diagram) and illustrated one example for SE imaging. In the chapters to come, we will see examples of more complicated PSD's. Of course, the PSD does not tell us all the parameters used in MR imaging, such as the field of view (discussed in the next chapter), but it offers an algorithm or prescription for performing the study.

Questions

14-1. The acquisition time depends on which of the following? (one or more)
(a) TE   (b) TR   (c) NEX
(d) Nx   (e) Ny

14-2. (a) Calculate the acquisition time for a multi-acquisition SE sequence with TR = 1500, NEX = 2, Ny = 256.
(b) Repeat (a) for single slice acquisition of 10 slices. Is this practical?

INTRODUCTION

A PSD (pulse sequence diagram) provides a timing algorithm for the sequence of events that is carried out during an MR study. However, the operator must specify the dimensions of the desired part of the body under study. This is the subject of this chapter; namely, the field of view (FOV). As we shall see shortly, there is a limitation as to how small we can make the FOV depending on the maximum strength of the gradients and the bandwidth of the received signals.

FIELD OF VIEW (FOV)

We're going to discuss the relationship between the following entities:

1. FOV
2. Bandwidth
3. Gradients

Understanding these concepts is important because these features have definite clinical applications.

Let's take an image with its x and y axes (Fig. 15-1). There is an FOV along the x axis.

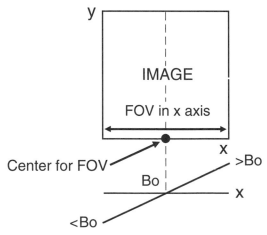

Figure 15-1. An image with axes x and y. The frequency-encode gradient G_x causes the center of the field of view (FOV) to have magnetic field strength B_0 and the right and left ends to have strengths greater and less than B_0, respectively.

Normally, we apply a gradient that increases as we move in the x direction (G_x). This means that we create magnetic inhomogeneities along the x axis in a *linear* fashion. Consequently,

1. at the center point of the FOV, the magnetic field will be B_0;
2. on the right side of the FOV, the magnetic field will be greater than B_0;
3. on the left side of the FOV, the magnetic field will be less than B_0.

The magnetic filed along the x-axis is B_x. The value of B_x is given by the linear equation:

$$B_x = (G_x) \cdot x$$

This equation shows that the value of the magnetic field at any point along the gradient (G_x) is the slope of the gradient (G_x) times the distance x along the x-axis (Fig. 15-2). Let's multiply both sides of the equation by the gyromagnetic ratio γ:

$$\gamma \cdot B_x \cdot x = \gamma(G_x) x$$

Recall that (γB_x) is the **Larmor equation**, which relates the magnetic field strength to the frequency:

$$\text{frequency}_x = \gamma B_x$$

This equation states that the frequency of oscillation at any point along the x-axis is proportional to the magnetic field strength at that point; i.e.,

$$f_x = \gamma B_x$$

or

$$f_x = \gamma(G_x) x$$

In other words, the frequency at any point along the x-axis is proportional to the slope of the gradient (G_x) multiplied by the position along the x-axis.

Let's see what happens at each end of the FOV (Fig. 15-3). At the right-side end of the FOV (i.e., at x = FOV/2), the frequency is maximum (call it f_{max}) because the G_x gradient, and

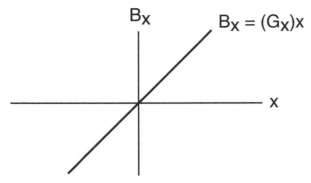

Figure 15-2. The gradient G_x describes a linear equation $B_x = G_x \cdot x$. Therefore, at $x = 0$, no net magnetic field is added to the system, whereas at a positive value of x, a positive value of magnetic field is added to the main field.

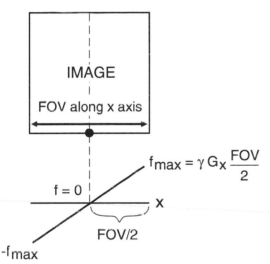

Figure 15-3. At each end of the FOV, the frequency f_x (which is proportional to gradient strength G_x) is maximal. This relationship is given by $f_x = \gamma \cdot G_x \cdot x$, where $x = FOV/2$ for f_{max}.

therefore the magnetic field strength, is maximum.

The formula for frequency is:

$$f_x = \gamma(G_x)(x)$$

Now, for f_{max}, the distance along the x-axis is ½ FOV. So,

$$f_{max} = \gamma(G_x) FOV/2$$

Remember this is after we subtract the *center* frequency. Therefore, these measurements are centered around the zero frequency. At the opposite end of the gradient, we have $-f_{max}$

$$-f_{max} = -\gamma(G_x) FOV/2$$

What is the **range of frequencies**? The frequency range is from $-f_{max}$ to $+f_{max}$, i.e.,

$$\text{freq. range} = -f_{max} \rightarrow +f_{max}$$
$$= \pm f_{max} = 2 f_{max}$$

Another term for the range of frequencies is **bandwidth (BW)**. Thus,

$$BW = \pm f_{max} = 2 f_{max}$$

If we take the frequency at the right-most side of the image and at the left-most side of the image, we get the range of frequencies, or the bandwidth. We already know that, for maximum frequency,

$$f_{max} = \gamma(G_x) FOV/2$$

Because

$$BW = 2 f_{max},$$

we can conclude that

$$BW = \gamma \cdot G_x \cdot FOV$$

We therefore see a dependent relationship between the *field of view, bandwidth,* and *gradient strength.* Let's now solve the equation for the FOV in the x-direction:

$$FOV_x = \frac{\text{Bandwidth}}{\gamma(G_x)}$$

This equations shows that the FOV is directly proportional to the bandwidth and that the FOV is inversely proportional to the gradient. Hence, if one wishes to decrease the field of view, one can use either 1) a stronger gradient, or 2) a lower bandwidth.

To ↓ FOV:
1. ↑ Gradient
2. ↓ Bandwidth

There are limits as to how strong you can make the gradient and there are also limits as to how low you can make the bandwidth.

Question: *What is the minimum FOV possible?*

Answer: *It is the minimum bandwidth divided by the maximum gradient:*

$$FOV\ min = \frac{BW_{min}}{\gamma G_{max}}$$

G_{max} and BW_{min} are specific for each machine. For example, for a GE Signa 1.5 T scanner,

maximum gradient strength = 10 mT/meter
minimum bandwidth = ± 4 kHz = 8 kHz.

Thus, the minimum FOV is approximately:

8 kHz/(42.6 MHz/T × 10 mT/m) ≅ 2 cm.

Conversely, to increase the FOV, we can

1. increase the BW or
2. decrease the gradient

To ↑ FOV:
1. ↓ Gradient
2. ↑ Bandwidth

Key Points

We have discussed the interesting relationship between the FOV, BW, and gradients:

$$FOV = BW/(\gamma \cdot G)$$

As we saw, there is a limit as to how small one can make the FOV depending on the minimum allowable BW and the maximum possible gradient strength:

$$FOV_{min} = BW_{min}/(\gamma \cdot G_{max})$$

Selecting a smaller FOV may cause an aliasing (or wraparound) artifact, depending on the size of the structure being imaged. More on this in Chapter 18.

Questions

15-1.   If the minimum FOV = 40 cm for a frequency-encoding gradient G_x = 5mT/m, what would the minimum FOV be for a stronger G_x = 10mT/m? (i.e., does a stronger Gx reduce or increase the minimum FOV?)

15-2.   What is the minimum FOV for a maximum sampling interval of $\Delta Ts = 10\ \mu s$ (i.e., without encountering aliasing) and a maximum frequency gradient of 10 mT/m?
Hint: BW = $1/\Delta Ts$
(a)   47 cm   (b)   23.5 cm
(c)   47 mm   (d)   23.5 mm

15-3.   If the amplitude of a phase-encoding gradient Gy is 0.1 mT/m and its duration is 2 ms, what is the phase shift of the transverse magnetization from a tissue that is 20 mm = 2 cm from the center of the FOV?
Hint: $\Delta\phi = 360° \times \gamma \times Gy \times$ duration × position, where γ = 42.6 MHz/T

15-4.   The minimum FOV can be reduced by:
(a)   increasing the gradient strength
(b)   decreasing the bandwidth
(c)   increasing the sampling interval
(d)   all of the above
(e)   only (a) and (b)

15-5.   T/F Reducing the FOV minimizes wraparound artifacts (aliasing).

k-space...the final frontier!

INTRODUCTION

This chapter will summarize some concepts that we've already discussed and clarify some of the fine points of k-space. Remember that we have, up to this point, referred to the **Data space** as an "analog" k-space, and we said that the *Fourier transform* of the Data space is the image (Fig. 16-1).

This is, in fact, correct, but there is a problem with this concept: the *matrix* in the data space is very *asymmetric*. In the frequency encoding direction, the interval between two samples (i.e., the sampling interval ΔTs) is on the order of microseconds, so that the total time to take all the samples (i.e., the sampling time Ts) is on the order of milliseconds. The time intervals in the phase encoding direction, however, are each on the order of one TR (i.e., on the order of seconds). The total time to obtain all the data in the phase encoding direction is the scan time for one acquisition (on the order of minutes).

Thus, in the data space we have a matrix whose *x-axis* is on the order of *milliseconds*, and whose *y-axis* is on the order of *minutes*. This would give us a very asymmetric matrix. The true k-space is the same matrix as the data space,

but with a *different* **scale**. Recall that

$$FOV = \frac{Bandwidth}{\gamma \cdot Gradient} \qquad \text{(Eqn. 16-1)}$$

In the last chapter, we talked about the field of view (FOV). We derived Equation 16-1, showing the relationship between the FOV, bandwidth, and gradient strength. According to this formula, the FOV is equal to BW divided by the product of γ and G. We also know from a previous chapter that the bandwidth is inversely related to the sampling internal (ΔTs), i.e.,

$$BW = 1/\Delta Ts$$

From the following two formulas:

$$FOV = \frac{BW}{\gamma G}$$

and

$$BW = \frac{1}{\Delta Ts}$$

we can derive a new formula for the FOV:

$$FOV = \frac{BW}{\gamma G} = \frac{1}{\gamma G \Delta Ts}$$

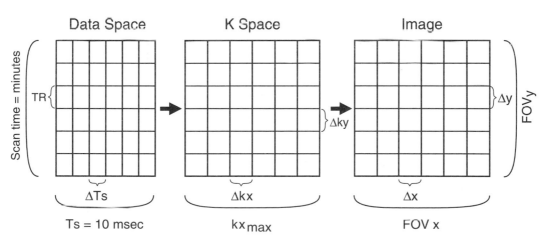

Figure 16-1.   The Data space (with axes ΔTs and TR) is in the time domain. k-space (with axes Δkx and Δky) is in the *spatial* frequency domain and is derived from the Data space. The Fourier transform of k-space is the image (with axes x and y), which is in the frequency domain.

To calculate this in terms of distance and time, we need to invert both sides of the previous formula to obtain:

$$\frac{1}{FOV} = \gamma \cdot G \cdot \Delta Ts$$

Now consider the FOV in the x and y directions. If we consider the FOV in the x direction, the formula tells us that we need to take the gradient strength and the sampling interval in the x-direction.

$$\frac{1}{FOV_x} = \gamma \cdot G_x \cdot \Delta t_x$$

The term $(\gamma\ Gx\ \Delta t_x)$ is denoted $\mathbf{\Delta k_x}$. If we now look back at the three diagrams at the beginning of the chapter, we see that (Δk_x) is the unit interval in k-space in the x-direction. Thus,

$$\Delta k_x = \gamma\ Gx\ \Delta t_x$$

Let's discuss the units of measurement in the above:

γ = gyromagnetic ratio = MHz/Tesla
G_x = gradient strength = milliTesla/meter
Δt_x = sampling interval = milliseconds

so

$$\Delta k_x = (MHz/T)(mT/m)(msec)$$
$$= (cycles/sec\ .\ T) \times (T/m) \times sec$$
$$= cycles/m$$

Thus, Δk_x has units of cycles/m or cycles/cm.

The main thing to remember is that Δk_x is 1/FOV in the x-direction.

$$\Delta k_x = 1/FOV_x$$

The above formula tells us that the interval in k-space is equal to 1/FOV in the x-direction (where the FOV, according to Equation 16-1, depends on the bandwidth and gradient strength in the x direction). This fact is shown diagrammatically in Figure 16-2.

From this, we can see a direct relationship between k-space and the image in that the interval in k-space has an inverse relationship to the FOV of the image. For example, if the FOV of the image is 10 cm, then

$$\Delta k_x = 1/FOV = 1/10cm = 1/0.1m$$
$$= 0.1\ cm^{-1}\ (cycles/cm)$$
$$= 10\ m^{-1}\ (cycles/m)$$

Therefore, with an FOV of 10 cm in the image, the pixel size of k-space is 0.1 cm^{-1} or 10 m^{-1} (remember that the unit of the axes in k-space is 1/distance or cycles/distance). The inverse of this is also true:

$$\Delta x = pixel\ size\ in\ the\ image$$
$$k_x = sum\ of\ the\ pixels\ in\ k\text{-}space$$

In summary:

$$\Delta x = 1/k_x, \Delta k_x = 1/FOV_x$$
$$\Delta k_x = \gamma \cdot G_x \cdot \Delta t_x, k_x = \gamma \cdot G_x \cdot t_x$$

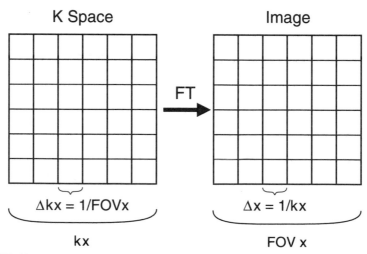

Figure 16-2. The FT of k-space is the image. There is a relationship between the axes in k-space and the image: $\Delta k_x = 1/FOV_x$, $\Delta x = 1/k_x$, where $FOV_x = N_x \cdot \Delta x$ and $k_x = N_x \cdot \Delta k_x$.

where Δx is the pixel size in the x-direction. In essence, this is how we figure out the pixel size in the image.

$$\Delta x = \text{pixel (x direction)} = \text{FOV}_x/\text{N}_x$$

This formula tells us that the pixel size in the x-direction is equal to the FOV divided by the number of pixels in the x-direction.

EXAMPLE:

1. Calculate the pixel size for the following situation:

    FOVx = 128 mm
    Nx = number of sampling points
       in the x direction = 128

    then

    pixel size in the x direction
       $= \Delta x = 128 \text{ mm}/128 = 1.0 \text{ mm}$

2. Calculate the dimensions in k-space for the above example:

    Δkx = pixel size in k-space = 1/FOVx.
    $\Delta kx - 1/128 \text{ mm} = 1/12.8 \text{ cm} \cong .08 \text{ cm}^{-1}$
       $= 8 \text{ m}^{-1}$
    $kx = 1/\Delta x = 1/1 \text{ mm} = 1 \text{ mm}^{-1} = 10 \text{ cm}^{-1}$
       $= 1000 \text{ m}^{-1} = 128 \Delta kx$

    The unit in k-space is

    Δkx = cycles/distance
    kx — cycles/distance

The measurement cycles/distance is called the spatial frequency.

Therefore,

---

k-space is in the spatial frequency domain.

This is different from the other frequency that we have discussed thus far. Before, we discussed the Fourier transform of a signal that varied with time, with the transform in the frequency domain. Spatial frequency is a different kind of frequency.

**The usual frequency = cycles/time
Spatial frequency = cycles/distance**

Therefore, when k-space is said to be in the "frequency domain," we are referring to the "spatial frequency domain," which, as we just saw,

is a mathematical manipulation of the *data space* (which is in the time domain).

Remember that the units of the axes in data space are time: milliseconds and minutes. In k-space, we have converted these axes into "spatial frequencies" that have units of cycles/distance, measured in cm^{-1} (cycles/cm) and meter^{-1} (cycles/meter). If we Fourier transform k-space, we get the desired image.

Mathematically, we could go straight from the data space, via a Fourier transform, directly to the image. We are simply renaming the variables (i.e., $\gamma \text{ G}_x \Delta t_x = \Delta k_x$). This renaming is known as an *algebraic manipulation*, but to go through this intermediate mathematical step in k-space allows us to work with a space that is *more symmetric*; now, the distance in the x-direction of k-space and the distance in the y-direction of k-space are roughly similar (as opposed to the difference between milliseconds and minutes in the x-direction and y-direction in the data space, respectively).

This same concept in the y-direction is somewhat harder to understand but the same principles hold; namely,

$$\Delta k_y = \frac{1}{\text{FOV}_y}$$

The interval ky in k-space is inversely proportional to the FOV in the y-direction.

$$k_y = \frac{1}{\Delta y}$$

The distance in k-space in the y-direction is inversely proportional to the pixel size of the image in the y-direction.

One more mathematical principle concerns the relationship between phase and frequency:

$$\theta = \int \omega \, dt$$

In other words, the phase θ is the integral of the frequency with respect to time, where ω (angular frequency) is given by the Larmor equation[a]:

$$\omega = \gamma B = \gamma \cdot G \cdot x$$

---

[a] You may have wondered why we have been using ω and f somewhat interchangeably in our equations, although these are two separate entities. This practice is all right as long as you keep the right units for the gyromagnetic ratio γ (i.e., MHz/T when dealing with f and 2π.MHz/T when dealing with ω).

In other words, the frequency ω is proportional to the magnetic field strength which is, in turn, proportional to the gradient strength multiplied by the distance. Thus,

$$\theta_y = \omega_y\, t_y = \gamma \cdot B_y \cdot t_y = \gamma \cdot G_y \cdot y \cdot t_y$$

or

$$\theta_y = (\gamma\, G_y\, t_y) \cdot y$$

Remember that:

$$\Delta k_y = \gamma\, G_y\, \Delta t_y \text{ and}$$
$$(k_y = \Delta k_y \cdot N_y) \text{ and } (t_y = \Delta t_y \cdot N_y)$$

so

$$k_y = \Delta k_y \cdot N_y = \gamma\, G_y\, \Delta t_y \cdot N_y$$

Therefore,

$$k_y = \gamma \cdot G_y \cdot t_y$$

so

$$\theta_y = (k_y)\cdot(y)$$

We thus have a very simple relationship between *phase* and *position* along the y direction:

$$\theta_y = (k_y) \cdot (y) = (\gamma\, G_y)(t_y)(y)$$

In the y-direction, the *gradient* at y depends on the position of y. In contrast, we always apply the same gradient in the x-direction regardless of what position the x direction is going (i.e., Gx is independent of x). However, in the y-direction, we apply different gradients at different points along the y-axis (Gy varies with y: it is 0 at y = 0 and gets progressively larger with increasing y).

Key Points

The true k-space is a mathematically manipulated variant of the data space, with axes referred to as "spatial frequencies." Therefore, k-space is in a "spatial" frequency domain. *Spatial frequencies* k_x and k_y are inversely proportional to *distance* (with units of cycles/cm). The Fourier transform of k-space is the desired image.

The spatial frequencies k_x and k_y are expressed as:

$$k_x = \gamma \cdot G_x \cdot t_x$$
$$k_y = \gamma \cdot G_y \cdot t_y$$

with units in cycles/cm.

Questions

16-1.   T/F   k-space can be thought of as a digital (in the spatial frequency domain) version of the data space (which is in the time domain).

16-2.   T/F   (a)   The axes in k-space are designated k_x and k_y.
(b)   The axes in k-space are in the frequency domain (with units 1/time or cycle/sec).

16-3.   T/F   Spatial frequencies have units 1/distance (cycles/cm)

16-4. Δk_x is equal to:
(a) $1/FOV_x$ (b) $\gamma\, G_x\, \Delta t_x$
(c) k_x/N_x (d)   all of the above
(e)   only (a) and (b)

16-5.   T/F   (a)   The center of k-space contributes to maximum image contrast.
(b)   The periphery of k-space contributes to image details.

17 Scan Parameters and Image Optimization

INTRODUCTION

In this chapter, we will discuss all the important parameters in MR imaging that the operator can control and adjust. We will then see how these changes influence the image quality. Every radiologist is comfortable with a particular set of techniques; therefore, "custom-made" techniques can be achieved only if the radiologist is aware of the parameters and tradeoffs that are involved.

PRIMARY AND SECONDARY PARAMETERS

Primary parameters are those that are set directly:

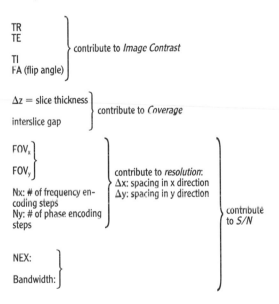

From the *primary* parameters above, we can get the *secondary* parameters (which are also used to describe the image):

1. S/N ratio
2. Scan time
3. Coverage
4. Resolution
5. Image contrast

Unfortunately, optimization of these parameters may involve some **trade-offs**. To gain some advantage with one parameter, we might have to sacrifice another parameter. Let's start out with the concept of signal to noise ratio.

Signal to Noise Ratio

What we want is signal. What we don't want is noise. Although we can't completely eliminate noise, there are ways to maximize the signal to noise ratio (SNR or S/N). SNR is given by

$$S/N \propto (Voxel\ Volume)\ \sqrt{(Ny)(NEX)/BW} \quad \text{(Eqn. 17-1)}$$

Therefore, S/N depends on:

1. Voxel Volume = $\Delta x \cdot \Delta y \cdot \Delta z$
2. Number of excitations = NEX
3. Number of phase encoding steps = Ny
4. Bandwidth = BW

Let's go through each parameter and see how SNR is affected.

VOXEL VOLUME

If we increase the voxel size, we increase the number of proton spins in the voxel and, therefore, increase the signal coming out of the voxel (Fig. 17-1). The voxel volume is given by

$$Voxel\ volume = \Delta x \cdot \Delta y \cdot \Delta z$$

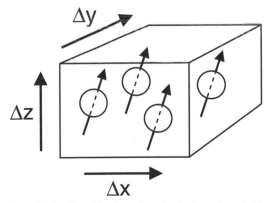

Figure 17-1. A voxel is a three-dimensional volume element with dimensions Δx, Δy, and Δz. The more spins in a voxel, the more signal. Therefore, increasing voxel size increases S/N.

where Δx = pixel size in the x direction, Δy = pixel size in the y direction, and Δz = slice thickness.

NEX (NUMBER OF EXCITATIONS OR ACQUISITIONS)

NEX stands for the number of times the scan is repeated. Let's say we have two signals (S1 and S2), corresponding to the same slice (with the same Gy). There is constant noise (N) associated with each signal ($N1 = N2 = N$). If we add up the signals (assuming $S_1 = S_2 = S$), we get

$$S_1 + S_2 = 2S$$

However, if we add up the noise, we get

$$N_1 + N_2 = (\sqrt{2}) N \text{ where } \sqrt{2} \approx 1.41$$

This formula does not make sense at first glance. Why do we get $\sqrt{2}$ N and not 2N? The answer has to do with a somewhat complicated statistical concept and the so-called random **Brownian motion** theory, which deals with the *spectral density* of the noise.

In a simplistic approach, think of the noise as the **variance** (σ^2) of a Gaussian distribution (σ = **standard deviation**). Then, for the sum of the two noise distributions, the variance is additive and given by

$$\sigma_1{}^2 + \sigma_2{}^2 = \sigma^2 + \sigma^2 = 2\,\sigma^2$$

from which the standard deviation is calculated to be

$$\sqrt{(2\sigma^2)} = (\sqrt{2})\,\sigma$$

This is where the $\sqrt{2}$ factor comes from. However, you don't need to know the underlying math—you just need to understand the concept. In summary:

$$\frac{S1 + S2}{N1 + N2} = \frac{2S}{\sqrt{2}\,N}$$

The resulting signal will be twice the original signal. The resulting noise, however, will be less—it will be the square root of 2 multiplied by the noise ($\sqrt{2}$ N).

In other words, if we increase the number of acquisitions by a factor of 2, the signal doubles and noise increases by $\sqrt{2}$, for a net $2/\sqrt{2} = \sqrt{2}$; thus, S/N increases by a factor of $\sqrt{2}$.

$$\therefore \uparrow \text{NEX by a factor of } 2 \rightarrow \uparrow \text{S/N}$$
$$\text{by a factor of } \sqrt{2}$$

Think of the NEX as an *averaging* operation that causes "smoothing" and improvement in the image quality by increasing the signal to a greater degree (e.g., factor 2) relative to the increase in the noise (e.g., factor 2).

NY (NUMBER OF PHASE-ENCODING STEPS)

The same concept holds for Ny. That is, similar to NEX, there is a 41% ($\sqrt{2}$) increase in S/N when Ny is doubled. As with NEX, when the number of phase-encode steps doubles, signal doubles and noise increases (randomly) by $\sqrt{2}$ (for a net $\sqrt{2}$ increase in S/N).

BANDWIDTH

An inverse relationship exists between BW and SNR. If we go to a wider bandwidth, we include more noise, and the SNR decreases. If we decrease the bandwidth, we allow less noise to come through, and the SNR increases.

$$\uparrow \text{BW} \Rightarrow \downarrow \text{SNR}$$
$$\downarrow \text{BW} \Rightarrow \uparrow \text{SNR}$$

To be exact, decreasing the BW by a factor of 2 causes the SNR to improve by a factor of $\sqrt{2}$.

In general, decreased bandwidth causes the following:

1. Increased S/N ratio
2. Increased chemical shift artifact (more on this later)
3. Longer TE (which means less signal due to more T2 decay). Remember that

$$\text{Bandwidth} = 1/\Delta Ts = N/Ts$$

Therefore, a longer sampling time (Ts), which is necessary for a decreased bandwidth, results in a longer TE. With a long TE, increased T2 dephasing results in decreased signal. However, the contribution from reduced noise due to a lower bandwidth outweighs the deleterious effect of reduced signal due to greater T2 decay from increased TE.

4. Decreased number of slices. This decrease is caused by the longer TE. Remember,

$$\text{\# slices} = TR/(TE + Ts/2 + To)$$

where Ts is the total sampling (readout) time and To is the "overhead" time. A narrower bandwidth is usually used on the second echo of a T2 weighted dual echo image because, with the second echo, we have a longer TE and we are able to afford the longer sampling time. On the first echo, however, we can't afford to use a narrower bandwidth because we can't afford to lengthen the TE. However, we probably don't need the smaller bandwidth anyway because we already have enough SNR on the proton density weighted first echo of a long T2, double echo image. A typical Ts for a 1.5 T scanner is 8 msec, resulting in a BW (for a 256 matrix) of

$$BW = N/Ts = 256/8 = 32 \text{ kHz}$$
$$= \pm 16 \text{ kHz} = 125 \text{ Hz/pixel}.$$

A typical "Variable Bandwidth" option includes:

1. A wide bandwidth (± 16 kHz) on the first echo, and
2. A narrow bandwidth (± 4 kHz) on the second echo, thus increasing SNR and counteracting T2 decay effects.

Question: *How does the gradient affect the BW?*
Answer: *Recall from Chapter 15 that the field of view (FOV) is given by*

$$FOV = BW/\gamma\, Gx \quad or \quad Gx = BW/\gamma\, FOV$$

For a given FOV, increasing the gradient Gx causes increased BW and, therefore, decreased SNR.

SNR in 3D Imaging

In 3D imaging, we have the same factors contributing to SNR, plus an additional phase encoding step in the z direction (Nz):

$$3D \text{ SNR} \propto (\text{Voxel Volume})\sqrt{(Ny)(Nz)(NEX)/BW}$$
$$\text{(Eqn. 17-2)}$$

From this equation, you can see why SNR in 3D imaging is higher than in 2D imaging. Specifically,

$$SNR (3D) = \sqrt{Nz} \cdot SNR (2D)$$

Another way to look at SNR is to say that SNR depends on only two factors:

1. Voxel size
2. Total sampling time

Sampling time (Ts) is the time that we sample the signal. Therefore, it makes sense that the more time we spend sampling the signal, the higher the S/N ratio will be. Let's look again at the formula for SNR (in 2D imaging):

$$S/N \propto (\text{Voxel Volume})\sqrt{(Ny)(NEX)/BW}$$

Recall that

$$Ts = Nx/BW$$

or

$$1/BW = Ts/Nx$$

so

$$S/N \propto (\text{Voxel Volume})\sqrt{(Ny)(NEX)(Ts)/Nx}$$

We know that Ny = number of phase encoding steps, which is the number of times we sample the echo corresponding to a particular phase encoding gradient Gy, and that NEX is the number of times we repeat each phase encoding step. In essence, the factor

$$T = Ts \cdot Ny \cdot NEX$$

is the *total sampling time* of all the echoes received for a particular slice. Thus,

$$S/N \propto \frac{(\text{Voxel Volume})}{\sqrt{total\ sampling\ time\ of\ all\ signals}}$$

In summary, SNR can be increased by doing the following:

1. Increasing TR
2. Decreasing TE
3. Using a lower BW
4. Using volume (i.e., 3D) imaging
5. Increasing NEX
6. Increasing Ny
7. Increasing the voxel size

Resolution

Spatial resolution (or pixel size) is the minimum distance that we can distinguish between two points on an image. It is determined by

$$pixel\ size = FOV/\# \text{ of pixels}$$
$$\uparrow Ny \rightarrow \text{Better Resolution}$$

If we increase the number of phase encoding steps, what happens to S/N ratio? Obviously, *better resolution usually means poorer SNR*. However, if we look at Equation 17-1, it appears that by increasing Ny, the SNR should increase! What's the catch? The catch is, we are keeping the FOV constant while increasing Ny. Take, for example,

$$\text{pixel size along y-axis} = \Delta y = FOV_y/N_y$$

By increasing Ny, we are making the pixel size smaller. Now, recall that

$$\text{voxel volume} = \Delta x \cdot \Delta y \cdot \Delta z$$
$$= FOVx \cdot FOVy \cdot \Delta z/Nx \cdot Ny$$

Incorporating this information into Equation 17-1 gives us another way of expressing SNR:

$$SNR = (FOV_x/Nx)\,(FOV_y)\,\Delta z\,\sqrt{\frac{NEX}{(Ny)(BW)}} \quad \text{(Eqn. 17-3)}$$

This formula allows us to better separate the factors affecting SNR. From this, we can conclude the following:

1. If we keep FOV constant and increase Ny, we will decrease SNR.

    $\uparrow$ Ny, FOV constant $\Rightarrow$ $\downarrow$ SNR

2. If we increase Ny and increase FOV, thus keeping pixel size constant, then we will increase the SNR. Yet the resolution doesn't change. What is the tradeoff here? The answer is the acquisition time, which is proportional to Ny.

    $\uparrow$ FOV, pixels fixed $\Rightarrow$ $\uparrow$ SNR, $\uparrow$ Time

3. If we increase slice thickness Δz, we get more SNR, but also more partial volume artifact.
4. If we increase NEX, we get more SNR at the expense of longer acquisition time. For 3D imaging, the previous equation (Eqn. 17-3) is modified to:

$$SNR\ (3D) = (FOV_x/Nx)\,(FOV_y)\,(FOV_z)\,\sqrt{\frac{NEX}{(Ny)(Nz)(BW)}}$$
$$\text{(Eqn. 17-4)}$$

Basically, if we want better spatial resolution in a *given* acquisition time, we have to sacrifice SNR. Let's consider a few examples.

1. What happens if we increase the number of pixels with the FOV constant?

(a) Increase resolution
(b) Decrease S/N ratio (refer to Eqn. 17-3)

    Therefore, as we decrease the pixel size, we increase the resolution and decrease the SNR
(c) Increase scan time (number of pixels increases in phase encode direction)

2. What happens if we decrease the FOV and keep the number of pixels constant?
(a) Increase the resolution
(b) Decrease S/N ratio
(c) Potentially increase aliasing artifact

3. How do we determine the pixel size (resolution)?

    It is determined by dividing the FOV by the number of encoding steps.

EXAMPLE:

For FOV = 250 mm and a 256 × 256 matrix
Nx = Ny = 256
Pixel size (x) = FOV_x/Nx = 250/256 $\cong$ 1 mm in x direction.
Pixel size (y) = FOV_y/Ny = 250/256 $\cong$ 1 mm in y direction.

In the x direction, there are two ways of increasing resolution (for a given FOV):

1. Increase Nx by reducing the sampling time ΔTs (i.e., by increasing the BW) and keeping the total sampling time Ts fixed (recall that Ts = Nx $\cdot$ ΔTs). The advantage here is no increase in TE; the trade-off is a reduction in SNR (due to increased BW).
2. Increase Nx by lengthening Ts and keeping ΔTs (and thus BW) fixed. Here, the SNR does not change, but the trade-off is an increased TE (due to a longer Ts) and less T1 weighting.

ACQUISITION TIME

The acquisition time or scan time, as we have seen previously, is given by

$$\text{Scan Time} = TR \cdot Ny \cdot NEX$$

where Ny is the number of phase encoding steps (in the y direction).

For fast spin echo (FSE) imaging, the above is modified to

$$\text{FSE Time} = TR \cdot Ny \cdot NEX/ETL$$

where ETL = echo train length (4, 8, 16, 32).

For 3D imaging, the scan time is given by

$$time (3D) = TR \cdot Ny \cdot Nz \cdot NEX$$

where Nz is the number of phase encoding steps (partitions) in the z direction. In other words,

$$time (3D) = Nz \cdot time (2D)$$

Multiplication by such a large number (e.g., Nz = 32 to 64 or 128) might at first seem to result in an excessively long scan time for 3D imaging, but the TR used in 3D gradient echo imaging is approximately 100 times smaller (order of 30 ms) compared with the TR used in conventional spin echo imaging; we can perform a 3D scan in a reasonable time. Recently, 3D fast spin echo imaging (discussed in Chap. 19) has also become feasible.

EXAMPLES:

1. Calculate the acquisition time of an SE sequence with TR = 3000 msec, Ny = 256, and NEX = 1.
   Solution: Scan Time = 3000 × 256 msec = 768 sec = 12.8 min.

2. Calculate the acquisition time of an FSE sequence with the above parameters and an echo train length (ETL) of 8
   Solution: Scan Time = $\dfrac{12.8 \text{ min}}{8}$ = 1.6 min

3. (a) Calculate the acquisition time of a 3D gradient echo with TR = 30 ms, Ny = 256, NEX = 1, and Nz = 60.
   Solution: Scan Time = 30 × 256 × 1 × 60 msec = 460.8 sec = 7.68 min.
   (b) If TR = 300 in the previous example, then the scan time = 76.8 min = 1 hour and 16.8 min., which is, obviously, impractical. Hence, 3D techniques use gradient echo sequences employing a very short TR.

TR

What happens if we increase or decrease TR?

1. Increasing TR:
   (a) increases SNR (according to the T_1 recovery curve)
   (b) increases coverage (more slices)
   (c) decreases T1 weighting
   (d) increases proton density and T2 weighting
   (e) increases scan time

2. Decreasing TR:
   (a) decreases SNR
   (b) decreases coverage
   (c) increases T1 weighting
   (d) Decreases proton density and T2 weighting
   (e) Decreases scan time

Sometimes an MR technologist will find that, for a certain TR, the required coverage cannot be achieved. Therefore, to increase the coverage, he or she might increase the TR. However, in so doing, T1 weighting is decreased, which may be an undesirable effect.

COVERAGE

Coverage is the distance covered by a multislice acquisition. It depends on the number of slices and on the slice thickness and the interslice gap (Fig. 17-2). Because

$$\text{\# of slices} = TR/(TE + Ts/2 + To)$$

then

$$\text{coverage} = TR/(TE + Ts/2 + To)$$
$$\times \text{(slice thickness + gap)}$$

where Ts is the sampling time and To is the "overhead" time, as we've discussed in previous chapters.

Let's summarize:

1. Coverage is increased if we:
   (a) increase slice thickness
   (b) increase interslice gap
   (c) increase TR or decrease the last TE (i.e., increase TR/TE ratio)
   (d) decrease sampling time Ts (resulting in a lower TE), i.e., increase the bandwidth
2. Coverage is decreased if we:
   (a) increase TE
   (b) increase Ts

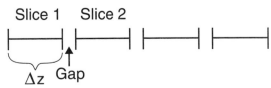

Figure 17-2. Coverage is determined by slice thickness Δz and by the interslice gap. Coverage = # slices × (Δz + gap).

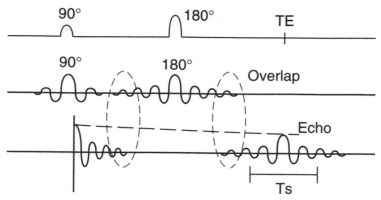

Figure 17-3.   To avoid overlapping of the FID and the side lobes of the 180° pulse, you need to increase TE. This increase is one cause of lengthening the minimum TE.

(c)   increase echo train length (ETL) in FSE imaging (due to longer final TE)

3.   Increasing interslice gap causes:
   (a)   increased coverage
   (b)   decreased "cross-talk" artifact
   (c)   increased SNR (due to increasing effective TR by reducing cross-talk)
   (d)   decreased detection of small lesions (which may lie within the gap)

TE (ECHO TIME)

Question: What happens if we increase or decrease TE?
Answer:

1.   By increasing TE, we:
   (a)   increase T2 weighting
   (b)   increase dephasing and thus decrease SNR (according to the T2 decay curve)
   (c)   decrease number of possible slices (decrease coverage), because

$$\text{\# of slices} \approx TR/TE$$

   (d)   no change in scan time (unless, of course, the coverage is not adequate and either longer TR or extra acquisitions are required)

2.   The reverse is true for decreasing TE:
   (a)   decrease T2 weighting and increase T1 or proton density weighting.
   (b)   increase SNR (less dephasing). However, if TE is reduced by reducing Ts

(i.e., increasing BW), SNR may be reduced!
   (c)   increase coverage
   (d)   no change in scan time

Question: What causes lengthening of TE?
Answer:

1.   TE should be long enough so that the side lobes of the 180° pulse do not interfere with the side lobes of the FID or the echo (Fig. 17-3). Remember that we need a Fourier transform of the RF pulse with a square shape to be able to get ideal contiguous slices. To do this, the RF must be a sinc wave (sinc $t = \sin t/t$) with as many side lobes as possible. This, in turn, will lengthen the 90° and 180° RF pulse.

2.   If TE is so short that it allows interference between the 180° RF pulse and the FID, an FID artifact (or zipper artifact) will appear along the zero frequency line.

Question: How can TE be shortened?
Answer:

1.   One way is to decrease the sampling time Ts. However, this results in a higher bandwidth and therefore a lower SNR (Equation 17-1).

2.   There is a limit as to how short TE could be. The factors limiting minimum TE include
   (a)   duration of RF pulse (especially the 180° pulse)
   (b)   duration of FID

(c) Ts or BW (which influence the SNR)

3. TE can also be shortened by switching to a gradient echo sequence because a 180° refocusing pulse is no longer used.

Contrast on a spin echo technique can be summarized:

Table 17-1

	TR	TE
T_1W	Short	Short
PDW	Long	Short
T_2W	Long	Long

TI (INVERSION TIME)

As we saw in Chapter 7, inversion recovery sequences employ an additional 180° pulse before the 90° pulse.

Advantages

1. Can suppress various tissues by selecting the appropriate TI. More specifically, as we saw in Chapter 7, if

$$TI = .693\ T_1\ (tissue\ x)$$

then tissue x is "nulled" or "suppressed."

2. **STIR** (Short TI Inversion Recovery) sequences suppress fat by selecting

$$TI = .693\ T_1\ (fat)$$

Since at 1.5 Tesla, T_1 of fat is approximately 200 msec, then to null fat, we must select

$$TI = .693 \times 200 \cong 140\ msec.$$

3. **FLAIR** (Fluid-Attenuated Inversion Recovery) sequences suppress fluid by selecting

$$TI = .693\ T_1\ (fluid)$$

This sequence is used, for example, in the brain to suppress CSF to increase the conspicuity of periventricular hyperintense lesions such as MS plaques. Since at 1.5 Tesla, T_1 of CSF is approximately 3600 msec, then to null CSF, we have to select

$$TI = 0.693 \times 3600 \cong 2500\ msec$$

Disadvantages

1. Decreased SNR
2. Decreased coverage (by a factor of about 2 due to the presence of the extra 180° pulse)

Key Points

In this chapter, we discussed the important and practical factors that influence the quality of MR imaging. To improve the quality of the images, it is crucial to have a firm grasp of the parameters that, directly or indirectly, affect the scan. We introduced the primary and secondary parameters that are used to determine MR images (refer to the *Introduction* in this chapter). In a nutshell, the name of the game is "trade-offs." Often, one cannot gain advantage in one area without sacrificing another.

Questions

17-1. For a TR = 1000 ms, 1 NEX, and a 256 × 256 matrix, calculate the scan time for:
(a) a single slice
(b) 10 slices (performed one at a time)
(c) 10 slices performed using a multislice (multiplanar) acquisition

17-2. Calculate the maximum number of achievable slices for a TR = 1000 msec, TE = 80 ms, sampling time Ts = 20 ms, and "overhead-time" $T_0 = 10$.

17-3. The concept of variable bandwidth: in order to improve SNR, the lowest possible BW is selected. Suppose that the BW is halved:

(a)   How is the SNR affected?

(b)   What happens to chemical shift artifacts?

(c)   How does this affect the maximum number of slices?

17-4.   The SNR is proportional to the square root of:

(a)   BW/Nx · NEX

(b)   BW/Ny · NEX

(c)   Ny · NEX/BW

(d)   Ny · BW/NEX

17-5.   The SNR in 3D imaging is equal to the SNR in 2D imaging times the factor:

(a) N_z (b) $\sqrt{N_z}$

(c) N_y (d) $\sqrt{N_y}$

17-6.   The acquisition time in 3D imaging is equal to that in 2D imaging times the factor:

(a) N_z (b) $\sqrt{N_z}$

(c) N_y (d) $\sqrt{N_y}$

17-7.   SNR can be increased by:

(a)   increasing NEX

(b)   decreasing BW

(c)   increasing Ny

(d)   increasing voxel volume

(e)   increasing TR

(f)   decreasing TE

(g)   all of the above

(h)   only (a)–(d)

17-8.   Increasing Ny leads to:

(a)   better resolution

(b)   increased SNR (fixed FOV)

(c)   increased SNR (fixed pixels)

(d)   increase scan time

(e)   all of the above

(f)   only (a), (c), (d)

(g)   only (a), (b), (d)

17-9.   For a 128 square matrix and an FOV of 25 cm, the pixel size is about:

(a)   0.5 mm   (b)   1 mm

(c)   1.5 mm   (d)   2 mm

17-10.   The acquisition time of a single acquisition gradient echo sequence with TR 30, TE 10, NEX 2, Ny 256 for acquiring 15 slices is about:

(a)   15.36 sec   (b)   153.6 sec

(c)   230.4 sec   (d)   15360 sec

(e)   230400 sec

17-11.   Increasing TR leads to an increase in all the following EXCEPT:

(a)   scan time   (b)   SNR

(c)   T1W   (d)   T2W

(e)   coverage

17-12.   Coverage is increased by increasing all of the following EXCEPT:

(a)   slice thickness

(b)   interslice gap

(c)   TR   (d)   BW   (e)   TE

17-13.   Increasing TE leads to a decrease in all of the following EXCEPT:

(a)   T2W   (b)   signal

(c)   coverage   (d)   SNR

17-14.   Minimum TE can be reduced by:

(a)   reducing the duration of the RF pulses

(b)   reducing the sampling time Ts

(c)   increasing the bandwidth

(d)   using a sequence that doesn't use 180° pulses (as in gradient echo)

(e)   all of the above

17-15.   In STIR, TI should be set to:

(a)   1.44 T_1 (fat)

(b) $(1/\sqrt{2})$ T_1 (fat)

(c) $\sqrt{2}$ T_1 (fat)

(d)   0.693 T_1 (fat)

(e)   (1/0.693) T_1 (fat)

17-16.   In FLAIR, TI should be set to:

(a)   0.693 T_1 (fluid)

(b)   (ln 2) T_1 (fluid)

(c) $(-1/ln\ 0.5)$ T_1 (fluid)

(d)   all of the above

18 Artifacts in MRI

INTRODUCTION

MR imaging, as with any other imaging modality, has its share of artifacts. It is important to recognize these artifacts and to have the tools to eliminate or, at least, minimize them. There are many sources of artifacts in MRI. These are summarized as follows:

1. Image Processing Artifacts
   (a) Aliasing
   (b) Chemical shift
   (c) Truncation
   (d) Partial volume
2. Patient-related Artifacts
   (a) Motion artifacts
   (b) Magic angle
3. RF-related Artifacts
   (a) Crosstalk
   (b) Zipper artifact
   (c) RF feedthrough
   (d) RF noise
4. External Magnetic Field Artifacts
   (a) Magnetic inhomogeneity
5. Magnetic Susceptibility Artifacts
   (a) Diamagnetic, paramagnetic, ferromagnetic
   (b) Metal

6. Gradient-related Artifacts
   (a) Eddy currents
   (b) Non-linearity
   (c) Geometric distortion
7. Errors in the Data
8. Flow-related Artifacts

Let's discuss this list in more detail.

IMAGE PROCESSING ARTIFACTS
Aliasing (Wraparound)

Refer to the discussion on *undersampling* in Chapter 12.

SPIN ECHO IMAGING

Let's say we're studying the abdomen (Fig. 18-1). If the field of view only covers part of the body, we know that we may get **aliasing** (wraparound), but what causes the aliasing?

We have a gradient in the x-direction (Gx), with a maximum frequency (f_{max}) at one end of the field of view, and a minimum frequency $(-f_{max})$ at the other end of the FOV. These are the **Nyquist** frequencies (discussed in Chapter 12). Any frequency higher than the maximum frequency allowed by the gradient cannot be detected correctly.

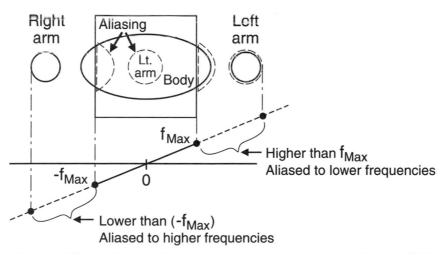

Figure 18-1. For a given FOV and gradient strength, the maximum frequency f_{max} corresponds to the edges of the FOV. Any part outside the FOV will experience a higher frequency. The higher frequencies outside the FOV may be aliased to a lower frequency inside the FOV. This will cause a wraparound artifact.

The gradient doesn't stop at the end of the FOV. The gradient is going to keep going because we still have magnetic fields outside the space designated by the FOV. The parts of the body outside the FOV (in this case, the arms) will be exposed to certain magnetic field gradients. One arm will receive a magnetic field that will generate a frequency higher than f_{max} for the FOV. It may be twice the frequency of f_{max}—twice the intended Nyquist frequency. The computer cannot recognize these frequencies above (f_{max}) or below ($-f_{max}$). They will be recognized as a frequency within the bandwidth. The higher frequency will be recognized as a lower frequency within the accepted bandwidth.

For example, if the higher frequency were 2 kHz higher than (f_{max}), it would be recognized as 2 kHz higher than ($-f_{max}$), and therefore its information would be "aliased" to the opposite side of the image—the side of the FOV that corresponds to the lowest frequencies (Fig. 18-1).

The part of the body and arm on the left side of the patient that are outside the FOV, and are exposed to a higher magnetic field, will have spins oscillating at a frequency higher than (f_{max}). Thus, it will be identified as a structure on the right side of the patient—that side of the image associated with lower frequencies.

Likewise, the arm and body outside the FOV on the right side of the patient will experience spins oscillating at frequencies lower than ($-f_{max}$) and will also be incorrectly recognized by the computer. For example, if the lower frequency were 2 kHz lower than ($-f_{max}$), it would be recognized as 2 kHz lower than (f_{max}), and its information would be "aliased" to the opposite side of the image—the side of the FOV that corresponds to the higher frequencies. This process is also called "**wraparound**"—the patient's arm gets "wrapped around" to the opposite side.

The computer can't recognize frequencies outside the bandwidth (which determines the FOV). Any frequency outside of this frequency range is going to get "aliased" to a frequency that exists within the bandwidth. The "perceived" frequency will be the actual frequency minus twice the Nyquist frequency.

$$f \text{ (perceived)} = f \text{ (true)} - 2f \text{ (Nyquist)}$$

Fig. 18-18 contains examples of wraparound.

3D IMAGING

Wraparound artifact can also be seen in 3D imaging in all three directions.

1. It can be seen along the x and y directions, as with SE.
2. It can also be seen along the slice-select (phase encoded) direction at each end of the slab (e.g., the last slice is overlapped on the first slice as in Fig. 18-19).

EXAMPLE:

Suppose the frequency bandwidth is 32 kHz ($\pm$16 kHz). This means that if we're centered at zero frequency, the maximum frequency $f_{max} = +16$ kHz and minimum frequency ($-f_{max}$) $= -16$ kHz (Fig. 18-1). If we have a frequency in the arm (outside the FOV) of +17 kHz, the perceived frequency will be:

$$f \text{ (perceived)} = +17 \text{ kHz} - 2 \text{ (16 kHz)} = -15 \text{ kHz}$$

Now, the arm, which is perceived as having a frequency of -15 kHz (rather than +17 kHz), will be recognized as a structure with a very low frequency—only 1 kHz faster than the negative end frequency of the bandwidth—and will be identified on the opposite side of the image—the low frequency side.

Remedy:

How do we solve this problem?

1. Surface Coil:

   The simplest way is to devise a method where we don't get any signal from outside the field of view. With the patient in a large transmit/receive coil that covers the whole body, we will receive signal from all of the body parts in that coil—and those parts outside the field of view will result in aliasing. But if we use a **coil** that only covers the area within the field of view, we will only get signal from those body parts within the maximum frequency range—and no aliasing will result. This type of coil is called a **surface coil**. We also use a surface coil to increase the signal to noise ratio.

2. Increase FOV:

   If we double the FOV to include the entire area of study, we can eliminate aliasing. To do so, we have to use a weaker gradient. The maximum and minimum frequency range will cover a larger area and all the body parts in the FOV will be included within the frequency bandwidth; therefore, no aliasing will result (Fig. 18-2). To maintain the resolution, double the matrix with a weaker gradient (Gx). The maximum and minimum frequency range will still be the same as the stronger gradient. They will just be spread out over a wider distance. Remember, to increase the field of view, we have to use a weaker gradient.

3. Oversampling:
   Two types are discussed:

   (a) Frequency oversampling (no frequency wrap, or NFW)
   (b) Phase oversampling (no phase wrap, or NPW)

Frequency Oversampling (NFW)

Frequency oversampling eliminates aliasing caused by **undersampling** in the frequency encoding direction (refer to the sampling theorem in Chapter 12). **Oversampling** can also be performed in the phase encode direction by increasing the number of phase encoding gradients.

Phase Oversampling (NPW)

We can double the field of view to avoid aliasing and, at the end, discard the unwanted parts when the image is displayed (Fig. 18-3). This is called "**no phase wrap**" (NPW) by some manufacturers. It is also called "**phase oversampling**" by other manufacturers. Because Ny is

doubled, NEX is halved to maintain the same scan time. Thus, the SNR is unchanged. (The scan time might be increased slightly because **overscanning** performs with slightly more than ½ NEX.)

4. Saturation Pulses:
   If we saturate the signals coming from outside the FOV, we can reduce aliasing.
5. 3D Imaging:
   In 3D imaging, if we see this artifact along the slice-select axis, we can simply discard the first and last few slices.

Chemical Shift Artifact

The principle behind the chemical shift artifact is that the protons from different molecules precess at slightly different frequencies. For example, look at fat and H_2O. A slight difference exists between the precessional frequencies of the hydrogen protons in fat and H_2O. Actually, the protons in H_2O precess slightly faster than those in fat. This difference is only 3.5 parts per million (ppm). Let's see what this means by an example:

EXAMPLE 1:
Consider a 1.5T magnet. The precessional frequency is as follows:

1. Frequency $= \omega_0 = \gamma B_0$
   $= (42.6 \text{ MHz/T}) (1.5T)$
   $\approx 64 \text{ MHz} = 64 \times 10^6 \text{ Hz}$
2. 3.5 ppm $= 3.5 \times 10^{-6}$
3. $(3.5 \times 10^{-6}) (64 \times 10^6 \text{ Hz}) \cong 220 \text{ Hz}$

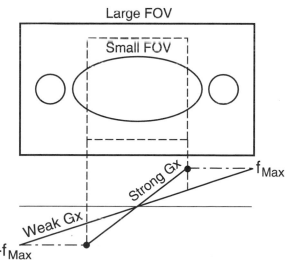

Figure 18-2. To avoid aliasing, increase the FOV.

Acquire data but
eliminate from image

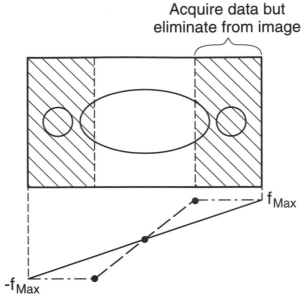

Figure 18-3. In No Phase Wrap, aliasing is avoided by doubling the FOV in the y direction and, at the end, discarding the unwanted part of the image.

In other words, at 1.5 Tesla, the difference in precessional frequency of the hydrogen protons in fat and in H_2O is 220 Hz.

EXAMPLE 2:

We now have a 0.5T magnet. The precessional frequency of protons in a 0.5T magnet is 1/3 of a 1.5T magnet. The frequency difference is then

$$1/3 \ (220 \ Hz) = 73 \ Hz$$

Therefore, at 0.5 Tesla, the difference in precessional frequency of the hydrogen protons in fat and in H_2O is only 73 Hz. In other words, if we use a **weaker magnet**, we will get **less chemical shift**.

How does this affect the image? Chemical shift artifacts are seen in the orbits, along vertebral endplates, in the abdomen (at organ/fat interfaces), and anywhere else fatty structures abut watery structures. In a 1.5T magnet, the sampling time (Ts) is usually about 8 msec. Let's take 256 frequency points in the frequency encoding direction.

$$BW = N/Ts$$
$$= 256/8 \ msec$$
$$BW = 32 \ kHz$$

These formulas show that the entire frequency range (i.e., bandwidth) of 32 kHz covers the whole length of the image in the x-direction. Because we have the FOV of the image in the x-direction divided into 256 pixels, each pixel is going to have a frequency range of its own,

32 kHz = 256 pixels

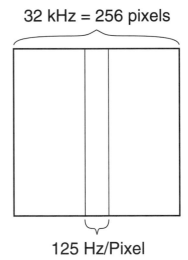

125 Hz/Pixel

Figure 18-4. At 1.5T with a BW of 32 kHz and 256 pixels, there will be about 125 Hz/pixel (32 kHz/256 = 125 Hz), i.e., there is 125 Hz of information in each pixel. This may be a better way of describing the BW of a scanner because there is no ± confusion.

i.e., each pixel has its own bandwidth:

$$Bandwidth/pixel = 32 \ kHz/256$$
$$\therefore BW/pixel = 125 \ Hz$$

(This representation of BW on a "per pixel" basis is used by Siemens and Picker. It has the advantage of less ambiguity than the ± 16 kHz designation, should the "±" be deleted.) Thus, each pixel contains 125 Hz of information (Fig. 18-4). Stated differently, the pixel "**bin**" contains

125 Hz of frequencies. Now, because fat and H_2O differ in the precessional frequency of hydrogen by 220 Hz at 1.5 Tesla, how many pixels does this difference correspond to?

pixel diff = 220 Hz/125 Hz/pixel ≈ 2 pixels

This means that fat and H_2O protons are going to be **misregistered** from one another by about 2 pixels (in a 1.5T magnet using a standard ± 16 kHz bandwidth). (Actually, it is *fat* that is misregistered because position is determined by assuming the resonance property of water.) If pixel size Δx = 1 mm, this then translates into 2 mm misregistration of fat.

MATH: For the mathematically interested reader, it can be shown that

$$\text{Chem shift} = \frac{3.5\,\gamma\,B}{BW/Nx} \text{ (in pixels)}$$

$$= \frac{3.5 \times \gamma\,B}{BW/Nx} \times \frac{FOV}{Nx}$$

$$= \frac{3.5\,\gamma\,B \times FOV}{BW} \text{ (in mm)}$$

where γ = 42.6 MHz/T, B is the field strength (in Tesla), BW is the bandwidth (in Hz), and FOV is the field of view (in cm).

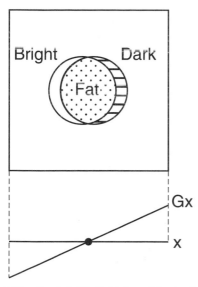

Figure 18-5. Chemical shift effect between fat and water causes a bright band towards the lower frequencies (due to overlap of fat and water at lower frequencies) and a dark band towards the higher frequencies (due to subtraction of fat and water signals).

Let's now consider chemical shift artifact visually (Fig. 18-5). Remember that H_2O protons resonate at a higher frequency compared with the hydrogen protons in fat. With the polarity of the frequency-encoding gradient in the x-direction set such that higher frequencies are toward the right, H_2O protons are relatively shifted to the right (towards the higher frequencies) and fat protons are relatively shifted to the left (towards the lower frequencies). This shifting will result in overlap at lower frequency and signal void at higher frequency. This in turn leads to a *bright band* toward the lower frequencies and a *dark band* toward the higher frequencies on a T1 or proton density-weighted conventional spin echo image. (On a T2W CSE, fat is dark so the chemical shift artifact is reduced. Unfortunately, on a T2W FSE [fast spin echo—see Chapter 19], fat is bright and the chemical shift artifact is seen.) We will see this misregistration artifact anywhere that we have a fat/H_2O interface. Also remember that this fat/H_2O chemical shift artifact only occurs in the frequency encoding direction (in a conventional spin echo).

EXAMPLE: VERTEBRAL BODIES:
With frequency encoding direction—in this case going up and down (and "up" having higher frequency)—the fat in the vertebral body would be misregistered down, making the lower endplate bright due to overlap of water and fat, and the top endplate dark due to water alone (Fig. 18-6). If we increase the pixel size, the misregistration artifact will increase.

Figure 18-20 contains examples of chemical shift artifact.

Question: What factors increase chemical shift artifact?
Answer:

1. *A stronger magnetic field strength.*
2. *A lower BW:*
   If we decrease the bandwidth, we have a lower bandwidth per pixel and fewer frequencies/pixel. As an example, if instead of 32 kHz, we have a 16 kHz bandwidth, then

$$\text{bandwidth/pixel} = 16 \text{ kHz}/256$$
$$= 62.5 \text{ Hz/pixel}$$

Now, each pixel covers 62.5 Hz, but the chemical shift is still 220 Hz. Consequently,

$$220 \text{ Hz}/62.5 \text{ Hz/pixel}$$
$$\cong 4 \text{ pixel misregistration.}$$

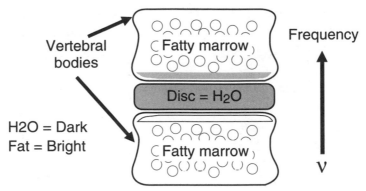

Figure 18-6. Chemical shift artifact in the vertebral endplates produces a dark band in the inferior endplates and a bright band in the superior endplates (assuming the frequency-encode direction to be upward).

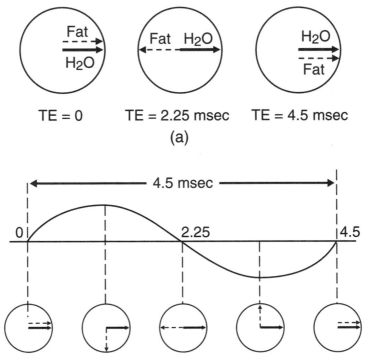

Figure 18-7. Chemical shift effect of the second kind. Fat and water protons get in and out of phase at various values of TE. Specifically, they are in phase at TE of 0, 4.5 msec, 9 msec, and out of phase at TE of 2.25 msec, 6.75 msec, and so on. This effect can be represented graphically by a sine function.

Decreasing bandwidth results in increased chemical shift artifact.

This is one of the side effects of selecting a lower BW on your scanner. Unfortunately, the chemical shift due to field strength and that due to BW are independent and additive; thus, higher field-low BW techniques have the worst chemical shift artifact.

3. Smaller pixels:
    If we keep the BW of 32 kHz and the FOV the same but increase the number of frequency encoding steps to 512 (instead of 256), the pixel bin will have half as many frequencies:

    $$\text{pixel bin} = 32 \text{ kHz}/512$$
    $$= 62.5 \text{ Hz/pixel}$$

    again leading to a greater chemical shift as above (i.e., 4 pixels instead of 2).

Solution—How can you fix chemical shift artifacts?

1. Get rid of fat using fat suppression. If there is no signal from fat, there can be no chemical shift. This can be done with a spectroscopic "fat sat" pulse or a STIR sequence.
2. Increase pixel size by keeping FOV the same and decreasing Nx (*tradeoff:* deteriorates resolution).
3. Lower the magnet's field strength (not practical!).
4. Increase bandwidth (*tradeoff:* lowers SNR).
5. Switch phase and frequency directions. This will just change the direction of the chemical shift.
6. Use a long TE (causes more dephasing and less signal from fat).

CHEMICAL SHIFT OF THE "SECOND KIND"

This phenomenon applies to gradient echo techniques (see Chapters 20 and 21). As discussed previously, fat and water protons precess at slightly different frequencies in the transverse plane (220 Hz at 1.5 T). Because water precesses faster, it gets 360° *ahead* of fat after a short period of time. Thus, there will be times (TE) when fat and water spins will be totally in phase and times when they will be 180° out of phase. At 1.5 Tesla, fat and water are in phase every 4.5 msec. This number is derived by the following:

$$\text{frequency difference between fat and water} = 220 \text{ Hz}$$
$$\text{period} = 1/\text{frequency} = 1/(220 \text{ Hz})$$
$$= .0045 \text{ sec} = 4.5 \text{ msec}$$

In Fig. 18-7, fat and water are in phase initially at TE = 0, go out phase at TE = 2.25, and are back in phase at TE = 4.5. In general, at 1.5T,

fat and H_2O go in and out of phase every 2.25 msec. This is called a **chemical shift effect of the second kind**.

Boundary Effect

If the selected TE is 2.25, 6.75, 11.25, 15.75 msec, and so on, fat and water protons will be out of phase and a dark boundary will be seen around organs that are surrounded by fat (such as the kidneys and muscles). This result is called the **boundary effect,** which is the result of chemical shift of the "second kind." This type of imaging is referred to as "**out of phase**" scanning, referring to the fact that at these TEs, fat and water spins will be 180° out of phase. This phenomenon does not just occur along the frequency encoding axis (like with the chemical shift artifact of the first kind) because it is a result of fat and water protons phase cancellation in all directions. (Boundary effect does not occur in conventional SE techniques because of the presence of the 180° refocusing pulse, which is absent in gradient-echo techniques.)

Remedy:

1. Make fat and H_2O in phase by picking appropriate TE.
2. Switch phase and frequency.
3. Increase the BW (*tradeoff:* decreases SNR).
4. Use fat suppression.

Truncation Artifact (Gibbs Phenomenon)

This artifact occurs at high contrast interfaces (e.g., skull/brain, cord/CSF, meniscus/fluid in the knee) and causes alternating bright and dark bands which may be mistaken for lesions (e.g., pseudo syrinx of the spinal cord or pseudo tear of the knee meniscus).

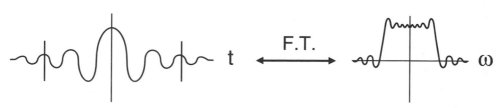

Figure 18-8.   Truncation artifact causes a ring-down effect because the FT of a truncated sinc function has ripples at its edges.

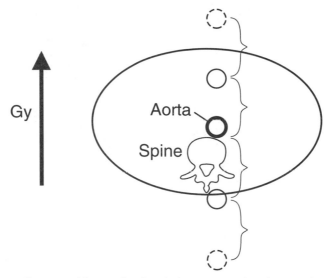

Figure 18-9.   Ghost artifacts are equidistant replica of a pulsating structure, such as the aorta, along the phase direction.

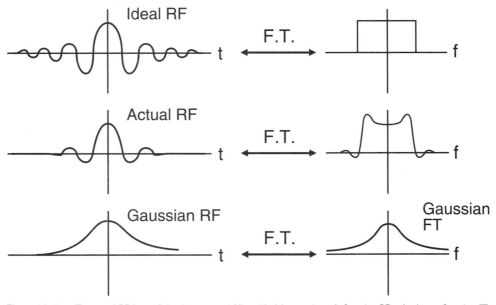

Figure 18-10.   The actual RF has a finite time span, yielding side lobes or rings. A Gaussian RF pulse has a Gaussian FT.

The cause is inability to exactly approximate a steplike change in the signal intensity due to a limited number of samples or sampling time. The ripples in Figure 18-8 are responsible for the parallel bands seen at such sharp interfaces. This artifact is seen mostly in the phase direction (because we typically have few pixels and lower resolution in phase compared to frequency). Incidentally, the correct term is "truncation artifact." "Gibbs phenomenon" refers to the infi-nitely thin discontinuity that still persists with an infinite number of pixel elements.

Figure 18-21 contains examples of truncation artifact.

Remedy:

1.   Increase sampling time to reduce the ripples (remember, a wider signal in time domain means a narrower one in frequency domain).

2. Decrease pixel size:
   (a) increasing the number of phase encodes, or
   (b) decreasing the FOV

Partial Volume Artifact

This artifact has the same concept as CT. To reduce it, decrease the slice thickness (Δz). Figure 18-22 contains an example of partial volume artifact.

PATIENT-RELATED ARTIFACT

This artifact is caused by voluntary or involuntary patient motion, and by the patient's anatomy. Pulsating motion in vessels is also an interesting source of motion related artifacts. (More on this on later chapters.)

Motion Artifact

Motion artifact is caused by the patient's (voluntary or involuntary) movements (**random**) or by pulsating flow in vessels (**periodic**). We only get motion artifacts in the *phase encoding* direction.

Question: Why is motion artifact only seen in the phase-encode direction?
Answer: The reason is twofold:

1. First of all, motion along any magnetic field gradient results in abnormal phase accumulation which mismaps the signal along the phase encode gradient.

2. Also, there is a significant asymmetry in the data space (see Chapter 13) so that it takes much less to sample the signal via frequency encoding (on the order of milliseconds) than to do a single phase-encode step (on the order of seconds). Thus, most motions experienced during clinical MRI are much slower than the rapid sampling process along the frequency-encode axis. This disparity between frequency and phase encoding periods allows motion artifacts to be propagated mainly along the phase-encode axis. Motion artifacts along the frequency-encode axis may occur, but they are insignificant (at best, they may cause minimal blurring).

PERIODIC MOTION

Periodic motion is caused by pulsating or periodic motion of vessels, heart, or CSF. In the example in Figure 18-9 (also Fig. 18-23), with a cross section of the body through the aorta, and with the phase encoding in the AP direction, we will get "ghost" artifacts of the aorta equally separated. The artifacts become fainter with increasing distance from the original structure. The separation SEP between the "ghosts" is given by:

$$SEP = \frac{(TR)\,(Ny)\,(NEX)}{T(motion)}$$

Another way of expressing this is

$$SEP = Acquisition\ Time/T(motion)$$

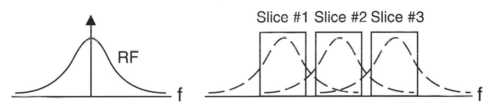

Figure 18-11. Side lobes of the FT of RF pulses (such as in the case of Gaussian curves) may overlap, causing crosstalk.

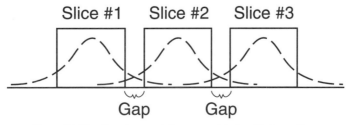

Figure 18-12. To reduce crosstalk, gaps are introduced between slices.

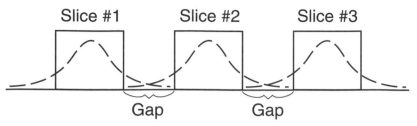

Figure 18-13.   The larger the interslice gap is, the less crosstalk is observed.

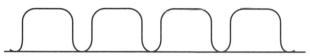

Figure 18-14.   The closer the profile of the RF pulse (actually its FT) is to a rectangle, the better we can achieve contiguous slices without encountering crosstalk.

where T(motion) is the period of motion of the object (in this case, the aorta).

EXAMPLE:

The aorta pulsates according to the heart rate. If the heart rate is

$$HR = 60 \text{ beats/minute} = 60 \text{ bpm}$$
$$= 1 \text{ beat/second}$$

then the period of motion = T (motion) = 1 second.

This means that we have a pulsation every 1 second. For example, if we have a TR = 500 msec = 0.5 sec, NEX = 1, Nx = 256, then

$$SEP = 0.5 \times 256/1 = 128/1 = 128 \text{ pixels.}$$

Therefore, we get two ghosts in the image. If the heart rate is 120 bpm, then we get

$$SEP = 128/.5 = 256 \text{ pixels}$$

and only one ghost.

$$\frac{(TR)\,(Ny)\,(NEX)}{T(motion)}$$
$$= \text{Separation between ghosts (in pixels)}$$

If we multiply this by pixel size, we get the distance between the "ghosts." Therefore, if we increase TR, number of phase encoding steps, or NEX, we can increase the separation of ghosts so that they won't be so numerous within the body part we're studying. More rapidly pulsating flow (i.e., shorter period) also causes more separation. If the FOV is too small, the "ghost" images outside the FOV might get "aliased" into the FOV. The ghosts may be dark or bright depending on the phase of the pulsating structure with respect to the phase of the background. (If

they are in phase, they'll be bright and, if out of phase, dark).

Remedy:

1. Use spatial presaturation pulses to saturate inflowing protons and reduce the artifacts.
2. Increase separation between ghosts by increasing TR, Ny, or NEX (which is tantamount to increasing scan time).
3. Swap phase and frequency: while this only changes the direction of the artifacts, it does allow differentiation between a true lesion and an artifact.
4. Use cardiac gating.
5. Use flow compensation.

RANDOM MOTION

Random motion is caused by the patient's voluntary or involuntary movements (e.g., breathing, changing position, swallowing, tremors, coughing). It causes blurring of the image (Fig. 18-24). We may get parallel bands in the phase encoding direction as well. Although this may simulate truncation artifacts, it is different in that truncation causes *fading* parallel bands.

Remedy:

1. Patient instruction: Don't move! (probably the most useful remedy)
2. Respiratory compensation (RC) (uses chest wall motion pattern to reorder scan and minimize motion)
3. Use of glucagon in the abdomen to reduce artifacts due to bowel peristalsis
4. Sedation

5. Pain killers
6. Faster scanning (FSE, GRE, EPI, etc.); sequential 2D rather than 3D scanning.

CSF FLOW EFFECTS

Dephasing of protons due to CSF motion may sometimes simulate a lesion. Flow compensation techniques can reduce this effect (Fig. 18-25). Examples include the following:

1. Pseudo aneurysm of basilar artery due to pulsatile radial motion of CSF around it.
2. Pseudo MS plaques in the brain stem due to CSF flow in the basal cisterns.
3. Pseudo disc herniation, again secondary to CSF flow.

Remedy:

1. Be certain that "lesions" are seen on all pulse sequences (artifacts tend to only be seen on one image).
2. Use cardiac gating.
3. Use flow compensation.

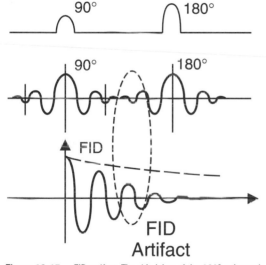

Figure 18-15. FID artifact. The side lobes of the 180° pulse and the FID may overlap, causing a zipper artifact at zero frequency along the phase direction.

Magic Angle Artifacts

In imaging the joints, if a tendon is oriented at a certain angle (55°) relative to the main magnetic field, then the tendon appears brighter on T1 and PD weighted images, but normal on T2 weighted images (Fig. 18-26). This artifactual increased intensity might potentially be confused with pathology.

Collagen, which is responsible for the majority of tendon composition, has an **anisotropic** structure. This anisotropic structure has properties that vary with the direction of measurement and is responsible for dependence of T2 of tendons on their orientation. (**Isotropic** structures, however, have properties independent of their orientation.)

At the magic angle, the T2 of the tendon is slightly increased. This increase is negligible when TE is long. However, when TE is short (as in T1 or PD weighted images), the result is increased signal intensity. The mathematics behind this T2 prolongation has to do with some of the mathematical terms in the Hamiltonian going to zero at $\theta = 55°$.

MATH: This "**magic angle**" effect is the solution to the equation

$$3(\cos\theta)^2 - 1 = 0 \rightarrow (\cos\theta)^2 = 1/3$$
$$\text{or } \cos\theta = \sqrt{1/3}$$

which is calculated to be $\theta \approx 55°$. The above equation comes from a complicated mathematical theory dealing with the so-called **dipolar Hamiltonian**.

RF-RELATED ARTIFACTS
Crosstalk

We have already discussed this issue in previous chapters. The problem arises from the fact that the Fourier transform of the RF pulse is not

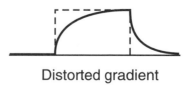

Figure 18-16. Eddy currents result from rapid on and off switching of the gradients and cause distortion in the gradient profile and thus the image.

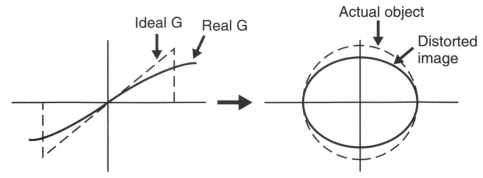

Figure 18-17. Nonlinearities in the gradient cause distortion in the image. For instance, a circle may appear elliptical.

a perfect rectangle but rather has side lobes (Fig. 18-10). We shall use a simpler version of the RF profile as in Figure 18-11. If we consider two adjacent slices, there will be an overlap in the FT of their RF pulses (Fig. 18-11). Crosstalk causes the effective TR per slice to decrease (due to saturation of protons by the RF signals for adjacent slices). Thus, more T1 weighting will result (this is particularly problematic for PD- and T2-weighted images). Also, due to reduced effective TR, the SNR will decrease.

In short, crosstalk causes increased T1 weighting and decreased SNR.

Remedy:

1. Gaps can be introduced between adjacent slices (Fig. 18-12).
2. Two acquisitions with 100% gaps can be interleaved.
3. The RF pulse can be lengthened to achieve a more rectangular pulse profile.

Let's discuss these in more detail:

1. If we increase the gap between slices, we reduce crosstalk (Fig. 18-13). The *trade-off* is an increase in the unsampled volume and the increased potential for missing a small lesion located within the gap.
2. It doesn't matter which way we order the slices (we can do slice #1, then slice #3, then slice #2, etc.). Adjacent slices still will be sharing a certain frequency range and cause crosstalk. The only way to eliminate crosstalk is to do two separate sequences each with a 100% gap, such as:

    First sequence: odd slices 1,3,5,7, ...
    Next sequence: even slices 2,4,6,8, ...

This is the technique of "true" interleaving. Interleaving within a *single* sequence will not totally eliminate crosstalk, although it might reduce it somewhat. The interslice gap in this case is usually 25% to 50% of the slice thickness and a simple sequence is performed. Interleaving in the true sense, however, will double the scan time because it employs two separate sequences. Figure 18-27 demonstrates the value of introducing gaps in reducing crosstalk effects.

CONTIGUOUS SLICES

The RF pulse on newer scanners more closely approximates a rectangular wave (Fig. 18-14). With this feature, we may have a 10% to 20% interslice gap without significant crosstalk. However, with reduced interslice gap, we reduce coverage and need more slices. Remember, we are talking trade offs again.

RF Zipper Artifact

This artifact is one form of **central artifacts** (the other form is RF feedthrough, discussed later). They are referred to as **zippers** due to the formation of a central stripe of alternating bright and dark spots along the *frequency*-encode axis (at zero phase) as in Figure 18-28. Two sources of zipper artifacts are discussed here:

FID ARTIFACTS

FID Artifacts occur due to overlapping of side lobes of the 180° pulse with the FID, before it has had a chance to completely decay (Fig. 18-15). This overlapping causes a "zipper" artifact along the *frequency*-encode direction.

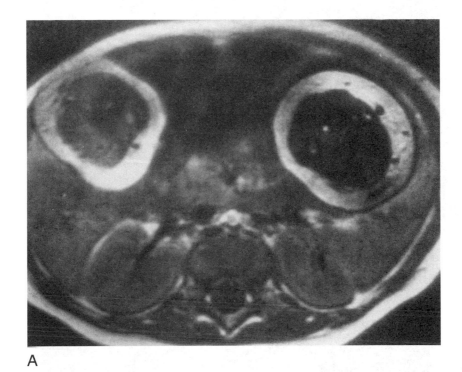

A

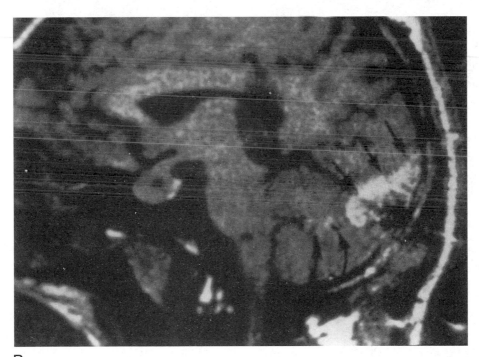

B

Figure 18-18.   Wraparound artifact. **(a)** Wraparound of the patient's arms. **(b)** Wraparound of the patient's nose.

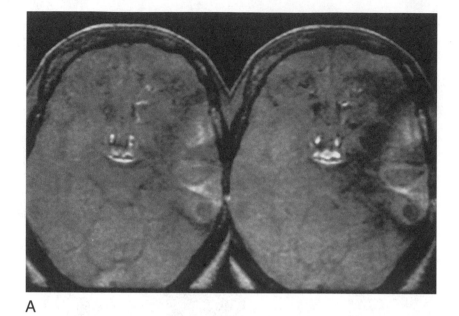

A

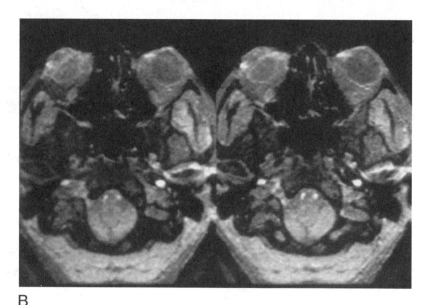

B

Figure 18-19.   Wraparound in 3D. The artifacts in the proximal slice **(a)** are caused by wraparound of the distal slice **(b)**.

Remedy:

1. Increase the TE (increases the separation between the FID and the 180° RF pulse).
2. Increase slice thickness (Δz). This in effect results from selecting a wide RF bandwidth which narrows the RF signal in time domain, thus lowering chances for overlap.

SIMULATED ECHO

This artifact also appears as a narrow or wide-band noise in the center along the *frequency-*encoding axis. The mechanism is similar to FID artifacts. In this case, imperfect RF pulses of adjacent slices or imperfect 90° − 180° − 180° pulses of a dual-echo sequence form a simulated echo that may not be phase-encoded, thus ap-

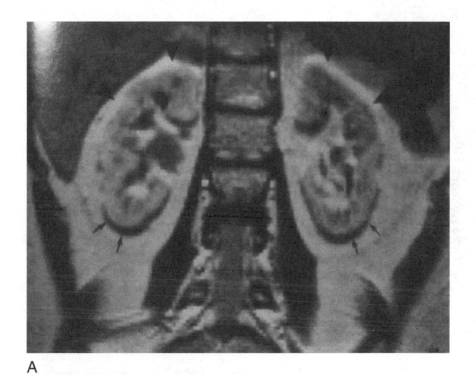

A

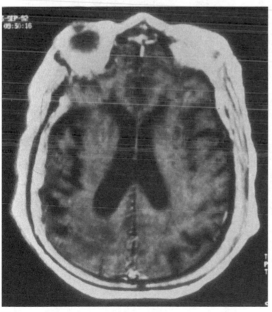

B

Figure 18-20.   Chemical shift artifact. **(a)** Dark and bright bands are seen along frequency-encode direction at kidney-fat interfaces. **(b)** Pseudo subdural hematoma due to chemical shift artifact at brain-fatty marrow interface.

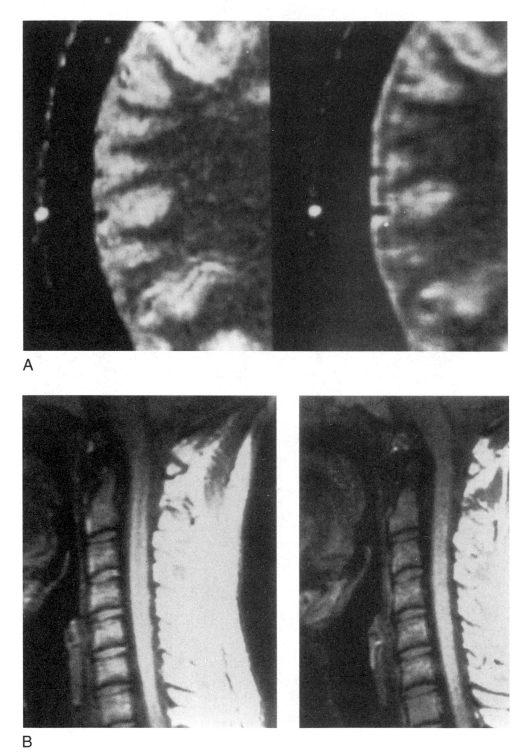

Figure 18-21. Truncation artifact: **(a)** at skull-brain interface; **(b)** producing a pseudo syrinx; **(c)** producing a pseudo meniscal tear.

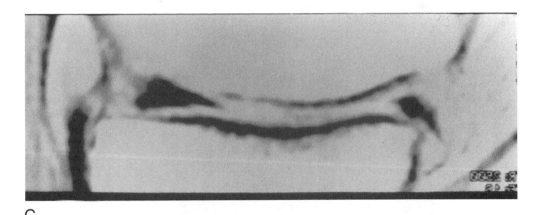

C

Figure 18-21.   Continued.

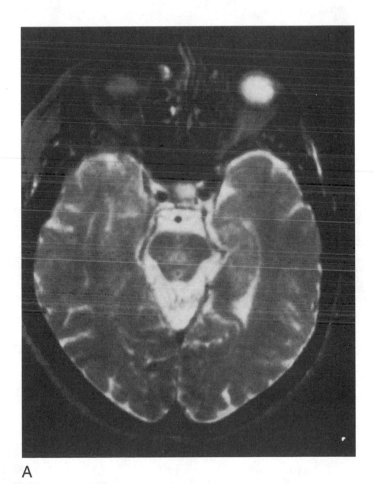

A

Figure 18-22.   Partial volume artifact. The apparent lesion in the brain stem in **(a)** is due to partial increase in volume of CSF in the interpeduncular cistern **(b)**.

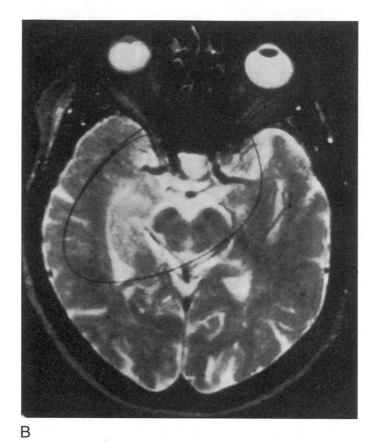

B

Figure 18-22.   Continued.

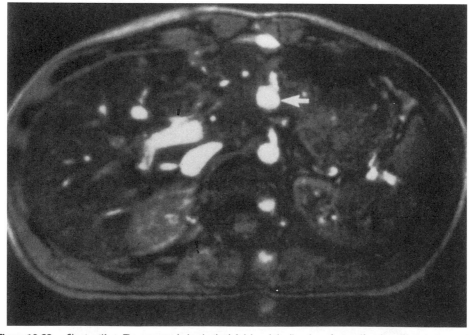

Figure 18-23.   Ghost artifact. The apparent lesion in the left lobe of the liver is a ghost artifact from the pulsating aorta.

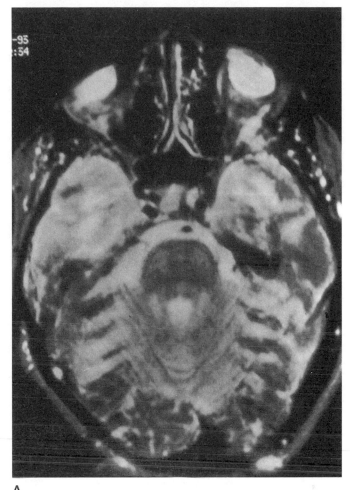

A

Figure 18-24. **(a)** Patient motion can cause pseudo lesions as in the brain stem. **(b)** Repeat study with less motion.

pearing in the central line along the frequency encode axis.[a]

Remedy:

1. Use spoiler gradients.
2. Adjust the transmitter.
3. Call the service engineer.

RF Feedthrough Zipper Artifact

This artifact occurs when the *excitation* RF pulse is not completely gated off during data acquisition and "feeds" through the receiver coil. It appears as a "zipper" stripe along the *phase-encoding* axis at *zero* frequency (Fig. 18-29).

---

[a] For more details, see Stark DD, Bradley WG. Magnetic resonance imaging. Vol. 1. 2nd ed. St. Louis: Mosby, 1992.

Remedy:

Alternate the phase of the excitation RF pulses by 180° on successive acquisitions; the averaged phase-alternated excitations will essentially eliminate RF feedthrough.

RF Noise

RF noise is caused by unwanted *external* RF noise (e.g., TV channel, a radio station, a flickering fluorescent light, patient electronic monitoring equipment). It is similar to RF feedthrough except that it occurs at the specific frequency (or frequencies) of the unwanted RF pulse(s) rather than at zero frequency (Fig. 18-30).

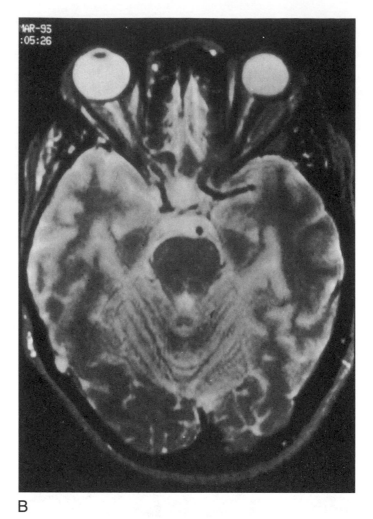

B

Figure 18-24. Continued.

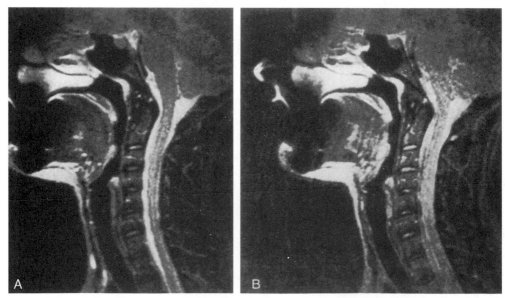

Figure 18-25. The flow compensation technique **(a)** reduces CSF motion artifacts **(b)**.

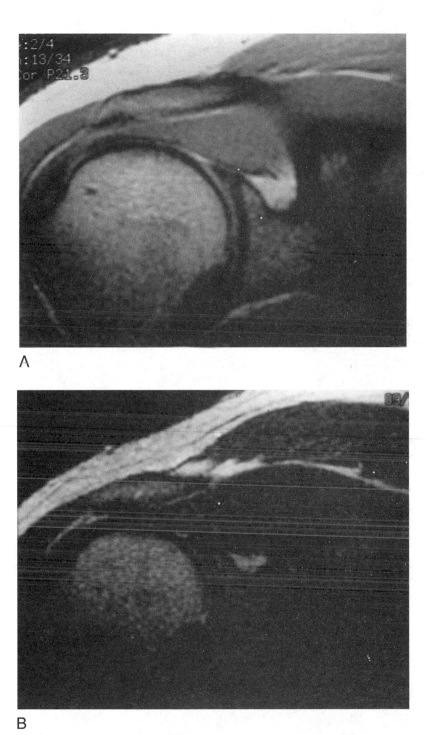

A

B

Figure 18-26.   Magic angle artifact causes increased signal in the supraspinatus tendon on a PDW image **(a)**. The tendon appears normal on the corresponding T2W image **(b)**.

Remedy:

1. Improve RF shielding.
2. Remove monitoring devices if possible.
3. Shut the door of the magnet room!

EXTERNAL MAGNETIC FIELD ARTIFACTS

Artifacts related to B_0 are usually caused by magnetic inhomogeneities. These nonuniformities are usually due to improper shimming or environmental factors and can lead to image distortion (Fig. 18-31). They can be reduced in spin echo and fast spin echo imaging by using 180° refocusing pulses. They can be a source of image inhomogeneity when a fat suppression technique is used.

In gradient echo (GRE) imaging, small spatial nonuniformities cause **moiré fringes** (zebra pattern) due to the overlay of the primary image and aliased overlay.

Remedy:

Appropriate **shimming coils** (**auto shimming**) can minimize the problem.

MAGNETIC SUSCEPTIBILITY ARTIFACTS

As discussed in Chapter 2, all substances get magnetized to a degree when placed in a magnetic field, and their **magnetic susceptibility** (denoted by the Greek symbol χ) is a measure of how magnetized they get.

There are three types of substances—each with a different magnetic susceptibility—commonly dealt with in MRI: paramagnetic, diamagnetic, and ferromagnetic. These substances were described in Chapter 2 and are briefly reviewed here:

1. **Diamagnetic** substances with no unpaired electrons have negative magnetic susceptibility χ (i.e., $\chi < 0$ and $\mu = 1 + \chi < 1$). They are basically nonmagnetic. The vast majority of tissues in the body have this property. Figure 18-32 contains an example.
2. **Paramagnetic** substances contain unpaired electrons and have a small positive χ (i.e., $\chi > 0$ and $\mu > 1$) and are weakly

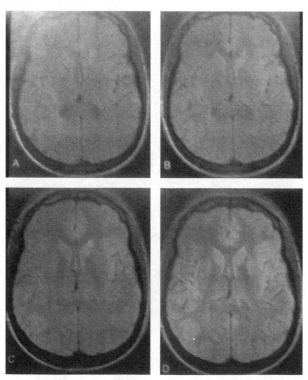

Figure 18-27.   Crosstalk effect before (**[a]–[b]**) and after (**[c]–[d]**) an increase in the interslice gaps.

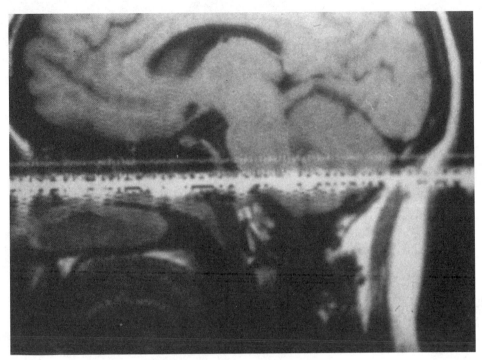

Figure 18-28.   Zipper artifact at zero phase.

attracted by the external magnetic field. The rare-earth element **gadolinium** (Gd) with seven unpaired electrons is a strong paramagnetic substance. Gd is a member of the **lanthanide** group in the periodic table. The rare-earth element **dysprosium** (Dy) is another strong paramagnetic substance that belongs to this group. Certain breakdown products of hemoglobin are paramagnetic: deoxyhemoglobin has four unpaired electrons, and methemoglobin has five. Hemosiderin, the end-stage of hemorrhage, contains, in comparison, more than 10,000 unpaired electrons. It is in a group of substances referred to as **superparamagnetic** with magnetic susceptibilities 100 to 1000 times stronger than paramagnetic substances. Figure 18-33 demonstrates paramagnetic effect of deoxyhemoglobin.

3. **Ferromagnetic** substances are strongly attracted by a magnetic field and have a large positive χ, even larger than that of superparamagnetic substances. Three types of ferromagnets are known: iron (Fe), cobalt (Co), and nickel (Ni). Figures 18-34 and 18-35 contain examples of this type of artifact.

Susceptibility artifacts in MRI occur at interfaces of differing magnetic susceptibilities, such as at tissue-air and tissue-fat interfaces (examples include paranasal sinuses, skull base, and sella). These differences in susceptibilities leads to a distortion in the local magnetic environment, causing dephasing of spins with signal loss and mismapping (artifacts). Ferromagnetic substances (such as metallic clips and foreign bodies) with their large susceptibilities lead to substantial field distortion and artifacts.

Question: Which MR technique is least sensitive to magnetic susceptibility effects?
Answer: In decreasing order, gradient echo (GRE), followed by conventional spin echo (CSE), followed by fast spin echo (FSE). FSE is least sensitive to magnetic susceptibility effects due to the presence of multiple refocusing 180° gradients. On the contrary, GRE is the most sensitive due to lack of a 180° pulse.

Figure 18-29. RF feedthrough causes a zipper artifact at zero frequency along the phase direction.

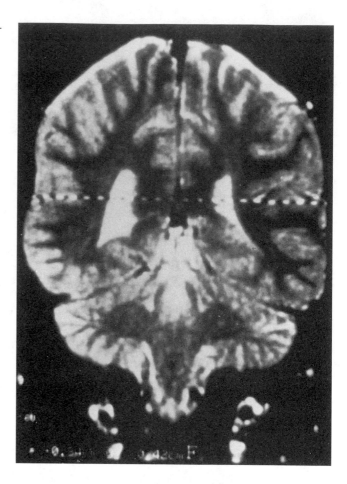

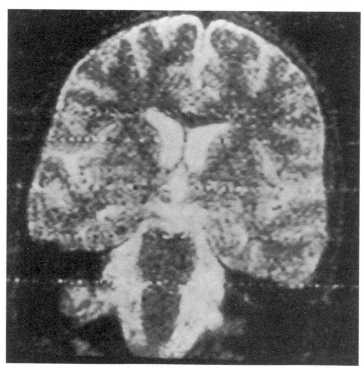

Figure 18-30. RF noise artifact.

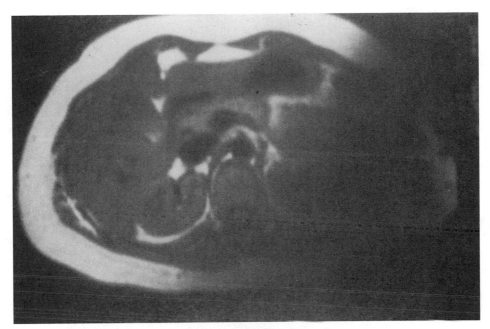

Figure 18-31.   Magnetic inhomogeneity artifact.

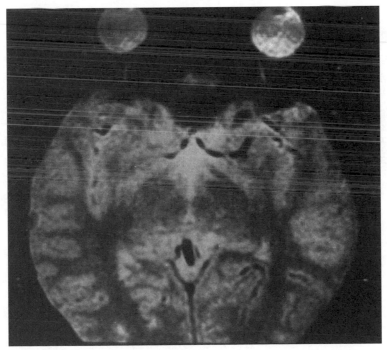

Figure 18-32.   Diamagnetic susceptibility artifact caused by air in the sphenoid sinus.

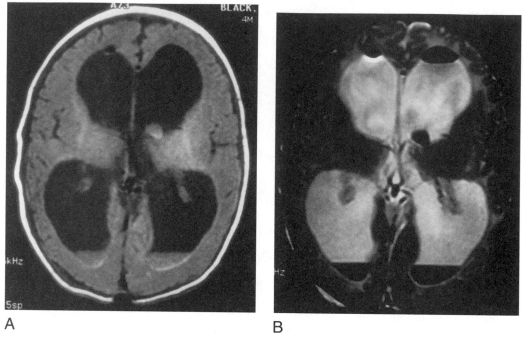

Figure 18-33. Paramagnetic effect of deoxyhemoglobin in the left lateral effect on T1W **(a)** and T2W **(b)** images.

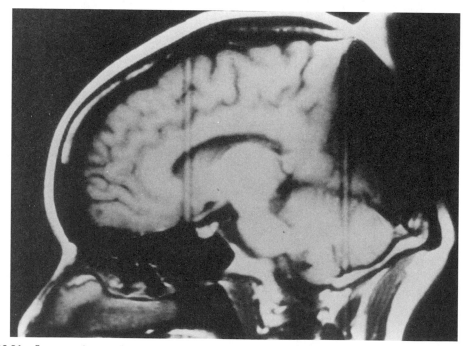

Figure 18-34. Ferromagnetic susceptibility artifact caused by local magnetic field distortions related to a metallic object (shunt reservoir).

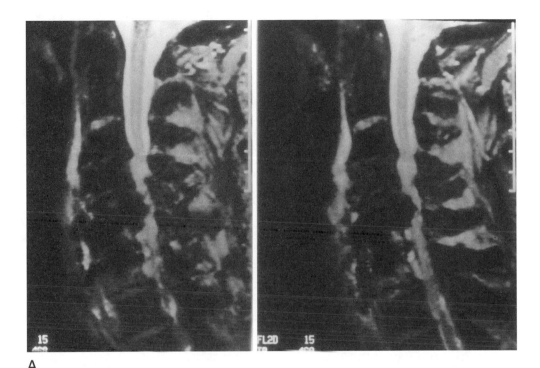

A

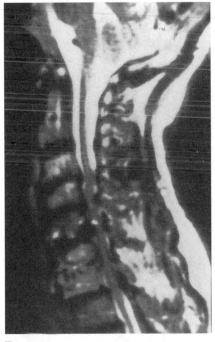

B

Figure 18-35.   Susceptibility artifacts from post surgical changes are more pronounced on gradient echo techniques **(a)** compared with spin echo and fast spin echo techniques **(b)**.

GRADIENT-RELATED ARTIFACTS
Eddy Currents

Eddy currents are small electric currents that are generated when the gradients are rapidly switched on and off (i.e., the resulting sudden rises and falls in the magnetic field produce elec-tric currents). These currents will result in a distortion in the gradient profile (Fig. 18-16) and in turn cause artifacts in the image (Fig. 18-36).

Nonlinearities

Ideal gradients are linear. However, as in other aspects of life, there is no such thing as an ideal gradient. These nonlinearities cause local magnetic distortions and image artifacts. The effect is similar to artifacts related to B_0 inhomogeneities.

Geometric Distortion

Geometric distortion is a consequence of gradient nonlinearities or gradient power drop-off. Figure 18-17 illustrates this concept. The real gradient has dampened peaks, causing image distortion (e.g., a circle may appear elliptical). An example is presented in Figure 18-37 where the abdomen has an exaggerated ovoid appearance. You need to call your service engineer to fix this.

ERRORS IN THE DATA

Errors in the data are caused by a single calculation error in processing the data related to the k-space of a single slice. The result is a crisscross striation artifact that is present across a single image and not present on any other image.

Remedy:

1. Delete the discrete error and average out the neighboring data.
2. Simply repeating the sequence solves the problem.

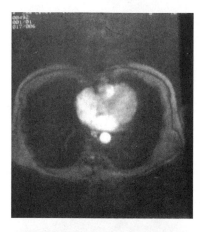
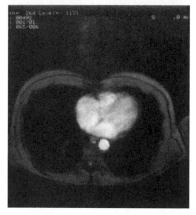

Figure 18-36.   Image distortions caused by eddy currents (top image) are reduced after proper correction (bottom image).

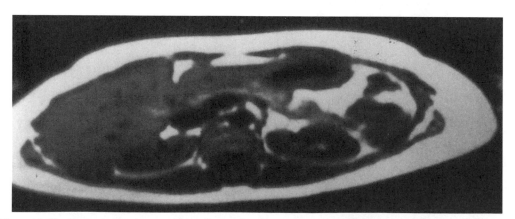

Figure 18-37.   Geometric distortion caused by gradient nonlinearities makes the abdomen have an exaggerated ovoid appearance.

FLOW-RELATED ARTIFACTS

Motion artifacts were discussed previously, including periodic flow artifacts. Other flow related phenomena are discussed in Chapters 25 and 26.

Key Points

In this chapter, we discussed the most common and important causes of potential artifacts in MR imaging that every MR radiologist should be aware of. For a list of these artifacts, refer to the introduction in this chapter. There are a few other less significant sources of artifacts which were not discussed in this chapter.

Questions

18-1.   Regarding chemical shift artifact:
(a)   protons in fat resonate at 3.5 ppm higher than protons in water
(b)   at 1.5 T it is about 220 Hz
(c)   at 1.5 T and for a 32 kHz BW and 256 × 256 matrix, it is about 2 pixels
(d)   all of the above
(e)   only (b) and (c)

18-2.   (a)   Determine the chemical shifts (in terms of numbers of pixels) for the following situations (assume 256 frequency-encoding steps):

B_0	.2 T	.5 T	1.0 T	1.5 T
BW				
50 kHz				
10 kHz				
4 kHz				

(b)   Repeat this table in terms of mm given an FOV = 24 cm = 240 mm.
(c)   What is your conclusion?

18-3.   Periodic motion causes "ghost" artifacts along the phase-encoding direction. The number of *pixels* between two consecutive ghosts is given by (SEP = separation)

$$SEP = TR . NEX . Ny/T$$
$$= Acq. \ time/T$$

where T = period of the oscillating motion.

(a)   Calculate SEP for the aortic ghosts (HR = 60 bpm, i.e. T= 1 sec) when TR = 200 ms = 0.2 sec, NEX = 1, Ny = 256.
(b)   What is the maximum number of ghosts you could potentially see along the phase-encoding axis in example (a)?
(c)   What is the effect of increasing NEX?

18-4.   Wraparound can be reduced by all of the following EXCEPT:
(a)   using a surface coil
(b)   decreasing the FOV
(c)   using presaturation pulses
(d)   using a no phase wrap option
(e)   using a no frequency wrap option

18-5.   Chemical shift in general can be represented by:
(a)   3.5 γ B . Nx/BW
(b)   3.5 γ B . FOV/BW
(c)   3.5 γ B/(BW . Nx)
(d)   both (a) and (b)

18-6.   T/F   Chemical shift artifact causes a bright band toward the higher frequency and a dark band toward the lower frequency at a water/fat interface.

18-7.   Chemical shift is decreased by all of the following EXCEPT:
(a)   lowering the bandwidth
(b)   using a fat suppression technique
(c)   using a lower field magnet
(d)   using a longer TE

18-8.   T/F   Fat and water protons get out of phase at TE of odd multiples of 2.25 msec.

18-9.   Truncation artifacts can be reduced by all of the following EXCEPT:
(a)   decreasing pixel size
(b)   increasing sampling time
(c)   increasing Ny
(d)   increasing FOV

18-10.   (a)   Calculate the separation (in pixels and mm) between aortic ghosts for TR 500, NEX 1, Ny 128, HR 80 bpm, and FOV 20 cm.
(b)   What is the maximum number of ghosts you could potentially see within the FOV?

18-11.   The number of ghost artifacts can be reduced by all of the following EXCEPT:
(a)   flow compensation
(b)   presaturation pulses
(c)   decreasing Ny
(d)   increasing TR

18-12.   Motion artifacts can be reduced by all of the following EXCEPT:
(a)   fast scanning   (b)   sedation
(c)   3D imaging
(d)   flow compensation

18-13.   CSF flow can lead to all of the following artifacts EXCEPT:
(a)   pseudo MS plaques in the brain stem

(b)   pseudo disc herniation
(c)   pseudo basilar artery aneurysm
(d)   pseudo syrinx

18-14.   T/F   Magic angle artifact demonstrates increased signal on proton density images in a tendon that is positioned perpendicular to the main magnetic field.

18-15.   Cross talk artifact can be reduced by all of the following EXCEPT:
(a)   increasing the gradient strength
(b)   increasing interslice gaps
(c)   double acquisition with 100% gaps interleaved
(d)   improving the RF profile

18-16.   Paramagnetic elements include all of the following EXCEPT:
(a)   gadolinium   (b)   cobalt
(c)   dysprosium
(d)   methemoglobin

18-17.   Truncation artifacts include:
(a)   pseudo meniscal tear
(b)   pseudo syrinx
(c)   pseudo MS plaques
(d)   all of the above
(e)   only (a) and (b)
(f)   only (a) and (c)

Part II   Fast Scanning

19 Fast Spin Echo

INTRODUCTION

In this chapter, we will discuss the elegant and cunning technique of fast spin echo. This technique was first proposed by Hennig et al.[a] and was called **RARE** (rapid acquisition with relaxation enhancement). However, it is commonly referred to as **fast spin echo (FSE)** or **turbo spin echo (TSE)**. Different manufacturers have different names for it (Table 19-1).

Consider the pulse sequence diagram in Figure 19-1. This pulse sequence can be used for either a conventional spin echo or a fast spin echo study.

CONVENTIONAL SPIN ECHO (CSE OR SE)

Let's first talk about a conventional spin echo study and again see how the lines in k-space are filled in. With a conventional spin echo, immediately after the 90° RF pulse, an **FID** (free induction decay) is formed. At a time TE after the first 90° pulse (time TE/2 after the first 180° refocusing pulse—17 msec in our example), we receive the first spin echo. We have a whole train of 180° refocusing pulses, after each of which we get another echo. Each echo is a multiple of 17 msec. Notice that each successive echo has less amplitude as a result of T2 decay.

In a conventional spin echo sequence, we often get two echoes, i.e., we apply two 180° RF pulses and get back an echo from each pulse, each with a different TE. However, we *could* have as many echoes as we want in a conventional spin-echo sequence. In our example, we have an 8-echo sequence, all easily occurring within the time of one TR.

With each TR in a conventional spin echo, we have a single phase-encoding step. Each of the echoes following each 180° pulse is obtained after a single application of the phase-encoding gradient in conventional spin echo. Each echo

has its own k-space, and each time we get an echo, we fill in one line of k-space (Fig. 19-1).

In conventional spin echo, each k-space will generate a different image, i.e., we'll get a first echo image, a second echo image, and so on, with eight 180° pulses generating eight echoes. We'll have eight different k-spaces and eight different images. If we had 256 different phase-encoding steps, we would do this 256 different times. The scan time would be

Scan Time
$$= (TR)(number\ phase\text{-}encodes)(NEX)$$

Within the scan time, we'll get eight images, one of each TE echo. If we were only interested in the last echo image, we wouldn't have to bother with filling in the k-spaces for the first seven echoes. However, the first seven echoes come "free." We don't save any time by not doing them because we have to wait out the time it takes to get to the last echo anyway. In a dual echo conventional SE sequence, the first echo is always "free"—it doesn't cost any time. (However, as we shall see later, that isn't true with Fast Spin Echo).

Thus, for each k-space in conventional spin echo, we repeat the TR 256 times (each at a different phase-encoding gradient) and fill in the k-space for each echo with 256 different lines. For an eight echo train, we get eight different images.

FAST SPIN ECHO (FSE)

By using the same example, we can see how FSE works. Fast Spin Echo is a very elegant way of manipulating the conventional spin echo technique to save time. Again, we'll start with a train of eight echoes (ETL = 8). However, now we will only have one k-space. We'll fill this

---

[a] Hennig J et al. RARE imaging: a fast imaging method for clinical MR. Magn Reson Med 1986;3:823–833.

Table 19-1

Manufacturer	Name
GE, Picker, Hitachi, Toshiba	Fast Spin Echo (FSE)
Siemens, Philips	Turbo Spin Echo (TSE)

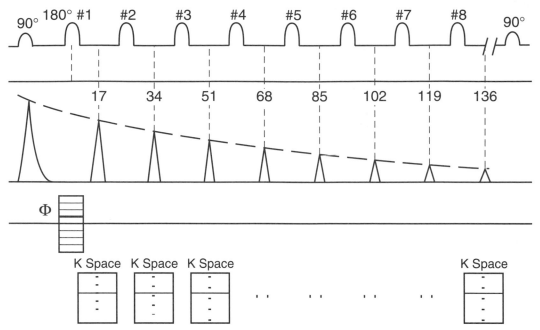

Figure 19-1. A spin-echo PSD with eight echoes. The echo spacing (ESP) is 17 msec.

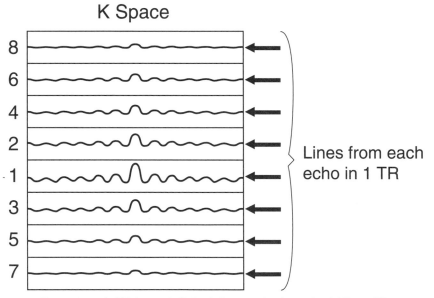

Figure 19-2. In FSE, k-space is filled eight lines at a time in one shot (within one TR).

k-space eight lines at a time (Fig. 19-2). Instead of having eight separate k-spaces, one for each echo, we will have one k-space using the data from all eight echoes.

Within the time of 1 TR (one "shot"), we will get eight lines, one from each echo, in the single k-space. With the next TR, we'll accumulate 8 more lines, one from each echo, and we'll also put them into the same k-space (Fig. 19-3).

For each shot/TR, we will fill in another eight lines into the single k-space. Because we have a total of 256 lines in k-space, and because during each TR we are filling in eight lines of k-space at a shot, then we only have to repeat the process

32 times (i.e., 256/8 = 32) to fill 256 lines of k-space.

In conventional spin echo, it took one TR for each line of k-space. Therefore, in a conventional spin echo study, we have to repeat the TR 256 times. In this manner, we have cut the time of the study by a factor of eight.

EXAMPLE:
Acquisition time of conventional SE sequence with TR = 3000, Ny = 256, NEX = 1 is

SE time = (TR) (number of phase-encoding steps)(NEX)
= (3000)(256)(1) msec
= 12.8 minutes

This time for the FSE sequence with TR = 3000 is

FSE time = (TR)(number of phase-encoding steps/ETL)
(NEX)
= (3000)(256/8)(1) msec
= 1.6 minutes

In this example, we have shortened the time of the study from 12.8 minutes to 1.6 minutes, a factor of eight times faster than the conventional spin echo study.

ECHO TRAIN LENGTH (ETL)

ETL refers to the number of echoes used in FSE. The ETL can be even (e.g., GE scanners) or odd (e.g., Siemens scanners) and ranges typically from 3 to 32. The time interval between succes- sive echoes (or between 180° pulses) is called the **echo spacing (ESP)**. A typical ESP is on the order of 16–20 msec at typical high field BW of 32 kHz (±16 kHz).

Figure 19.4 is an example. Let's say we want an image with contrast reflecting a TE of approxi- mately 100 msec. In FSE, the only TEs we can choose are integral multiples of the echo spacing (ESP = 17 msec in our example). This is called the "**Effective TE**" (TE_{eff}). We will see shortly that this is *not* a true TE. Therefore, in our exam- ple, TE_{eff} = 102 msec (= 6 × 17 msec).

Remember that the center of k-space has max- imum signal, and as we go out to the edges of k-space, we get less and less signal. Therefore, if we divide k-space into 8 slabs of 32 lines each (one slab for each echo), the *center slab* will be assigned to the sixth echo, i.e., the echo corre- sponding to the chosen effective TE = 102 msec (Fig. 19-5).

In FSE, before *each* 180° pulse, we place a different value of the phase-encoding gradient. For the 180° pulse before the echo we choose as the effective TE (in this case, 102 msec), we use a phase-encoding gradient with the lowest strength. Each subsequent phase-encoding step will have a gradient with more and more ampli- tude. This increase will result in the most signal coming from the echo at 102 msec (because this signal is obtained with a minimum phase

K Space

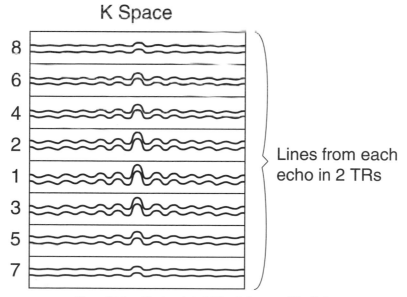

Lines from each echo in 2 TRs

Figure 19-3. After two shots, 16 lines in k-space will be filled.

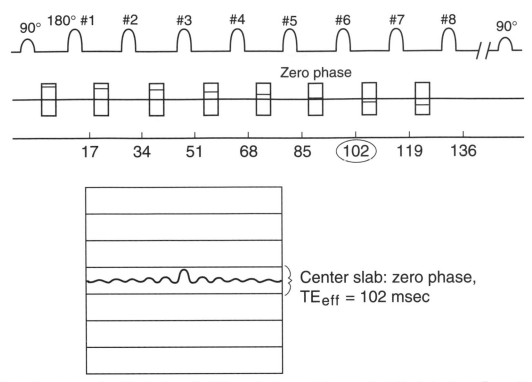

Figure 19-4. An example of FSE with effective TE of 102 msec. The phase gradient corresponding to this echo in minimum. The associated echo is placed in the center row of k-space.

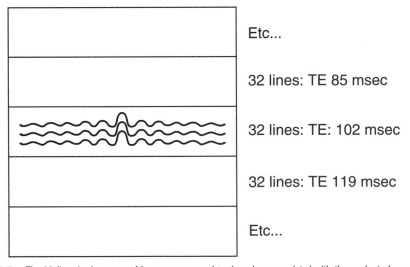

Etc...

32 lines: TE 85 msec

32 lines: TE: 102 msec

32 lines: TE 119 msec

Etc...

Figure 19-5. The 32 lines in the center of k-space correspond to the echoes associated with the weakest phase gradients.

gradient) and decreasing signal from all the other echoes because their signals are obtained with increasing phase-encoding gradients (Fig. 19-6).

In the next TR, we again pick a phase-encoding step for the sixth echo which will be close to zero gradient and all the other phase-encoding steps will be close to their previous respective

gradient values, so that again the maximum signal during this TR will be obtained from echo 6 (TE 102 msec) and progressively weaker signals will be obtained from the other echoes.

The signals from the sixth echo (from the first TR to the 32nd TR) will all be placed in the center of k-space (Fig. 19-5). The signals from the other echoes will be placed in the other slabs. The echoes that experience progressively greater phase-encoding gradients (and therefore less signal) fall into slabs further away from the center slab, and those echoes experiencing the weakest phase-encoding gradients (and therefore having more signal) are placed closer to the center slab. k-space is organized so that the greatest amount of signal comes from the center of k-space and the least amount of signal comes from the periphery of k-space.

Therefore, if we choose an echo train length of 8 echoes, we will have 8 slabs in k-space, with each slab containing 32 lines from 32 shots. Echo slab corresponds to a different echo. Let's see what the echo looks like (Fig. 19-6).

Because the center slab belongs to the lowest phase-encoding gradient, it will have the least amount of dephasing. The signal received at TE = 102 msec will have the greatest amplitude. As we go farther away from 102 msec in either direction, the signal amplitude will get progressively smaller because the phase-encoding gradients get progressively larger.

By definition, the maximum signal comes at the effective TE time. But we still get echoes from the other TEs that do not help our contrast. The signal from these other echoes are all in the same k-space. Even though the respective signal amplitudes from the other TEs are progressively smaller, the further away in time they are from the TE_{eff}, they still contribute to the contrast from the TE_{eff}. This is why it is called an "**effective TE**" and not a true TE.

In a way, what we are doing is *averaging* the echoes, although it is a *weighted average*. By appropriately picking the slabs, we put most of the *weight* on the echo corresponding to 102 msec (the effective TE), and less weight on the other echoes. As we go away from the center slab of k-space, we are reducing the weighting, i.e., we are reducing the contribution of the data on that slab to the effective echo.

The previous example gives us a long TR/long TE, which is a T2-weighted image. Now we want to do a proton density weighted image with a long TR/short TE and an effective TE of approx 30 msec (Fig. 19-7). In this case, we would assign the center slab of k-space to correspond to the second echo, i.e., TE = 34 msec. The echo with maximum magnitude will be at a TE of 34 msec, and the magnitude of the signal would fall off progressively with subsequent echoes. This is because, now, the second echo will be assigned the weakest phase-encoding gradients, and the subsequent echoes will have progressively stronger phase-encoding gradients.

Remember that with the effective TE of 34 msec, we are still getting the cumulative signal from the entire echo train of 8 echoes. So even information from an echo corresponding to a TE of 136 msec (8 × 17=136) is contributing to the signal of the effective TE of 34 msec, which we don't want. Therefore, for a T1-weighted study, we usually pick a smaller echo train length such as 4. With an ETL of 4, we would only do four phase-encoding steps. Thus, k-space would only have 4 slabs, and the longest

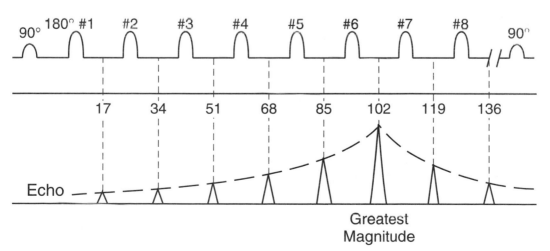

Figure 19-6. The echo corresponding to eff. TE of 102 msec has the largest peak.

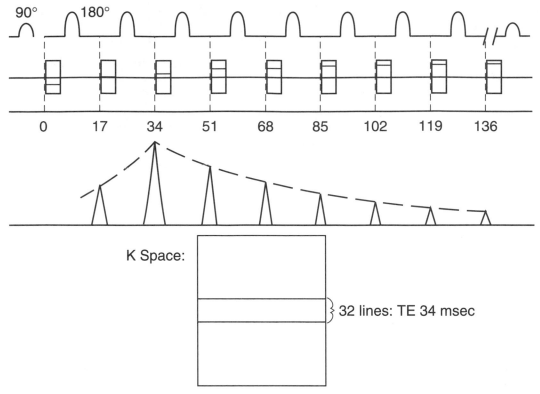

Figure 19-7. Another example with eff. TE of 34 msec. Here, the largest echo corresponds to TE of 34 msec.

echo contributing to the contrast of the shortest effective TE (e.g., 17 msec) would be the echo at 68 msec (4 × 17 = 68). This will eliminate the T2 effect on a T1-weighted image caused by the signal contribution of the longer echo times.

Question: *What happens to the time it takes to do a fast spin echo study when we decrease the ETL from 8 to 4?*
Answer: *The time of the study will be reduced only by a factor of 4, rather than by a factor of 8.*

Question: *If we have an ETL of 8, how many lines of k-space do we fill in with each TR?*
Answer: *We fill in 8 lines of k-space with each TR, each line going to a separate slab within k-space.*

Question: *How many times do we have to repeat the TR to fill up k-space with 256 lines?*
Answer: *In general, we have to repeat it by the following ratio:*

$$\frac{Ny}{ETL} = \frac{number\ of\ phase\text{-}encoding\ steps}{Echo\ train\ length}$$

Remember that scan time is calculated by the following formula:

$$Scan\ time\ (FSE) = \frac{(TR)(Ny)(NEX)}{ETL}$$

The numerator of the formula is the same as for a conventional spin echo study:

$$Scan\ time\ (CSE) = (TR)(Ny)(NEX)$$

The difference in fast spin echo is that the numerator is divided by the echo train length. So, in the case of an 8 ETL study, the number of times we would have to repeat the TR (i.e., the number of shots) to complete 256 lines in k-space would be

$$256/8 = 32$$

In the case of a 4 ETL study, we would fill four lines of k-space with each TR. The number of times we would have to repeat the TR to complete 256 lines in k-space is now

$$256/4 = 64\ times$$

EXAMPLE 1:

1. Consider a T2-weighted study with TR = 3000 msec, Ny = 256 and NEX = 1, and let's compare the scan time between CSE and FSE (using a TE_{eff} = 102 msec and an ETL = 8).

$$\text{Scan time (FSE)} = \frac{(TR)(Ny)(NEX)}{ETL}$$
$$= (3 \sec)(256)(1)/8$$
$$= 1.6 \text{ minutes}$$
$$\text{Scan time (CSE)} = (TR)(Ny)(NEX)$$
$$= (3 \sec)(256)(1) = 12.8 \text{ minutes}$$

2. Repeat the above for a T1-weighted study with TR = 500 and FSE using ETL = 4

$$\text{Scan time (FSE)} = (TR)(Ny)(NEX)/ETL$$
$$= (0.5 \sec)(256)(1)/4 = 32 \sec$$
$$\text{Scan time (CSE)} = (TR)(Ny)(NEX)$$
$$= (0.5 \sec)(256)(1) = 128 \sec$$
$$= 2 \text{ minutes, 8 seconds}$$

TRADE-OFFS

What are the *trade-offs* of FSE Imaging?

1. Slice coverage:

    As we increase the echo train length to increase the speed of the exam, we also *decrease* the *number of slices* we can do in a study (Fig. 19-8). In one TR, with an 8 ETL, we can fit in so many slices. If we use the same TR, but now use an echo train length of 16, it will take twice as long to receive the echo (i.e., 16 × 17 msec = 272 msec), because now we have to accumulate data from 16 echoes (each a multiple of 17 msec). Because the time it takes to accumulate 16 lines of k-space is double the time it takes to accumulate 8 lines, we can fit in only half the number of slices into one TR.

Therefore, the trade-off is that we decrease the number of slices as we increase the echo train length.

$$\uparrow ETL \rightarrow \uparrow \text{ speed}$$
$$\leftrightarrow \downarrow \text{ coverage } (\downarrow \text{ \# slices})$$

One way to get around this is to *increase TR*. Although increasing TR increases scan time, we save so much time by using a long ETL compared to conventional spin echo that we can afford a longer TR. We don't need to be limited anymore to a TR of 3000 msec. We can go up to 4000–6000 msec, get more coverage, and still save time.

Let's say we need a coverage of 15 5-mm slices with a 2 mm gap to cover an area of interest (like the brain):

EXAMPLE 2:

Let's choose TR = 3000 msec, ETL = 8, NEX = 1, Ny = 256

The number of slices we can do in any TR depends on the length of the longest echo (we'll leave out sampling time for now):

$$\text{number of slices} \leq TR/TE$$

In the case of an ETL of 8, the longest echo is 136 msec (17 × 8 = 136). So,

$$\text{number of slices} \leq TR/TE$$
$$= 3000 \text{ msec}/136 \text{ msec} \cong 22 \text{ slices}$$

This formula is regardless of TE_{eff} we pick. The scan time for this example would be

$$\text{Scan time} = \frac{(TR)(Ny)(NEX)}{ETL}$$
$$(3000 \text{ msec})(256)(1)/8 = 1.6 \text{ min}$$

Therefore, we can do 22 slices in 1.6 minutes with an ETL of 8.

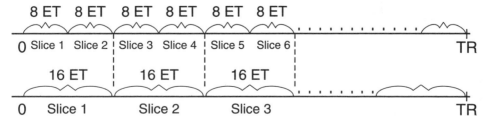

Figure 19-8. Increasing the ETL causes a reduction in coverage (number of slices).

EXAMPLE 3:

Let's now chose a different ETL:

$$ETL = 16, NEX = 1, Ny = 256, TR = 3000 \text{ msec}$$

With an ETL of 16 (since echoes are multiples of 17 msec), the longest echo would be 272 msec (16 × 17 = 272). So,

$$\text{the number of slices} = TR/TE$$
$$= 3000 \text{ msec}/72 \text{ msec} \cong 11$$
$$\text{Scan time} = \frac{(TR)(Ny)(NEX)}{ETL}$$
$$= \frac{(3000)(256)(1)}{16} \cong 0.8 \text{ min}$$

With an ETL of 16, we can do only 11 slices, but in 0.8 minutes. The scan is faster, but we have limited coverage, and we have not accomplished the minimum of 15 slices we needed for the exam.

EXAMPLE 4:

To increase the coverage with an ETL of 16, let's now increase the TR:

$$TR = 4500, ETL = 16, Ny = 256, NEX = 1$$

Now,

$$\text{number slices} \le TR/TE$$
$$= 4500/72 \text{ msec} \cong 16 \text{ slices}$$
$$\text{scan time} = \frac{(TR)(Ny)(NEX)}{ETL}$$
$$= \frac{(4500)(256)(1)}{16} \cong 1.2 \text{ min}$$

Even though we have limited coverage with an ETL of 16, we resorted to increasing the TR to 4500 msec, which allowed us a coverage of 16 slices (enough to cover the 15 slices we needed for the exam), and we were still able to keep the scan time below the scan time required for an ETL of 8.

Sometimes, you'll look at a scan and find that it took twice as long to do the study than you thought it would. What happens sometimes is that the technologist will try to get a coverage that is too wide for the TR chosen. If nothing is corrected, the machine will "default" to performing *two* separate acquisitions to provide the coverage, thus making the exam twice as long. With a simple calculation to allow either increasing the TR slightly or increasing slice thickness slightly, you could more efficiently rectify the situation.

MULTI-ECHO FSE

Consider the case of 8 echoes again. With conventional spin echo, we would have 8 k-spaces and the first seven echoes would come "free." That's not true for fast spin echo. Every single one of the echoes is used to fill in a line in a k-space. If we want to do double echo imaging, we have twice as many lines in k-space to fill (in 2 k-spaces). Thus, we either have to 1) give up half of the echoes per ETL, in which case the scan time is going to be doubled, or 2) repeat the scan twice, and again the scan time is increased. Therefore, regardless of the way we do it, it's going to cost us time.

In FSE, the first echo is no longer "free!"

There are three ways to get a double echo image with FSE:

1. Full echo train
2. Split echo train
3. Shared echo

Full Echo Train

In a full echo train, all echoes in the train contribute to the image. Thus, the full ETL is completed for Effective TE_1 before Effective TE_2 is performed. In other words, two separate concatenated sequences are acquired. For example, for an ETL of 8 and a 256 × 256 matrix (Fig. 19-9), 32 echo trains would be required to fill k-space (8 × 32 = 256).

Split Echo Train

In a split echo train, the first half of the echo train contributes to the image with Effective TE_1 and the second half to Effective TE_2 (thus, two k-spaces are created). For example, for an ETL of 8 (Fig. 19-10), only 4 echoes would be applied to each Eff. TE. Therefore, 64 trains would be required to fill k-space (4 × 64 = 256).

Shared Echo

In a shared echo approach, the first and last echoes in the train are emphasized for TE_1 and TE_2, respectively, and the echoes in between are shared for both images. This approach has the advantage of shorter ETL compared with a full

Full Echo Train

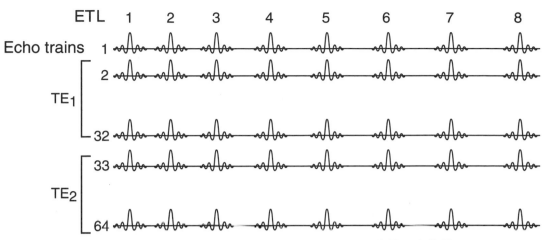

Figure 19-9. In a full echo train, the entire echo train is completed for eff. TE1 and eff. TE2.

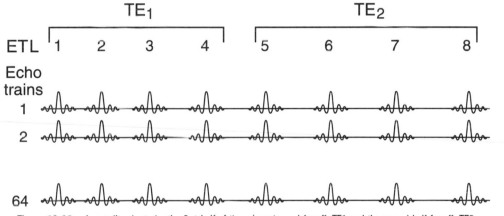

Figure 19-10. In a split echo train, the first half of the echoes is used for eff. TE1 and the second half for eff. TE2.

or split echo train approach, allowing more slices to be acquired for a given TR [since the number of slices is roughly determined by TR divided by the product of ESP and ETL, i.e., # slices $\cong$ TR/(ETL $\times$ ESP)].

In Figure 19-11, an ETL of 5 is used and four lines of k-space are filled per TR, three of which are the same for the first and second echo images. (Thus, there is some overlap of the "information" in the two images, compared to the four split echo approach.) Filling four echoes per pass provides the same efficiency as a split echo approach, i.e., 64 echo trains will be required to fill k-space (4 $\times$ 64 = 256). However, the shorter ETL allows 60% more slices to be acquired in the same time. Let's prove this mathe-

matically:

slices (ETL = 5) $\div$ # slices (ETL = 8)
$$= (TR/5 \times ESP) \div (TR/8 \times ESP)$$
$$= 8/5 = 1.6 = 100\% + 60\%.$$

A variant of the shared echo approach is the so-called "**keyhole**" imaging. In this technique, k-space is covered completely on the first image, but only the central portion (e.g., 20%) of k-space is covered on subsequent images, providing most of the contrast (recall that the center of k-space contains most of the signal). This approach has a disadvantage in that the high spatial frequency outer portion (e.g., 80%) of k-space is shared information; however, it has the advantage of speeding up the subsequent

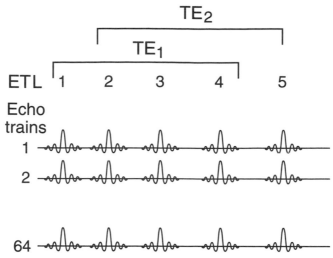

Figure 19-11. In a shared echo approach, the first and last echoes are emphasized for TE1 and TE2, respectively, and the rest are shared between the two echoes. In this example, the ETL is 5 and the central three echoes are shared.

imaging by a factor of 5 (100% ÷ 20% = 5). Thus, keyhole imaging is useful when fast repetitive imaging of the same slice is required, e.g., for perfusion imaging.

Each of the previous methods has its advantages and disadvantages. The advantages of the full echo train approach are full flexibility in selecting the TE_{eff} and the ETL for both the first and the second echoes; the disadvantage is more contrast averaging.

The disadvantage of the split echo approach is that the effective TE_2 is constrained in the second half of the echo train. For example, for an ETL of 16 and ESP of 17 msec, the minimum Eff. TE_2 is 9 × 17 = 153 msec, which might be longer than desired. The advantage is less contrast averaging and crisper images. In general, the split echo train is used for ETLs of eight or less, whereas the full echo train is used for ETLs greater than eight.

The advantage of the shared echo approach is increased coverage (number of slices). The disadvantage is an overlap of information between the two echo images.

Advantages of FSE

1. The scan time is decreased (which allows faster scanning).
2. The S/N ratio is maintained because we still have 256 phase-encoding steps.

3. The increased speed allows for high-resolution imaging in a reasonable amount of time. An example is 512 × 512 imaging through the internal auditory canals with very long TR.
4. Motion artifacts will be less severe. Because the 180° pulses are evenly spaced, there is a natural **even-echo rephasing** effect. For instance, CSF motion artifacts are much less severe on FSE than on CSE images.
5. The rephasing from the multiple 180° pulses leads to less distortion from metallic objects on FSE images (see Chapter 18. Also see the discussion below on magnetic susceptibility).
6. Similarly, FSE images are much more tolerant of a poorly shimmed magnet than are CSE images.

Disadvantages of FSE

1. Reduced coverage, i.e., decreased number of slices.
2. Contrast averaging ("k-space averaging") so that:

   (a) **CSF is brighter on proton density weighted FSE images**. This is caused by the effect of averaging all the echoes into a single k-space. We are still contributing data from very long TEs into the proton density image, even though the weighting is toward the lower TE. Therefore, we will have some T2 effect (i.e., bright CSF) on a short TE_{eff}. To alleviate this problem, either use a shorter echo train length (to exclude longer TEs) or a higher BW (to decrease ESP and the minimum effective TE).

(b) *Pathology*: **MS plaques and other lesions at the brain-CSF interface may be missed on FSE.** CSF appears brighter on FSE proton density images (as discussed above) and, therefore, the distinction between CSF and periventricular high intensity plaques is more difficult. As in (a), to alleviate this problem, use a shorter ETL, which helps exclude longer TEs in the echo.

3. **Magnetization Transfer (MT or MTC) effect in FSE.** MTC is inadvertently present in FSE. This is caused by the presence of multiple, rapid 180° pulses containing off-resonant frequencies. When MT (discussed in more detail in Chapter 24) is *intentionally* produced, an RF pulse 500–3000 Hz off the bulk water resonance saturates protein-bound water in the broad peaks on either side of the bulk phase water peak. Because the 180° pulses are rapid (in the time domain), they have a broad BW (in the frequency domain), thus containing frequencies off the bulk water resonance frequency. These frequencies suppress protein-bound water like a fat saturation pulse suppresses fat.

4. **Normal intervertebral discs are not as bright on T2 weighted FSE images compared to CSE.** This is caused by the MT effects in FSE previously discussed. They diminish the contrast between desiccated (usually dark) and normal (usually bright) discs.

5. **Magnetic susceptibility effects will be less than with CSE.** This is caused by decreased dephasing from closely-spaced (refocussing) 180° pulses that leave little time for spins to dephase as they diffuse through regions of magnetic nonuniformity. In FSE, the signal loss is minimized

because of the rephasing effects of multiple 180° pulses. Therefore, T2-weighted FSE images are less sensitive to magnetic susceptibility effects of hemorrhage (e.g., deoxyhemoglobin and hemosiderin) than are T2-weighted CSE images.

6. **Fat is bright on T2 weighted FSE images.** This is due to suppression of diffusion-mediated susceptibility dephasing caused by the closely-spaced 180° pulses[b]. You could do a *fat-saturated* FSE to decrease the intensity of fat.

EXAMPLE:
Performing a fat-sat T2W FSE sequence of the knee to suppress fat in the marrow will allow bone marrow edema to stand out against a dark marrow background. This technique increases the sensitivity of detecting bone bruises (contusions) by about 30%[c].

OTHER FEATURES OF FSE

More recent versions of FSE with high performance gradients allow other options, such as higher BWs, flow compensation, and 3D FSE.

Higher BWs cause a reduction in the sampling time Ts and thus ESP, allowing a lower minimum effective TE. Therefore, the previously hyperintense CSF on supposedly PDW images can now be made isointense to white matter. Use of a split (versus full) echo train also minimizes unwanted T2 contributions by only averaging the first four echoes of an eight echo train. (This is the same principle that allows T1W FSEs to be performed, i.e., higher BWs and shorter echo trains.)

Flow compensation is an added feature that is possible with high performance gradients; such gradients allow a higher maximum strength that can be applied over a shorter period. As a result, flow compensation with high performance gra-

---

[b] For more details, refer to Henkelman RM et al. Why fat is bright in RARE and fast spin-echo imaging. J Magn Reson Imaging 1992;2(5):533–540.

[c] For more details, see Kapelov SR, Teresi LM, Bradley WG, et al. Bone contusions of the knee: increased lesion detection with fast spin-echo MR imaging with spectroscopic fat saturation. Radiology 1993;189(3): 901–904.

dients do not place a large time burden on the cycle.

3D FSE

With the advent of **high performance gradients** (see Chapter 27), three dimensional FSE (3D FSE) imaging in reasonable scan times is now a reality. This imaging is particularly useful for the brain, cervical spine, and lumbar spine where bright CSF (T2 weighted) images are required in more than one plane. Whereas 3D T1W images have been available for some time (e.g., MP RAGE [Siemens], 3D SPGR [GE], 3D RF spoiled FAST [Picker]), 3D T2W images have not been available until recently. This is now possible with 3D FSE.

The basic idea in 3D imaging (3D techniques in connection with gradient echo imaging is discussed in Chapter 20) is to have a phase-encoding gradient not only in the y direction but also in the z direction (Fig. 19-12). Therefore, the multiple slices in 2D FSE are replaced by multiple slabs. **Crusher gradients** (see Chapter 14) are applied before and after every 180° pulse (which is slice selective). Each echo is first phase encoded, then sampled, and finally phase *unwound* (i.e., a **rewinder gradient** is applied—see Chapter 21). Consequently, the scan time will be

$$T \text{ (3D FSE)} = (TR \times NEX \times Ny \times Nz)/ETL$$

where Ny and Nz are the number of phase-encoding steps along the y and z axes.

High performance gradients have higher maximum strengths and thus allow a significant reduction in the gradient duration. This in turn allows a larger ETL (decreasing scan time) and a reduction in minimum TE (increasing the coverage). Therefore, despite a significant increase in the acquisition time (compared to 2D FSE) caused by the addition of the Nz factor into the previous formula, the scan can still be performed in a reasonable time.

EXAMPLE:

What is the scan time for a T2-weighted 3D FSE technique with TR = 3000 msec, ETL = 64, NEX = 1, Ny = 256, and Nz = 32?

Answer:
$$T = 3 \text{ sec} \times 1 \times 256 \times 32/64 = 384 \text{ sec}$$
$$= 6 \text{ min, } 24 \text{ sec}$$

which is very reasonable.

Advantages of 3D FSE

1. Higher SNR (compared with 2D FSE)
2. High (1 mm) isotropic resolution
3. Less partial volume averaging (due to thinner slices)
4. Capability to perform high-quality reformation in any plane (due to ability to generate *isotropic* voxels)

3D-FSE

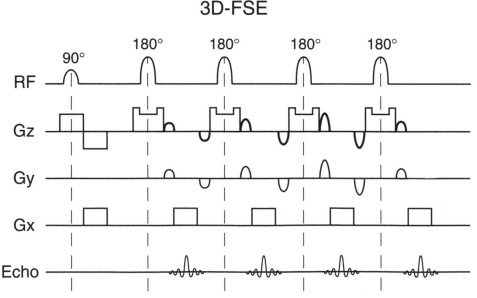

Figure 19-12.   A PSD for a 3D FSE. Phase encoding gradients are applied along both y and z axes.

5. Lower crosstalk (for slab-interleaved approaches)
6. Reduced magnetic susceptibility and field inhomogeneity artifacts (compared with 3D gradient echo techniques)

GRADIENT AND SPIN ECHO (GRASE) TECHNIQUE

Another new fast scanning technique called **GRASE (gradient and spin echo)** is a hybrid of GRE and FSE techniques. It is also called **Turbo GSE** or **TGSE**. In this technique, some of the spin echoes are replaced by gradient echoes. Contrast in GRASE reflects the relative number of gradient and spin echoes. This contrast leads to greater gradient-echo contrast and increased sensitivity to susceptibility effects. Because gradi-

ent echoes are produced by refocussing gradients without a 180° rephasing pulse, fewer 180° pulses are required. Because less time is required to produce a gradient echo (than an SE), the echo spacing (ESP) is reduced, potentially leading to longer echo trains and greater k-space coverage in the same acquisition time, allowing for larger matrices or longer TRs.

FAST IR

By adding a 180° inversion pulse prior to FSE, "fast IR" can be achieved. For more details, refer to the discussion on Fast FLAIR (Fast Fluid Attenuated Inversion Recovery) in Chapter 24. Fast STIR is similar to Fast FLAIR except that fat (instead of fluid) is nulled.

Key Points

Fast spin-echo (FSE) imaging provides almost all the advantages of conventional spin-echo imaging at a faster speed. The basic idea behind FSE is utilization of multiple 180° refocusing pulses, which allows filling multiple lines in k-space in one shot. The number of train of 180° pulses is called the ETL (echo train length). As a result, compared to conventional SE (CSE), the acquisition time T in FSE is reduced by a factor of ETL:

$$T (FSE) = T (CSE)/ETL$$

The increased speed also allows for other features not achievable by CSE techniques, such as high resolution imaging of, for example, the internal auditory canals with very long TRs and, more recently, three-dimensional imaging using FSE (3D FSE).

Questions

19-1. The scan time for FSE is given by:
(a) TR . NEX . Ny
(b) TR . Ny . ETL / NEX
(c) ETL/(TR . NEX . Ny)
(d) TR . NEX . Ny / ETL

19-2. Suppose TR = 3000, TE = 100, NEX = 2, Ny = 256.
(a) Calculate the scan time for CSE.
(b) Calculate the scan time for FSE with ETL = 8.

19-3. T/F Increasing ETL leads to increased speed and coverage.

19-4. Dual echo imaging in FSE can be achieved by:
(a) split echo train
(b) full echo train
(c) shared echo approach
(d) all of the above
(e) only (a) and (b)

19-5. Advantages of FSE include all of the following EXCEPT:
(a) increased speed
(b) decreased ferromagnetic susceptibility artifacts

(c)   decreased motion artifacts

(d)   increased number of possible slices

19-6.   Disadvantages of FSE compared to CSE include all of the following EXCEPT:

(a)   brighter CSF on Proton density weighted images

(b)   fat is brighter

(c)   increased magnetic susceptibility effects

(d)   normal intervertebral discs are not as bright

19-7.   Calculate the scan time for a 3D FSE technique with TR = 4000 msec, TE = 100 msec, Nx = 128, Ny = 256, Nz = 32, NEX = 1, ETL = 64.

Part I (Basic Principles)

INTRODUCTION

In this chapter, we will introduce the **gradient echo** (GRE) pulse sequence. It is also called **gradient recalled echo** (GRE), the reason for which will become clear later in the chapter. The major purpose behind the GRE technique is a significant reduction in the scan time. Toward this end, small flip angles are employed, which, in turn, allow very short TR values, thus decreasing the scan time. Consequently, such techniques are also referred to as **partial flip angle** techniques. One of the most important applications of GRE is the ability to employ three- dimensional (3D) imaging, thanks to the higher speed of GRE due to very short TRs. The major differences between GRE and spin-echo (SE) sequences will be explained in this chapter.

GRADIENT RECALLED
ECHO (GRE)

As mentioned in the introduction, the purpose of the GRE technique is to increase the speed of the scan. Recall that the scan time for "conventional" techniques is given by

$$\text{scan time} = TR \times Ny \times NEX \quad \text{(Eqn 20-1)}$$

where TR is the repetition time, Ny is the number of phase-encoding steps, and NEX is the number of excitations. Now, Ny is generally selected to yield a certain resolution (too small an Ny degrades the resolution) and NEX is chosen to yield a certain SNR (signal-to-noise ratio). Consequently, the only parameter in Equation 20-1 that can be controlled to reduce the scan time is TR.

In other words, we wish to select a TR that is as small as possible and still be able to receive a reasonable echo to create an image. If we use 90° RF pulses, then with very small TRs, the longitudinal magnetization is not given sufficient time to recover to a reasonable value, as depicted in Figure 20-1. This causes a significant reduction in the longitudinal magnetization and the subsequent transverse magnetization (Fig. 20-2). That is, the amplitude of the received signal will be diminished significantly (and, thus, SNR is deteriorated).

To rectify this problem, an RF pulse yielding a smaller flip angle α is used instead of the usual 90° RF pulse. This change causes incomplete flipping of the longitudinal magnetization into the x-y plane, producing transverse magnetization called M_{xy} (Fig. 20-3). In addition, the major component of magnetization remains along the z axis after the RF pulse (called M_z). Consequently, even with small TRs, there will be sufficient longitudinal magnetization at the time of the next cycle.

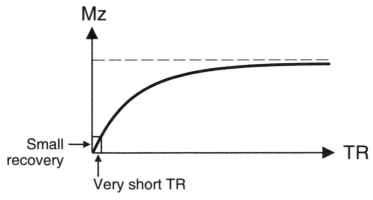

Figure 20-1. After a 90° pulse, longitudinal recovery after a short TR will be very small.

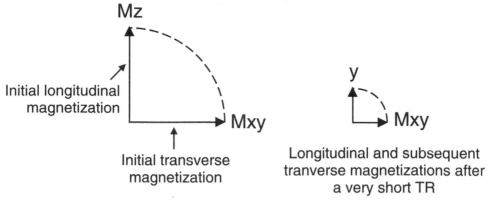

Figure 20-2.   (a) The initial longitudinal and transverse magnetizations. (b) After a short TR, the subsequent longitudinal and transverse magnetizations will be smaller.

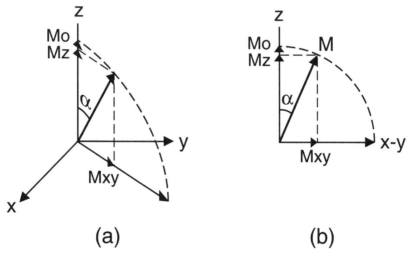

(a)   (b)

Figure 20-3.   If a small flip angle α is used, only a portion of longitudinal magnetization is flipped into the x-y plane and thus a portion of longitudinal magnetization will remain.

MATH: For the mathematically-oriented reader, the magnitude of the transverse and longitudinal magnetizations are given by

$$M_{xy} = M_0 \sin \alpha, \; M_z = M_0 \cos \alpha \quad \text{(Eqn. 20-2)}$$

right after the α RF pulse, where M_0 is the initial magnetization.

After this point, the process of recovery along the z axis and the process of dephasing in the x-y plane is exactly the same as in its spin-echo counterpart. There is, however, one major difference between GRE and SE sequences. In SE, a 180° refocussing pulse is used to eliminate dephasing caused by external magnetic field inhomogeneities. This pulse is not used in GRE imaging.

Question: *What is the reason for not using a 180° refocussing pulse in GRE?*
Answer: *Because we use a small flip angle in GRE, there would be a large component in the longitudinal axis at half the echo time (TE/2). (In SE imaging, however, this longitudinal component is insignificant at TE/2 because TE/2 is much smaller than T1 of the tissue.) Let's see what would happen to this longitudinal magnetization if we were to apply a 180° pulse. Although the application of a 180° pulse does yield rephasing in the x-y plane, it also causes M_z to invert and point south (Fig. 20-4). To recover this in-*

verted vector back in the north direction requires a long TR, which is clearly not the case in GRE. (The above is not a problem in conventional SE imaging because the longitudinal magnetization at TE/2 is very small and inverting it does not pose any significant loss of signal.)

Question: In the absence of a 180° pulse, how does one form an echo?

Answer: One way is to measure the FID instead. However, it's impractical to do so because the FID comes on at an inconvenient time. We need time to apply a phase-encoding gradient and prepare the signal for frequency encoding. We also need time to let the RF pulses and gradients die down before doing anything else. To this end, we will intentionally dephase the FID and rephase (or recall) it at a more convenient time, namely at TE. This is accomplished via a refocusing gradient in the x direction and is illustrated in Figure 20-5. This gradient has an initial negative lobe that intentionally dephases the spins in the transverse plane and thus eliminates the FID. It is then followed by a positive lobe that rephases the spins, thus restoring the FID in the form of a readable echo. The

area under the negative lobe is equal to half the area under the positive lobe. The refocusing occurs at the midpoint of the positive lobe. Figure 20-6 illustrates how the FID is refocused at TE. In other words, the FID is first eliminated and then recalled at time TE; hence the name gradient-recalled echo.

SLICE EXCITATION

The other difference between GRE and SE is that in GRE imaging, TR may be too short to allow for processing of other slices. For this reason, short TR GRE techniques may acquire only one slice at a time. This is referred to as *sequential* scanning. (In the next chapter, we will introduce variations of GRE that allow multi-planar imaging by lengthening the TR.) In other words, in a sequential mode (single-slice) GRE, the total scan time is given by

$$\text{scan time (GRE)} = \text{TR} \times \text{Ny} \times \text{NEX} \times (\text{\# of slices})$$
$$(\text{Eqn. 20-3a})$$

That is to say, acquisition of additional slices increases the scan time in a sequential mode GRE imaging.

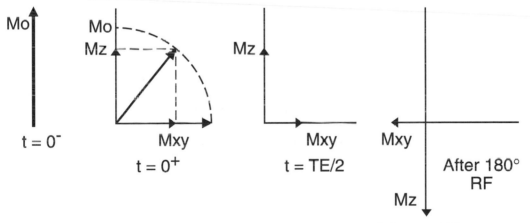

Figure 20-4.   After a partial flip angle, longitudinal recovery will no longer be small after a short TR (because partial flip retains a portion of initial longitudinal magnetization).

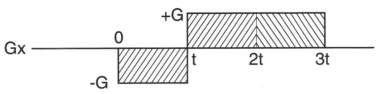

Figure 20-5.   Instead of using a 180° pulse, a bilobed gradient is used which has a negative lobe as well as a positive lobe of twice the duration.

In 3D GRE technique (see below), the scan time is given by

$$\text{Scan time (3D GRE)} = TR \times NEX \times Ny \times Nz$$
$$\text{(Eqn. 20-3b)}$$

where Ny and Nz refer to the number of phase-encoding steps in the y and z directions, respectively.

EXAMPLE:

Suppose TR = 50 msec, TE = 15 msec, α = 15°, NEX = 1, and Ny = 128. Then

$$TR \times NEX \times Ny = 50 \times 128 \times 1$$
$$= 6400 \text{ msec} = 6.4 \text{ sec}$$

Thus, it takes only 6.4 sec to obtain a single slice. If we were to obtain 10 slices, the scan time would be

$$\text{scan time (10 slices)} = 6.4 \times 10 = 64 \text{ sec}$$
$$= 1 \text{ min, 4 sec}$$

whereas acquisition of 20 slices would take

$$\text{scan time (20 slices)} = 6.4 \times 20 = 128 \text{ sec}$$
$$= 2 \text{ min, 8 sec}$$

which is twice as long.

MAGNETIC SUSCEPTIBILITY

The lack of a 180° refocussing pulse results in greater dephasing of spins compared with conventional spin echo. This in turn results in greater sensitivity to **magnetic susceptibility** effects. This increased sensitivity can be both problematic (e.g., increased artifact at the air-tissue interfaces) and advantageous (e.g., when searching for subtle hemorrhage), depending on the application.

STEADY-STATE TRANSVERSE MAGNETIZATION

There is one more major difference between GRE and SE pulse sequences. Whereas at the start of each cycle in SE imaging in which there is negligible component of magnetization M_{xy} in the x-y plane, this may not be the case in GRE imaging. In other words, GRE may only have **residual transverse magnetization** at the end of the cycle, which will be affected by the next RF pulse. This is because in GRE imaging, TR may be too short to allow for complete dephasing (i.e., T_2^* decay) of the spins in the transverse plane. (In contrast, in SE imaging, TR is long enough to allow complete dephasing of the spins in the x-y plane.) After a few cycles, this residual transverse magnetization reaches a **steady state**, referred to as M_{ss}. This scheme is illustrated in Figure 20-7 and is elaborated upon further in the next chapter.

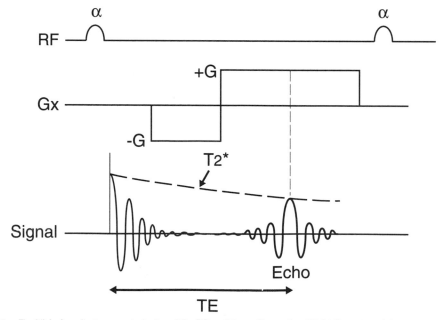

Figure 20-6. The bilobed gradient causes dephasing of the FID and its recalling at time TE (at the center of the positive lobe). Because there is no 180° rephasing pulse, the rate of decay is given by T2* (instead of T2).

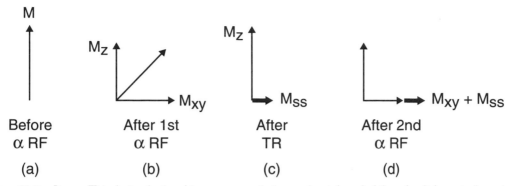

Figure 20-7. Because TR is short, a fraction of transverse magnetization remains at the end of the cycle which eventually reaches a steady state M_{ss}. This steady-state component is affected by the next RF pulse.

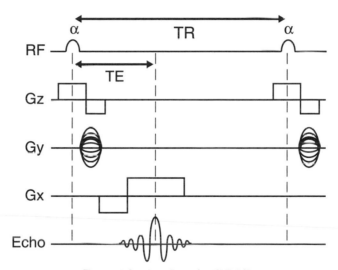

Figure 20-8. A gradient echo (GRE) PSD.

TISSUE CONTRAST

Figure 20-8 depicts a generic GRE pulse sequence diagram (PSD). There are three operator-controlled parameters that affect the tissue contrast: α, TR, and TE. Let's discuss how each of these plays a role in this matter.

First, consider a small flip angle α (e.g., 5° to 30°). As can be seen in Figure 20-9, a small flip angle results in a large amount of (persistent) longitudinal magnetization after application of the RF pulse. This result implies that complete recovery of the longitudinal magnetization to its initial value will take much less time than following the 90° RF pulse of a SE sequence. Consequently, given two tissues with different T1 values, a large difference will not exist between their respective T1 curves, and thus T1 recovery plays a minor role. This is better illus-

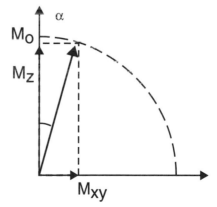

Figure 20-9. A small flip angle results in a large amount of longitudinal magnetization.

trated in Figure 20-10, in which tissue A's and tissue B's T1 curves are drawn for two different flip angles, 10° and 90°. The T1 curves for 10°

α start higher on the z axis owing to the fact that they are only partially flipped into the x-y plane. It can be inferred from this figure that the T1 differences between the two tissues is much less apparent for the smaller flip angle.

A small flip angle reduces T1 weighting.

A small α also implies a small transverse magnetization and thus a small steady-state component, reducing T2* weighting. As shown in Equation 20-2, M_{xy} is directly proportional to M_0; thus, tissue contrast is predominantly affected by proton density. This relationship is illustrated in Figure 20-11. In this diagram, tissue A (e.g., H_2O) has a higher proton density than tissue B (e.g., fat), i.e. $N(A) > N(B)$. At time TE, then, the difference between A and B is predominantly explained by their respective proton densities $N(A)$ and $N(B)$.

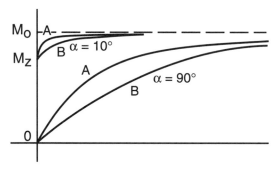

Figure 20-10. When the flip angle is small, it is difficult to discriminate the T1 contrast between two tissues. Thus, small α reduces T1 weighting.

A small flip angle yields proton density weighting.

Conversely, a large α (e.g., 75° to 90°) allows better differentiation of the T1 characteristics of the two tissues. This should be fairly obvious because in the extreme case when α is 90°, we are in a situation similar to SE, given that TR is not very small. However, if TR is very small, there won't be sufficient time for T1 recovery, thereby reducing T1 weighting (in this case, the large steady-state component that accumulates due to the large α increases T2* weighting—see later text).

A large flip angle (with a large TR) yields more T1 weighting.

For an intermediate α (e.g., 30° to 60°), the result is mixed contrast, although the gain in T1 weighting caused by larger flip angles tends to outweigh the gain in T2* weighting from increased steady state.

Next, consider the TR factor. If TR is very short (say a few tenths of a msec), then there won't be enough time for complete decay of transverse magnetization before the next α pulse. The residual transverse magnetization ($e^{-TR/T2*}$) will essentially all contribute to the next signal (at low flip angle). Thus, a short TR enhances T2* weighting. More simplistically, for TR < 3 T2* (say about 100 msec), contrast depends on T2*.

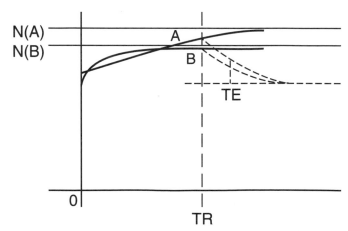

Figure 20-11. Small flip angles also result in small transverse magnetization, and thus poor T2* weighting and enhanced proton density weighting.

A short TR (with a small flip angle) increases T2* weighting.

Now, consider a long TR. Remember that "long" is a relative term; in GRE, a "long" TR is approximately several hundred milliseconds, which is commensurate with a "short" TR in SE! A long TR allows more recovery of the T1 curves and thus better differentiation of different T1 values. It also causes more T2* decay, reducing the steady-state component and thus reducing T2* weighting.

A longer TR enhances T1 weighting.

Finally, let's discuss the TE factor. This parameter's role in GRE is similar to the SE technique. That is, a short TE reduces T2* weighting and enhances T1 or proton density weighting.

A short TE reduces T2* weighting and increases PD or T1 weighting. A long TE enhances T2* weighting.

You might wonder what happens when these parameters are conflicting. For example, what contrast would a large TR and a small flip angle produce? The answer is that ultimately, one parameter is going to dominate. In this example, as described previously, a small α predominates and produces a PD weighted image. How about a short TR and a large α? This combination results in a mixed contrast that is proportional to the T2/T1 ratio of the tissues. (This is the contrast produced by a technique called steady state free precession (SSFP); see Chapter 21.)

MATH: Earlier in this book, we introduced a mathematical formula expressing the signal intensity (SI) with respect to TR, TE, T1, T2, and N(H); namely

$$SI = N(H) \, e^{-TE/T2} \, (1 - e^{-TR/T1}) \quad \text{(Eqn. 20-4)}$$

Now, with the addition of the flip angle α, this equation is modified as follows:

$$SI = N(H) \, e^{-TE/T2^*} \, (1 - e^{-TR/T1})$$
$$[\sin \alpha / (1 - \cos \alpha \, e^{-TR/T1})] \quad \text{(Eqn. 20-5)}$$

Equations 20-4 and 20-5 differ in several ways. The most obvious difference is the term in brackets containing the variable α. Also, note that T2 is replaced by T2* as is expected in GRE imaging (there is no 180° refocussing pulse).

Equation 20-5 is interesting in the extreme cases, namely at $\alpha = 0°$ and $\alpha = 90°$. When $\alpha = 90°$ (which is the case in SE), then $\sin \alpha = 1$ and $\cos \alpha = 0$, and the equation becomes

$$SI = N(H) \, e^{-TE/T2^*} \, (1 - e^{-TR/T1}) \quad \text{(Eqn. 20-6)}$$

which is the same as Equation 20-4 with T2 replaced by T2*, as expected.

When $\alpha \cong 0$ (i.e., very small) then $\cos \alpha \cong 1$ and $\sin \alpha \cong \alpha$, and Equation 20-5 becomes

$$SI \cong N(H) \, e^{-TE/T2^*} \, (1 - e^{-TR/T1}) \, [\alpha/(1 - e^{-TR/T1})]$$
$$= N(H) \, \alpha \, e^{-TE/T2^*} \quad \text{(Eqn. 20-7)}$$

which is dependent on the proton density N(H) as well as T2*.

SIGNAL-TO-NOISE RATIO (SNR OR S/N)

The SNR in a GRE technique is decreased per echo (as compared to SE) due to shorter TRs in GRE; however, more echoes are obtained in GRE per unit time, somewhat compensating for the former effect.

CHEMICAL SHIFT ARTIFACT OF THE SECOND KIND (DIXON EFFECT)

This phenomenon was discussed in Chapter 18 (MRI Artifacts) and applies only to GRE techniques. As discussed there, fat and water protons precess at slightly different frequencies in the transverse plane (220 Hz at 1.5 T). Immediately after the RF pulse, fat and water are both tipped (partially) into the transverse plane and are in phase. At various TEs later, fat and water spins will be in phase or out of phase. At 1.5 Tesla, fat and water get back into phase every 4.5 msec after the RF pulse. This number is derived by the following formula:

frequency difference between fat and water = 220 Hz

period = 1/frequency = 1/(220 Hz)
       = .0045 sec = 4.5 msec

Thus, fat and water are in phase initially at TE = 0, go out phase at TE = 2.25, and back in phase at TE = 4.5, etc. In general, at 1.5T, fat and H_2O go in and out of phase every 2.25 msec after the RF pulse (refer to Fig. 18-11). This is referred to as **chemical shift of the "second kind."**

If the selected TE is 2.25, 6.75, 11.25, 15.75 msec, etc., a dark boundary is seen around organs that are surrounded by fat (such as the kidneys and muscles). This is referred to as a **boundary effect,** which is not observed in SE imaging because of the presence of refocusing 180° pulses. This type of imaging is referred to as "**out of phase**" scanning, referring to the fact that at these TEs, fat and water spins will be 180° out of phase and cancel each other out.

To overcome this problem, we can do the following:

1. Make fat and H_2O in phase by picking appropriate TE.
2. Switch phase and frequency.
3. Increase the BW (*tradeoff:* decreases SNR).
4. Suppress fat.

The **Dixon method**[a] takes advantage of this phenomenon to create solely "water excitation" or "fat excitation" images. To understand how this is done, suppose that the signal intensities from fat and water is designated F and W, respectively. Then, the signal intensity of the image with fat and water in phase (I_{ip}) and out of phase (I_{op}) are given by

$$I_{ip} = W + F$$
$$I_{op} = W - F$$

Thus,

$$W = (I_{ip} + I_{op})/2$$
$$F = (I_{ip} - I_{op})/2$$

allowing only water (W) or fat (F) imaging. This is the method of Dixon.

---

[a] From Dixon WT. Simple proton spectroscopic imaging. Radiology 1984;153[1]:189–194.

THREE-DIMENSIONAL GE VOLUME IMAGING

Three-dimensional (3D) imaging with contiguous thin slices is feasible by using GRE techniques. This type of imaging is accomplished by an addition of a phase-encoding step (Nz) in the slice-select direction (z axis). Consequently, the total scan time is now

scan time = TR × Ny × NEX × Nz   (Eqn. 20-8)

where Nz is the number of phase-encoding steps in the z direction. Nz is usually a power of 2 (namely, 32, 64, 128), but because the addition of a phase-encoding step in the z direction may cause wrap-around artifacts in this direction as well, a few of the slices at each end are discarded and the number of slices displayed is slightly less (e.g., 28, 60, 120). This provides a **slab** of slices.

You may wonder how it is possible to achieve 3D imaging in a reasonable time given the large multiplicative factor Nz. The answer lies in the extremely short TR.

EXAMPLE:

Calculate the scan time for a 3D GRE technique in the C-spine with the following parameters:

TR 30/TE 13/α 5°/NEX 2/256 × 192/Nz 64
scan time = (TR)(NEX)(Ny)(Nz) = (30)(2)(192)(64)
= 737280 msec = 737.28 sec = 12 min, 17 sec.

A typical PSD is shown in Figure 20-12. The major difference here is the addition of an RF pulse for selection of a slab (i.e., a **slab-select gradient**), as well as application of phase-encoding steps in the z direction (i.e., **slice encoding**). This is depicted in Figure 20-13.

Volume imaging can be performed using **isotropic** (*cubic*, with $\Delta x = \Delta y = \Delta z$) voxels or **anisotropic** (noncubic) voxels. The advantage of the former is the ability to perform high-quality reformation in any plane of choice. 3D imaging is now also possible using newer FSE techniques that employ high performance gradients. More on this in a later chapter.

Advantages of 3D GRE

1. Rapid volume imaging of thin contiguous slices without crosstalk

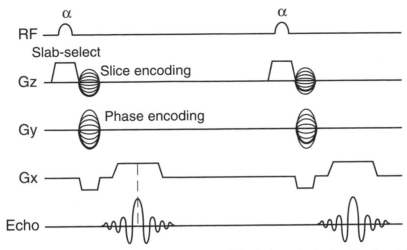

Figure 20-12. A PSD for 3D GRE. Phase encoding gradients are applied along both y and z directions. The slice select-gradient is also replaced by a *slab*-select gradient.

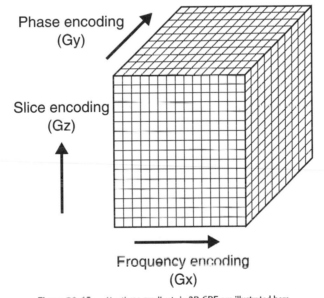

Figure 20-13. The three gradients in 3D GRE are illustrated here.

2. Reformation capabilities (especially if isotropic)
3. Increased SNR, because

$$SNR \propto \sqrt{Nz}.$$

Advantages of GRE
1. Increased speed
2. Increased sensitivity to magnetic susceptibility effects of hemorrhage (allowing better detection compared to SE)
3. Three-dimensional (3D) imaging (e.g., in the cervical spine) in a reasonable time
4. Imaging of flowing blood (i.e., MR Angiography)

Disadvantages of GRE
1. Decreased SNR caused by (a) small α, reducing the transverse magnetization, and (b) very short TR, not allowing sufficient recovery of the longitudinal magnetization
2. Increased magnetic susceptibility artifacts (caused by lack of a 180° refocussing pulse), most noticeable at air-tissue

interfaces such as in the region of the paranasal sinuses

3. Increased sensitivity to T2* decay caused by lack of 180° rephasing pulses (i.e., increased sensitivity to magnetic field inhomogeneities, intra-voxel dephasing, and magnetic susceptibility artifacts)

4. Compared with FID imaging, the GRE technique (which is really an FID-recalled technique) uses a longer TE, thus reducing the SNR caused by increased T2* decay

5. Introduction of chemical shift effects of the second kind, resulting in a dark band around organs with water-fat interfaces, such as the kidneys, liver, spleen, etc.

Key Points

1. The objective of GRE techniques is to reduce the scan time.

2. Scan time is proportional to TR; a very small TR is possible in GRE imaging.

3. Because a small TR does not allow reasonable recovery of the longitudinal magnetization (thus significantly diminishing SNR), a partial flip angle α (<90°) should be used.

4. Because TR may be too short to allow complete dephasing of the spins in the transverse plane, a residual transverse magnetization may remain before the next cycle.

5. A refocusing gradient (readout direction) is employed that eliminates the original FID and later *recalls* it at the echo time TE (hence the name gradient-*recalled* echo, or GRE).

6. Because TR may be too short to acquire other slices within one TR period, GRE techniques often perform one slice at a time. (In the next chapter we will discuss multiplanar GRE techniques.)

7. As a result, the scan time is also proportional to the number of slices obtained, i.e.,

scan time = TR × Ny × NEX × (# of slices)

8. The tissue contrast is a function of the flip angle α, the repetition time TR, and the echo time TE. A simplified way of presenting the results is summarized in Table 20-1.

Table 20-1

	Small	Large
α	↑ PDW	↑ T1W
TR	↑ T2*W	↑ T1W
TE	↑ PDW	↑ T2*W

Questions

20-1. T/F   The reason a 180° pulse is not used in GRE is to reduce the scan time.

20-2. T/F   In the absence of a 180° pulse, a bilobed refocussing gradient is used in GRE.

20-3. T/F   In general, GRE techniques use a partial flip angle because very short TRs are used to reduce the scan time.

20-4. T/F   GRE techniques often acquire one slice at a time.

20-5. T/F   A smaller flip angle increases PD weighting and reduces T1 weighting.

20-6. T/F   The longer the TR, the more T2* weighting will be achieved.

20-7. Calculate the scan time for a GRE with TR 30, NEX 1, Ny 256, for (a) a single slice and (b) 12 slices.

20-8. T/F   Magnetic susceptibility is less with GRE than with CSE.

20-9. T/F Regarding chemical shift of the second kind, at 1.5 T, fat and water protons get out of phase at TE = 4.5 msec, 9 msec, etc.

20-10. The SNR in 3D GRE is equal to the SNR in 2D GRE times the factor:
(a) N_z
(b) $\sqrt{N_z}$
(c) N_y
(d) $\sqrt{N_y}$

21 Gradient Echo

Part II (Fast Scanning Techniques)

INTRODUCTION

In the last chapter, the technique of gradient echo imaging was introduced. In this chapter, several gradient echo techniques will be discussed, including **GRASS** (gradient recalled acquisition in the steady state)/**FISP** (fast imaging with steady-state precession), **SPGR** (spoiled GRASS)/**FLASH** (fast low-angle shot), and **SSFP** (steady state free precession)/**PSIF** (opposite of FISP). Although every manufacturer uses a different acronym, the underlying concepts are the same. We will also discuss a multi-planar (MP) variant of these GRE techniques (e.g., MPGR/MP FISP, MPSPGR/MP FLASH). Finally, faster versions of these techniques are introduced (e.g., fast GRASS (FGR)/turbo FISP, fast SPGR (FSPGR)/Turbo FLASH) and their multi-planar versions (e.g., FMPGR/Fast MP FISP and FMPSPGR/Turbo MP FLASH).

NOMENCLATURE

Table 21-1 contains a summary of the important acronyms used by three major manufac-

turers: General Electric (GE), Siemens, and Picker. Also refer to the list of abbreviations in the Glossary. As an example, GE uses the prefix "*Fast*" and Siemens uses "*Turbo*" to denote similar fast scanning techniques, be it gradient-recalled echo or spin echo. (The acronyms are spelled out in the Glossary.)

GRASS/FISP

It was mentioned in the last chapter that, in contrast to SE, in GRE there may be **residual transverse magnetization** at the end of each cycle remaining for the next cycle. This residual magnetization reaches a steady state value after a few cycles and is denoted M_{ss}.

This residual, steady-state magnetization is added to the transverse magnetization created by the next α RF pulse and thus increases the length of the vector in the x-y plane (Fig. 21-1). This then yields more T2* weighting. In other words, tissues with a longer T2 have a longer M_{ss} than do tissues with shorter T2.

Actually, to preserve this steady state component, an additional step needs to be taken in the pulse sequence. A so-called "**rewinder**" **gradient** is applied in the phase-encoding direction at the end of the cycle to reverse the effects of the phase-encoding gradient applied at the beginning of the cycle (i.e., it "*unwinds*" the former effect). In other words, the rewinder gradient is nothing but the opposite

Table 21-1

GE	Siemens	Picker
GRASS	FISP	FAST
SPGR	FLASH	RF spoiled FAST
SSFP	PSIF	CE-FAST
FSPGR	turbo-FLASH	RAM-FAST

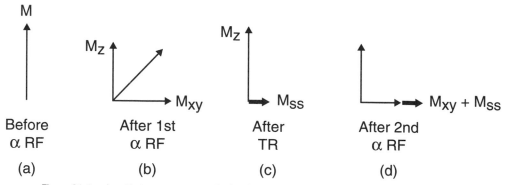

Figure 21-1. A residual transverse magnetization that reaches a steady state M_{ss} remains after a short TR.

GRASS Pulse Sequence Diagram

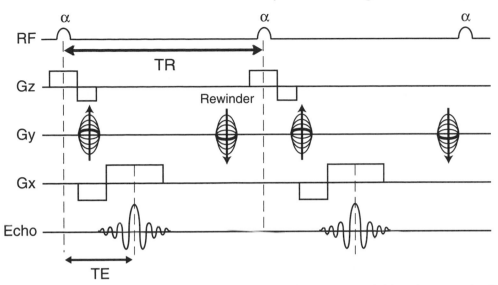

Figure 21-2. A PSD for GRASS/FISP. A "rewinder" gradient is applied along the y axis at the end of the cycle to reverse the effect of phase-encoding gradient.

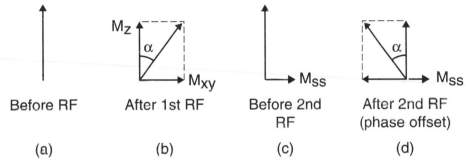

Figure 21-3. Spoiling of the steady-state transverse magnetization can be done via RF spoilers (as in SPGR), in which a phase offset is added to each successive RF pulse.

of the phase-encoding gradient (Fig. 21-2). For instance, if gradient +3 is applied for phase encoding, the rewinding gradient would be −3.

SPGR (SPOILED GRASS)/FLASH

The word "**spoiling**" refers to the elimination or "spoiling" of the steady-state transverse magnetization. There are various ways of accomplishing this task:

1. by applying RF spoiling
2. by applying variable gradient spoilers
3. by lengthening TR

RF Spoiling

RF spoiling is the method used in SPGR and is illustrated in Fig. 21-3. In this scheme, a phase offset is added to each successive RF pulse. This causes a corresponding phase shift in successive M_{ss} vectors. By maintaining a constant phase relationship between the transmitter and the receiver (achieved via a **phase-locked circuit**), successive M_{ss} vectors cancel each other out. A PSD for SPGR is shown in Figure 21-4. In this scheme, rewinder gradients are naturally not used because their purpose is to preserve the steady-state magnetization, thus defeating the purpose of spoiling.

SPGR Pulse Sequence Diagram

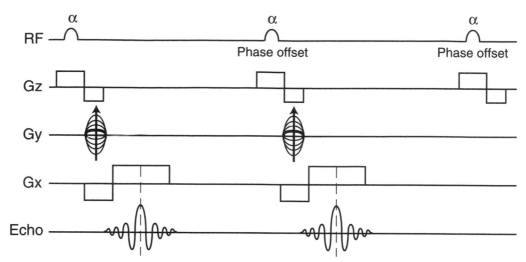

Figure 21-4. A PSD for spoiled GRE by using RF spoilers (as in SPGR).

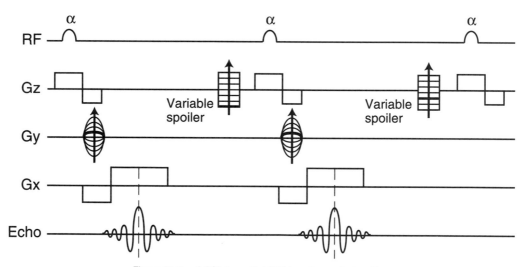

Figure 21-5. A PSD for spoiled GRE by using gradient spoilers.

Variable Gradient Spoilers

Spoiling can also be achieved by using gradient spoilers. This is accomplished by introducing an additional gradient with variable strengths from cycle to cycle (Fig. 21-5).

Lengthening TR

The last method to achieve spoiling of M_{ss} is by lengthening TR. When TR is sufficiently large (generally over 200 msec), there is enough time to allow complete dephasing of the spins in the transverse plane (because TR > T2). This is similar to the SE pulse sequence.

Question: For a long TR (e.g., 500 msec), what is the difference between GRASS (or FISP) and SPGR (or FLASH)?

Answer: There isn't any! A TR of 500 msec in GRASS effectively allows transverse magnetization to decay away over each cycle; i.e., it eliminates the steady state component (M_{ss}). Consequently, GRASS/FISP and SPGR/FLASH *would have similar properties for any given TE and α when TR is long.*

SPGR/FLASH—TISSUE CONTRAST

By eliminating the steady state component, only the longitudinal component affects the signal in the SPGR/FLASH technique. Thus, this technique lends itself to reduced T2* weighting and increased T1 weighting. This is true provided α is also relatively large. When α is small, however, the T1 recovery curves play a minor role, and proton density (PD) weighting is increased.

In SPGR, a long TR and a large α yield T1 weighting. A large TR and a small α yield PD or T2 weighted images depending on TE.*

SPGR (FLASH) Disadvantages

1. Increased dephasing caused by inhomogeneities in B_0
2. Increased magnetic susceptibility artifacts

3. Increased chemical shift artifacts (dark bands)

SSFP (STEADY STATE FREE PRECESSION)/PSIF

This technique is harder to comprehend. It yields heavily T2 (not T2*) weighted images. The PSD is shown in Figure 21-6. The idea here is that each α RF pulse contains some 90° and some 180° pulses embedded in it. Therefore, in Figure 21-6, α_1 acts like a 90° excitation pulse and α_2 like a 180° rephasing pulse. This yields a pulse sequence similar to SE whereby an echo is formed at α_3. Because it is difficult to read a signal and transmit α_3 at the same time, the echo is actually recalled 9 msec prior to α_3 by using an appropriate gradient. Note that the echo corresponding to α_1 is formed between α_2 and α_3. Interestingly, in this scheme, TE is larger than TR (and smaller than 2TR by 9 msec), which is somewhat counter-intuitive. The rewinder gradients are also shown in the diagram. The rewinder gradient is one cycle ahead of the

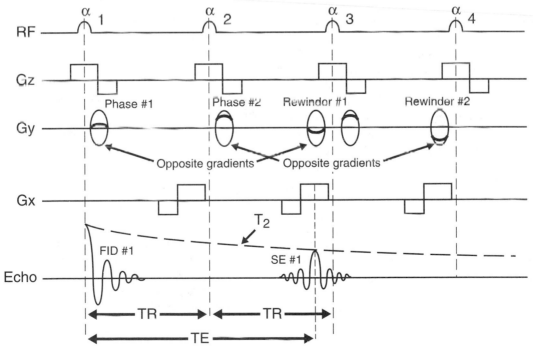

Figure 21-6. A PSD for SSFP/PSIF. Each α pulse contains some 180° pulse embedded in it that acts like a refocussing pulse. This in turn will result in a spin echo (SE) at the time of the next α pulse. Hence, contrast is determined by T2 (not T2*).

phase-encoding gradient due to the foregoing discussion. (In this technique, any two successive RF pulses can be employed to create a spin echo [SE]).

SSFP/PSIF—TISSUE CONTRAST

The SSFP sequence provides heavily T2 (not T2*) weighted images with increased scan speed without the use of dedicated excitation and rephasing pulses.

SSFP/PSIF Advantages

1. Decreased dephasing due to inhomogeneities in B_0 as compared to GRASS and SPGR
2. Decreased magnetic susceptibility artifacts as compared to GRASS and SPGR
3. Decreased chemical shift artifacts (dark bands) as compared to GRASS and SPGR

SSFP Disadvantages

1. Decreased SNR secondary to the use of longer TEs (TE > TR)
2. Increased sensitivity to nonstationary tissue

MULTI-PLANAR TECHNIQUES

The GRASS and SPGR sequences can be performed using a multi-planar technique by selecting a long TR (several hundred milliseconds). These are termed MPGR (multi-planar GRASS or multi-planar gradient recalled)/multi-planar FISP and MPSPGR (multi-planar SPGR)/multi-planar FLASH. As mentioned previously, this long TR causes spoiling of the steady-state component in the transverse plane, thus making GRASS and SPGR possess similar features.

We can still achieve both T1 and PD/T2* weighting depending on the flip angle α, as discussed previously. To reiterate, a small α yields PD weighting while a large α yields T1 weighting. More specifically, at small flip angles, MPGR and GRASS behave fairly similarly, whereas at larger angles, MPGR tends to be more T1 weighted than GRASS because MPGR uses a long TR.

Advantages of Long TR

1. Increased SNR, because the longitudinal magnetization has more time to completely recover.

2. Multi-planar scanning is feasible because a long TR allows acquisition of other slices during the dead time within one TR period (similar to SE).
3. It is also possible to perform multi-echo imaging (e.g., a short TE and a long TE) similar to multi-echo, multi-planar technique in SE. However, the second echo tends to get degraded in GRE secondary to rapid T2* decay.
4. A long TR, as discussed in Chapter 26, reduces **saturation effects** (seen with very short TRs caused by incomplete recovery of the longitudinal magnetization). Consequently, larger flip angles can be used. Although larger flip angles cause more saturation effects, the presence of a longer TR counterbalances it. Larger flip angles obviously increase the length of the transverse magnetization and thus the SNR.

FAST GRADIENT-ECHO TECHNIQUES

This topic might at first appear puzzling. Perhaps you are saying that you thought all GRE techniques were "fast." It is true that GRE techniques are generally faster than SE techniques, although the FSE (Fast Spin Echo)/TSE (Turbo Spin Echo) technique may be equally fast. However, there are additional methods that can further increase the speed of scanning. These methods are called Fast GRASS/Turbo FISP, Fast SPGR/Turbo FLASH, and so on.

The multi-planar variants of these methods are also available, referred to as Fast Multi-Planar GRASS/Turbo Multi-planar FISP, Fast Multi-planar Spoiled GRASS/Turbo Multi-planar FLASH, and so on. These render multiple slices with increased SNR in a rapid time period.

How can you make an already fast GRE technique faster? The answer lies in employing ultra short TRs and TEs to reduce the **sequence time**, i.e., the time it takes to excite, phase encode, and frequency encode. This is achieved by the use of the following:

1. Fractional echo
2. Fractional RF
3. Fractional NEX

Fractional Echo

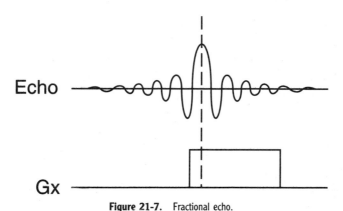

Figure 21-7.   Fractional echo.

Fractional RF

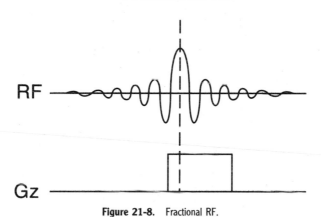

Figure 21-8.   Fractional RF.

4.   Reduction in the sampling time Ts (vis-à-vis by increasing the bandwidth)

The first three items are discussed in Chapter 23 on the new scanning features (Figs. 21-7, 21-8, and 21-9). Basically, by using a fraction of the echo and a fraction of the RF pulse, we can in effect decrease the echo time TE. Increasing the BW (bandwidth) from ±16 kHz (i.e., BW = 32 kHz) to ±32 kHz (i.e., BW = 64 kHz) results in a reduction of the sampling time Ts from 8 to 4 msec for 256 frequency-encoding steps Ny (Fig. 21-9). The trade-off here is a reduction in SNR because SNR is proportional to $1/\sqrt{BW}$. A wider BW allows more noise through, as shown in Figure 21-10. The sequence time is now given by

$$\text{sequence time} = TE + Ts/2 + T_o$$

Fractional NEX

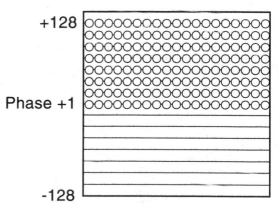

Figure 21-9.   Fractional NEX.

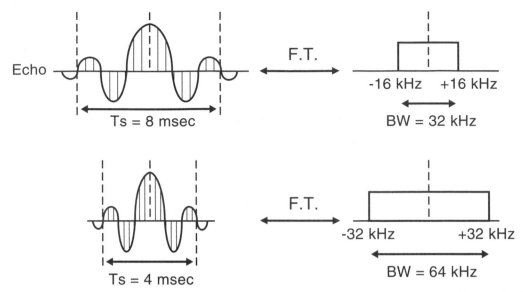

Figure 21-10. An increase in the BW results from a decrease in the sampling time Ts, thus allowing a reduction in TE. The trade-off is a decrease in S/N.

where T_o is the "overhead" time and Ts is the total sampling (readout) time. By minimizing TE and Ts, we can minimize the sequence time and thus reduce the minimum TR. Employing a fractional NEX decreases the overall scan time because the scan time is proportional to NEX.

In fast multi-planar techniques, a longer TR is used, but multiple slices are acquired within that TR period.

EXAMPLE:

1. Determine the scan time for obtaining 15 slices using Fast SPGR/Turbo FLASH (one slice at the time) when TR = 10 msec, TE = min, Ny = 256, NEX = 1:

$$\text{time} = (10)\,(256)\,(1)\,(15)$$
$$= 38400 \text{ msec} = 38.4 \text{ sec}$$

2. Determine the scan time for obtaining 15 slices using Multi-Planar Fast SPGR/Turbo FLASH (multi-slice) when TR = 100 msec, TE = min, Ny = 256, NEX = 1:

$$\text{time} = (100)\,(256)\,(1) = 25600 \text{ msec}$$
$$= 25.6 \text{ sec}$$

Applications

Useful in applications requiring very fast scanning such as the following:

1. Single breath-hold techniques in the abdomen

2. Imaging of a joint in motion (e.g., TMJ's)
3. Cine imaging of the heart
4. Temporal scanning of the same slice after contrast administration
5. Perfusion images after bolus injection of contrast

Disadvantages

1. Decreased SNR and CNR caused by ultra short TRs (less so in degree with multi-planar techniques)
2. Increased chemical shift artifacts of the second kind at very low TEs (namely at TE = 2.2 msec, 6.6 msec, etc.)

TISSUE-PREPARED FAST GRE TECHNIQUES

In fast GRE techniques, ultra short TRs are employed, so the tissue contrast may be suboptimal. To help improve the tissue contrast, a technique called magnetization preparation or **tissue preparation** is used (e.g., **MP-RAGE**). Before the α RF pulse (**prep time**), other RF pulses (180° and/or 90°) are applied to the tissue. This prep time allows the tissues to develop a certain contrast (T1 or T2 weighting, depending on the type of application).

Two types of tissue preparation methods are discussed:

1. IR Prepared (Inversion-Recovery Prepared)
2. DE Prepared (Driven-Equilibrium Prepared)

IR Prepared

First consider the **IR Prepared** method. In this scheme (Fig. 21-11), a 180° pulse is applied (prep time) before the α pulse. This method is similar to an inversion-recovery (IR) technique, providing increased T1 weighting and allowing suppression of various tissues depending on the prep time (Table 21-2).

DE Prepared

The second method is the **DE Prepared** technique. It employs a 90°—180°—90° pulse sequence similar to SE to provide T2-weighted contrast before the α pulse (Fig. 21-12). The longer the prep time, the more T2 decay occurs

and the more T2-weighted the tissue contrast becomes. In other words, tissues with longer T2s are degraded to a lesser degree compared with tissues with shorter T2s, thereby enhancing T2 contrast.

More specifically, referring to Figure 21-12, consider two tissues A and B with different T2 values (tissue A having a longer T2 than tissue B). After the first 90° pulse, both A and B will have similar transverse magnetization vectors. Right before the 180° pulse, tissue B (having a shorter T2) has decayed more than A and thus has a shorter vector in the transverse plane. After the 180° pulses, their direction is reversed by 180° in the transverse plane. The second 90° pulse causes these vectors to be *driven* to the longitudinal axis (hence the name *driven*-equilibrium), but with tissue A (having a longer T2) at a higher value than B. This allows the GRE sequence to start out with a bias towards tissues with longer T2s.

FLOW IMAGING

GRE scanning is generally performed one slice at a time (except in the multi-planar situation); therefore, each slice is an entry slice. Consequently, flow related enhancement (FRE) applies to every single slice, and vessels appear

Table 21-2

Suppressed Organ	Prep Time
liver	200–400 msec
spleen	400–500 msec
CSF	700–800 msec

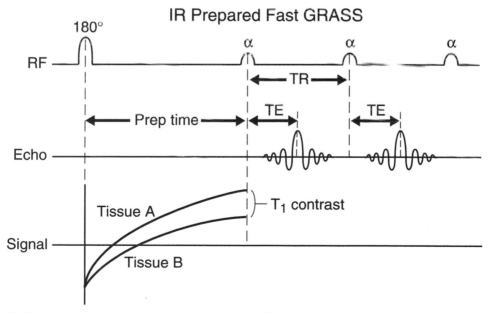

Figure 21-11. In an IR (inversion recovery) preparation technique, a 180° pulse is applied before the GRE sequence, allowing for better T1 discrimination of two different tissues. This will increase T1 weighting.

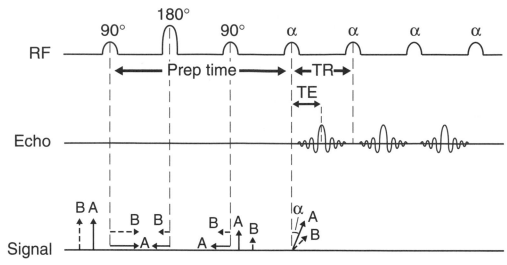

Figure 21-12. In a SE (spin echo) preparation technique, a 90°—180°—90° sequence (similar to SE) is applied before the GRE sequence, allowing better T2 discrimination. Refer to the text for more details.

bright on GRE images. The basic concept is that no saturated flowing protons enter the slice, so that flipping these protons yields maximum sig-nal. This is the basic concept behind 2D or 3D **time of flight** (**TOF**) MR angiography. This topic is discussed at length in Chapters 25–26.

Key Points

1. Several GRE techniques are available: GRASS/FISP, SPGR/FLASH, and SSFP/PSIF (see Table 21-1).

2. In GRASS, the residual transverse magneti-zation is preserved via a rewinder gradient, contributing to increased T2* weighting.

3. In SPGR/FLASH, the residual transverse magnetization is "spoiled" by introducing phase shifts in the successive RF pulses. This causes reduced T2* and increased T1 weighting.

4. Spoiling can also be accomplished via gradi-ent spoilers or by lengthening the TR.

5. In SSFP/PSIF, heavily T2 weighted images are obtained. Whereas GRASS/FISP and SPGR/FLASH represent gradient-recalled *FID* sequences, SSFP/PSIF represents a gra-dient-recalled *SE* (spin echo) sequence. In-terestingly, in this technique, TE is larger

than TR and usually is smaller than 2TR by 9 msec.

6. Multi-planar (MP) variants of the above are also available (e.g., MPGR/MP FISP, MPSPGR/MP FLASH, etc.) by employing a longer TR (over 200 msec).

7. Fast GRE techniques (e.g., FGR/Turbo FISP, FSPGR/Turbo FLASH, etc.) provide addi-tional speed. This is accomplished by using a fractional RF, fractional echo, and frac-tional NEX, as well as a wider BW (shorter sampling time Ts).

8. Combined fast and multi-planar GRE tech-niques (e.g., FMPGR , FMPSPGR/Turbo MP FLASH, etc.) render multiple slices with in-creased SNR in a fast mode.

9. The characteristics of GRASS/FISP, SPGR/ FLASH, and SSFP/PSIF are summarized in Table 21-3.

Table 21-3

GRE Technique	SNR	CNR	Comments
GRASS/FISP	highest	best possible T2*	preserves steady-state component
SPGR/FLASH	intermediate	best possible T1W	spoils steady-state component
SSFP/PSIF	lower	provides T2W	gradient-recalled SE; TR < TE < 2TR

Questions

21-1. Spoiling of the residual transverse magnetization can be accomplished by:
(a) gradient spoilers
(b) RF spoilers
(c) long TR
(d) all of the above
(e) only (a) and (b)

21-2. Fast GRE techniques may employ:
(a) fractional echo
(b) fractional RF
(c) fractional NEX
(d) narrow BW
(e) all of the above
(f) only (a)–(c)

21-3. T/F Spoiled GRE techniques increase T1 weighting.

21-4. T/F A rewinder gradient is applied in the phase encode direction to preserve the residual transverse magnetization M_{ss} (as in GRASS/FISP/FAST).

22 Echo Planar Imaging (EPI)

INTRODUCTION

In the last three chapters, we discussed some of the fast scanning techniques, namely the fast spin echo (FSE) technique and gradient-recalled echo (GRE) techniques along with their "fast" variants. In this chapter, we will discuss the echo planar imaging (EPI) technique, which is the fastest MRI technique available.

BASIC IDEA IN EPI

Unlike other fast scanning techniques that can be achieved via software updates, single shot EPI requires hardware modifications. More specifically, **high performance gradients** (discussed in Chapter 27) are needed to allow rapid on and off switching of the gradients. The basic idea is to fill k-space in one shot (single shot EPI) with readout gradient during one T2* decay (if longer, T2 blurring will occur) or in multiple shots (multishot EPI) by using multiple excitations. As we shall see shortly, single shot EPI allows oscillating frequency-encoding gradient pulses and complete k-space filling after a *single* RF pulse. Generally, gradient strengths of over 20 mT/m and gradient rise times of less than 300 μsec are required. Furthermore, extremely fast computers are needed to allow fast digital manipulations and signal processing. This is why EPI is still not widely used clinically.

TYPES OF EPI

Two main types exist: **single shot EPI** and **multishot EPI**. Earlier single shot EPI techniques used a constant phase-encode gradient. Newer techniques use a "blipped" phase-encode gradient, referred to as "blipped EPI."[a]

Single Shot EPI

In **single shot EPI**, all the lines in k-space are filled by multiple gradient reversals producing multiple gradient echoes in a *single* acquisition after a single RF pulse, i.e., in a single-measurement or "**shot**."

To achieve this, the readout gradient must be reversed rapidly from maximum positive to maximum negative $N_y/2$ times (e.g., 256/2 = 128 times) during a single T2* decay (e.g., 100 msec). Each lobe of the readout gradient above or below the baseline corresponds to a separate k_y line in k-space. Therefore, the number of phase-encode steps N_y is equal to the sum of the positive and negative lobes of the readout gradient. The area under the G_x lobe determines the FOV—the larger the area, the smaller the FOV will be. Apparently, single-shot EPI places tremendous demands on the gradients with respect to maximum strength G_{max} and minimum rise time t_{Rmin} (i.e., the maximum **slew rate** G_{max}/t_R) as well as on the ADC. In general, ADCs with maximum BWs on the order of MHz are required rather than kHz maximum BWs used for CSE.

In earlier EPI methods, the phase-encode gradient was kept on continuously (Fig. 22-1) during the acquisition, resulting in the zigzag coverage of k-space (Fig. 22-2). This led to some artifacts during Fourier transformation compared with conventional k-space trajectories. To rectify this problem, the phase-encode gradient was subsequently applied briefly during the time when the readout gradient was zero, i.e., when the k-space position was at either end of the k_x axis (Fig. 22-3). This method was referred to as "**blipped**" phase encoding as its duration was minimal (<200 μsec). Therefore, the same phase-encode gradient is applied briefly N_y number of times (e.g., 256 times). The technique was called "**blipped EPI**" and the k-space trajectory (Fig. 22-4) was much easier on the Fourier transformation.

As discussed previously, one of the problems with the single shot EPI is that any phase error tends to propagate through the entire k-space. (This is not a problem in CSE because of the presence of *rewinder gradients* which reset the phase at the end of each cycle.) The phase errors we are talking about here are not the ones caused

---

[a] For more details refer to Edelman RR et al. Echo-planar MR Imaging. Radiology 1994;192:600–612.

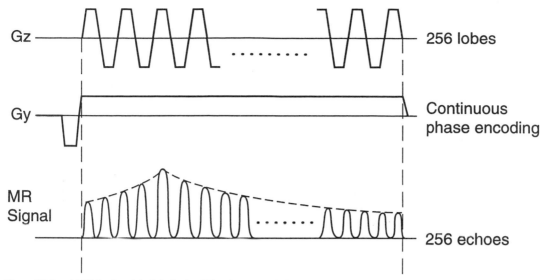

Figure 22-1. A PSD for the original single-shot EPI technique in which a constant phase-encode gradient is applied during readout. The G_x gradient has a sinusoidal shape caused by rapid on and off switching of the gradients.

K space trajectory

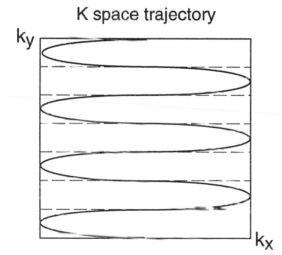

Figure 22-2. Single shot EPI with constant phase gradient allows traversal of k-space in a zigzag manner after a single RF pulse.

by motion (motion artifact is not a problem in the ultra fast EPI) but the errors arising from the variation in the resonating frequencies of protons (e.g., fat and water protons), which lead to mismapping along the phase-encode axis. Consequently, one of the technical problems of single shot EPI is magnetic susceptibility artifacts, particularly at air-tissue interfaces around the paranasal sinuses. Also, because of this phase error propagation along the phase-encode axis, chemical shift artifact in EPI is along the phase-encode axis rather than the frequency-encode axis, as in the case of CSE.

Multishot EPI

In **multi-shot EPI**, the readout is divided into multiple "shots" or segments (N_s), so that

$$N_y = N_s \times ETL$$

where ETL (echo train length) is the number of lines in each segment. Because k-space is segmented into multiple acquisitions, this technique is also called "**segmental EPI.**"

Advantages of Multishot EPI (compared with single shot EPI)

1. This technique places less stress on the gradients compared with single shot EPI.
2. Phase errors have less time to build up compared with single shot EPI, thus reducing diamagnetic susceptibility artifacts.

Disadvantages of Multishot EPI (compared with single shot EPI)

1. Multi-shot EPI takes longer to perform than does single shot EPI.
2. Because of this fact, multishot EPI is more susceptible to motion artifacts.

PULSE SEQUENCE DIAGRAM IN EPI

Figure 22-1 illustrates an example of the original EPI pulse sequence diagram. The major dif-

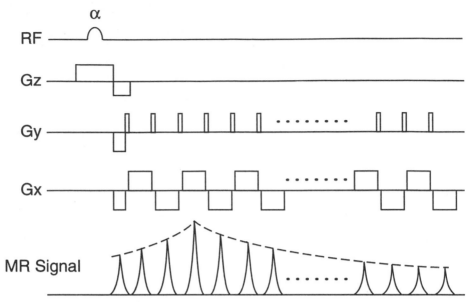

Figure 22-3. A PSD for blipped EPI. The phase-encode gradient is on briefly only while G$_x$ is zero (blipped phase encoding).

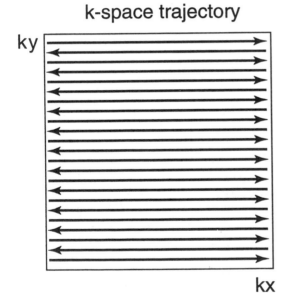

Figure 22-4. The k-space trajectory for blipped EPI in an odd-even manner, which is much easier on the Fourier transformation.

a constant phase-encoding gradient (remember that k-space is filled in one TR period). (The term TR may not be suitable here because each slice is obtained after a single RF pulse. However, TR could be defined as the time between successive slice select RF pulses.) The above scheme allows acquisition of raw data for each slice after a *single* RF pulse (unlike routine SE, where one RF pulse is needed for each phase-encoding step).

Figure 22-3 provides a PSD for blipped EPI in which the phase-encode gradient is applied briefly N$_y$ number of times when the readout gradient is zero.

k-SPACE TRAJECTORY IN EPI

Unlike conventional SE (CSE) in which data sampling is performed during a constant readout gradient, in earlier single shot EPI techniques, sampling was carried out during the readout gradient's alternating positive and negative lobes, which caused traversal of k-space in a zigzag or sinusoidal manner (Fig. 22-2). In the case of blipped EPI, k-space trajectory for even echoes is the opposite of that for odd echoes (Fig. 22-4). In multishot (segmental) EPI, data acquisition is carried out in multiple segments in an interleaved manner (Fig. 22-5). Spiral imaging in multishot EPI can also be formed (see Fig. 22-8) by using two oscillating gradients.

ference between this sequence and a conventional sequence is the application of a series of sinusoidal-shaped pulse sequences along the readout axis. This series requires rapid on and off switching of the gradients to achieve a train of positive and negative gradient pulses. It can be accomplished only with advanced hardware that can support such high performance gradients. The other difference is the application of

These trajectories are in contrast to CSE in which each line of k-space is filled during one TR period (and there are N_y number of such periods).

SCAN TIME IN EPI

Because the entire data acquisition for each slice is accomplished after a single RF pulse, the scan time for a single slice in single shot EPI is limited by T2* or T2 decay (on the order of 100 msec).

In general, if **ESP (echo sampling period)** is the time interval between two successive echoes, Ny is the number of lines in k-space, and NEX is the number of excitations (acquisitions), then for single shot EPI, the scan time is given by

T (single shot EPI) = ESP × N_y × NEX

For multishot EPI, the scan time is given by

$$T \text{ (multishot EPI) } = TR \times N_s \times NEX$$
$$= TR \times N_y \times NEX/ETL$$

which resembles the scan time for FSE (recall that $N_y = N_s \times ETL$).

CONTRAST IN EPI

Contrast in EPI depends on the **"root" pulsing sequence** (which is similar to preparation prepulses in GRE techniques). For instance, to achieve SE contrast, a 90°–180° SE root sequence is applied before the EPI module. Similarly, a partial flip RF pulse (<90°) before the EPI module provides gradient echo contrast. A 180°—90°—180° IR root prior to EPI provides inversion recovery contrast. In addition, diffusion gradients can be added for EPI-diffusion imaging.

Therefore, we can summarize the following:

1. SE-EPI (90°—180°—EPI) uses a 180° pulse to overcome external magnetic field inhomogeneities (Fig. 22-6). This technique provides T_1 and T_2 weighting. Because all the echoes in EPI are acquired with the *same* value of the phase-encode gradient, contrast in SE-EPI is determined from the temporal rephasing of the 180° RF pulse. Contrast in a T2W EPI is very similar to that of CSE, i.e., signal is determined by T2 decay and flowing blood is dark.

2. GRE-EPI (α°—EPI) does not employ the 180° pulse, thus providing T_2* weighting. This technique is faster and best suited for, say, cardiac cine imaging. Contrast here is determined by the time between the negative phase-encode gradient prepulse and the EPI readout module.

3. IR-EPI (180°—90°—180°—EPI) allows T1 contrast by applying a 180° inversion prepulse.

ARTIFACTS IN EPI
N/2 Ghost Artifacts

Even with blipped EPI, phase errors may result from the multiple positive and negative passes through k-space (i.e., alternating polarity of the readout gradient). "Ghost" artifacts of the main image may appear along the phase axis, not caused by motion as in CSE, but by eddy currents, imperfect gradients, field nonuniformities, or a mismatch between the timing of the odd and even echoes. Since the ghosts are derived from half the data (even or odd), they are called "**N/2 ghosts**."

k-space trajectory

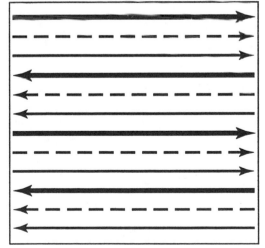

Figure 22-5. The k-space trajectory for multishot EPI. k-space is divided into multiple segments which are acquired in an interleaved manner.

Remedy:

Minimize eddy currents; proper tuning of the gradients.

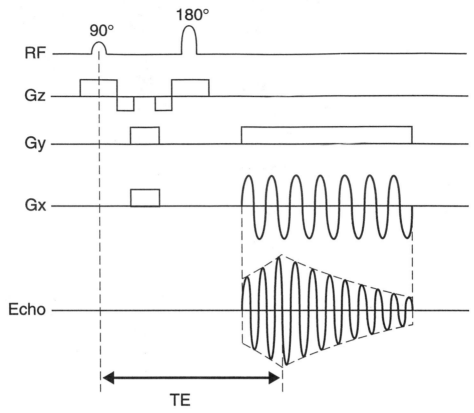

Figure 22-6. A SE-EPI PSD for the original EPI. A 90°–180° root pulsing sequence is applied before the EPI module.

Susceptibility Artifacts in EPI

Diamagnetic susceptibility effects in EPI may result in variations in frequencies and phase errors. This effect is reduced for multishot EPI because phase errors have less time to build up. An advantage of multishot EPI over FSE is that it has contrast much closer to CSE, so it has greater sensitivity to magnetic susceptibility effects such as hemorrhage compared with FSE.

Remedy:

Minimized by proper shimming, TE shortening, or use of multishot echo.

Chemical Shift Artifacts in EPI

Because of the presence of phase error propagation along the phase-encode axis, chemical shift artifacts in EPI occur along the phase-encode axis rather than along the frequency-encode axis seen in CSE. These artifacts are much more pronounced than with CSE, so an effective fat suppression technique is necessary.

Remedy:

Apply fat suppression.

FUNCTIONAL ECHO-PLANAR IMAGING
Diffusion Imaging

Diffusion is defined as the process of random molecular thermal motion (also referred to as Brownian motion) which plays an important role in, for example, cerebrovascular accidents. Diffusion-weighted SE EPI can be accomplished with a pair of diffusion gradients applied before and after the 180° pulse (Fig. 22-7) to dephase and eliminate signals caused by diffusing protons.

Perfusion Imaging

Because contrast in GE-EPI is T2*W, it is perfect for performing first pass "**perfusion**" sequences with gadolinium. Flowing blood is bright, as with conventional GRE, allowing for EPI-MRA.

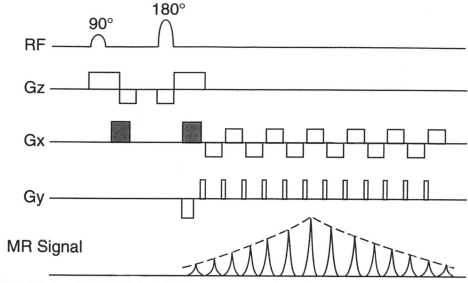

Figure 22-7. Diffusion-weighted SE-EPI. A pair of diffusion gradients is applied before and after the 180° pulse to dephase and eliminate signals from diffusing protons.

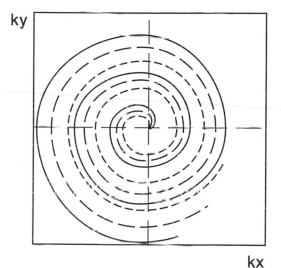

Figure 22-8. A spiral trajectory for multishot EPI using two oscillating gradients.

Advantages of EPI

1. Scan time is approximately 100 msec or less.
2. Cardiac and respiratory motion won't pose problems any longer.
3. Proton density, T_1, and T_2 weighted images free of motion artifacts can be achieved.
4. It allows studying organ function rather than merely depicting organ anatomy.

5. Resolution can be improved because time is not a significant factor.

Disadvantages of EPI

1. Because fat-water chemical shift artifacts (of the second kind [Dixon effect]) can be problematic with such short TEs, fat suppression with presaturation techniques is always required for EPI.
2. Because of rapid on and off switching of the gradients, there is a potential for generating an electric current or voltage in the patient, thus causing the sensation of an "electric shock" in the patient. This shock is caused by the well-known fact in electromagnetic theory that rapid changes in a magnetic field (i.e., dB/dt for the mathematically-oriented reader) induces an electric current (E) in a conductor (in this case the patient).
3. Potential for phase error (caused by slight variations in resonant frequencies) propagation exists. This effect is less for multishot EPI as there is less time for phase errors to build up.
4. Intrinsic nonuniformities in B_0 and diamagnetic susceptibility effects also result in variable resonance frequencies and increasing phase errors. Again, this effect occurs less in multishot EPI.

CLINICAL APPLICATIONS OF EPI

1. Cardiac and abdominal imaging free of motion artifacts in an extremely fast mode
2. Single breathhold imaging of the abdomen, providing T1W, T2W, or PDW
3. Anatomic, functional, or perfusion studies of the heart free of cardiac motion artifacts
4. Imaging the coronary arteries free of cardiac motion artifacts
5. Cine cardiac imaging within a single heart beat
6. Dynamic perfusion study of the myocardium after intravenous administration of gadolinium contrast to assess for ischemic regions
7. Dynamic perfusion studies of the brain
8. Diffusion imaging of the brain (by looking at the molecular diffusion of water). This is helpful in early diagnosis of acute cerebrovascular accidents (CVA) when routine images are unremarkable, and in distinguishing a CVA from other processes (e.g., neoplasm).

Key Points

Echo planar imaging (EPI) is the fastest MR technique currently available and is slowly becoming more and more clinically applicable. It employs a train of oscillating frequency-encoding gradients, thus rendering a sinusoidal k-space traversal after a single RF pulse. Consequently, each slice can be imaged in a matter of milliseconds (free of any motion artifact), and the entire study can be accomplished in a matter of seconds.

Questions

22-1. T/F   In single shot EPI, k-space is traversed in a zigzag fashion.

22-2. T/F   In multishot EPI, k-space is filled after a single excitation pulse.

22-3. Regarding multishot echo, all the following are true EXCEPT:
   (a) It places less stress on the gradients compared to single shot EPI.
   (b) Phase errors have less time to build up compared to single shot EPI.
   (c) It takes longer to perform than single shot EPI.
   (d) It is less susceptible to motion artifacts.

22-4. T/F   In blipped EPI, the phase encode gradient is constant during the acquisition.

22-5. T/F   Phase errors are eliminated with blipped EPI.

22-6. T/F   Contrast in EPI depends on the root pulsing sequence.

22-7. N/2 ghosts are generally seen with
   (a) constant phase EPI
   (b) blipped EPI
   (c) multishot EPI
   (d) none of the above

INTRODUCTION

In this chapter, we will discuss some of the more recent techniques used by newer MR scanners with more advanced software. The following is a summary of these features and their functions:

1. To increase speed
   (a) Fractional NEX
   (b) FSE
   (c) Fast gradient echo techniques
2. To reduce TE
   (a) Fractional echo
   (b) Fractional RF
3. To increase resolution (without time penalty)
   (a) Asymmetric FOV
4. To reduce aliasing
   (a) No phase wrap
   (b) No frequency wrap
5. To increase coverage
   (a) Phase offset RF pulses
6. To achieve contiguous slices
   (a) Contiguous slices
   (b) 3D acquisition
7. To achieve saturation
   (a) Spatial saturation
   (b) Spectral (chemical) saturation
8. To increase SNR
   (a) Low bandwidth

FRACTIONAL NEX (Fig. 23-1)

Also refer to Chapter 13.

Mechanism

1. Only a portion of k-space is used (e.g., 1/2 NEX, 3/4 NEX [actually, the number of phase encodes Ny is reduced not NEX]). Reconstruction is based on inherent symmetry of k-space along the phase axis.
2. Slightly more than half of k-space is used (called **overscan**) for phase correction.
3. The center of k-space is usually included because it contains the strongest signals.

Advantages

1. Increased speed (caused by reduced Ny)

Disadvantages

1. Decreased SNR
2. May increase artifacts

Applications

1. Used for localizer (scout) images
2. Used when speed is more important than SNR

FSE (FAST SPIN ECHO)

For more detailed discussion, refer to Chapter 19

Mechanism

1. Use of multiple 180° refocusing pulses
2. Filling the k-space with multiple lines per TR (per "shot")

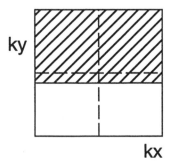
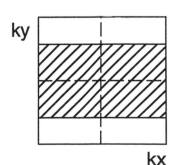

Figure 23-1. Fractional NEX.

3. Echo train length (ETL) denotes the number of 180° pulses (e.g., 2, 4, 8, 16, etc.)

Advantages

1. Reduces scan time by a factor of ETL (2, 4, 8, 16, etc.)
2. Spin echo contrast without reduction in SNR (SNR can actually be increased by using a very large TR)

Disadvantages

1. Reduced coverage (caused by the presence of long TEs)
2. CSF may be bright on PD images. This is a result of *weighted averaging* effect of later echoes. To reduce this undesirable effect, use a shorter ETL (e.g., ETL = 4), shorter TE (higher BW).
3. Fat is bright on T2WI because of elimination of diffusion-mediated dephasing caused by the closely-spaced 180° pulses as spins diffuse through regions of different magnetic field strength (e.g., fat and water).
4. Magnetic susceptibility effects (e.g., hemorrhage) are reduced because of decreased dephasing from closely-spaced (refocussing) 180° pulses, which leave little time for spins to dephase as they diffuse through regions of magnetic non-uniformity.

5. May increase heating as a result of rapidly changing gradients.

Applications

1. Fast scanning
2. High resolution (e.g., IACs)
3. Increase SNR with reasonable acquisition time
4. Single breath-hold technique
5. Isotropic T2W data set (e.g., 3D FSE)

FRACTIONAL ECHO (Fig. 23-2)

Mechanism

1. Only a fraction of the received echo is sampled (feasible because of the symmetry of the echo about TE and symmetry of k-space along frequency axis)

Advantages

1. TE can be reduced
2. SNR is improved in early echoes (less T2 decay)
3. Improves T1 weighting (reduces T2 effect)
4. May decrease flow artifacts and susceptibility effects

Applications

1. T1 weighted images
2. To reduce flow artifacts and magnetic susceptibility effects

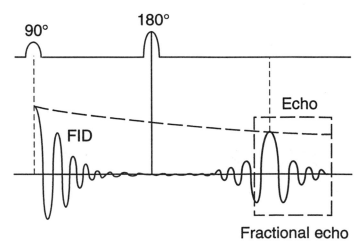

Figure 23-2. Fractional echo.

Fractional RF (90° or 180° or partial flip)

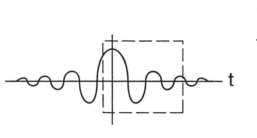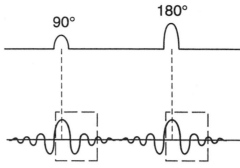

Figure 23-3. Fractional RF.

FRACTIONAL RF (90°, 180°, OR PARTIAL FLIP) (Fig. 23-3)

Mechanism

1. Same principles as in fractional echo (a fraction of the RF pulse is included in the pulse cycle because of the symmetry in the pulse)
2. TE can be reduced accordingly

Features

The features are similar to fractional echo.

ASYMMETRIC FOV (Fig. 23-4)

Mechanism

1. Rectangular FOV is used (FOV is typically reduced in phase direction because Ny is typically less than Nx)
2. May get square or rectangular pixels

Advantages

1. With rectangular FOV, we can obtain resolution of, say, 512 × 512 matrix in the time it takes to perform a 512 × 256 acquisition
2. Increases speed while maintaining resolution
3. Useful when the anatomy being imaged is asymmetric (smaller) in phase direction (e.g., the spine)

Disadvantages

1. Reduced SNR compared with full FOV
2. May cause wraparound in phase direction

Applications

1. Spine
2. Extremities

NO PHASE WRAP (PHASE OVERSAMPLING) (Fig. 23-5)

Mechanism

1. Doubles the number of phase encoding steps and the FOV
2. Discards one half of FOV at each end to maintain the specified FOV
3. NEX is reduced by one half to keep time constant

Advantages

1. Reduces or eliminates wraparound (aliasing)
2. No change in SNR or scan time

Disadvantages

1. If 1 NEX is used, scan time is doubled

Applications

1. Small FOV (may cause wraparound)
2. Extremities

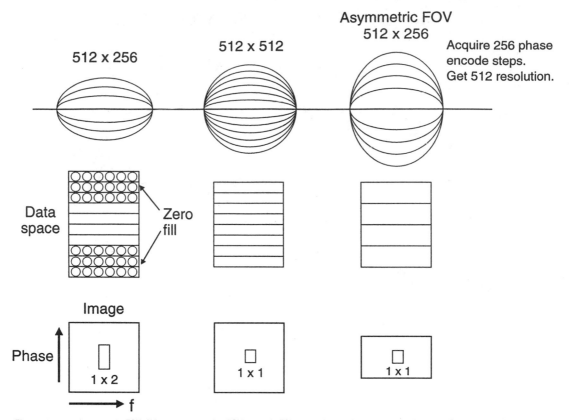

Figure 23-4. Asymmetric FOV. When a rectangular FOV is used, FOV typically is reduced in phase direction. By acquiring more phase-encode steps, a higher resolution can be achieved. In this example, you can acquire 256 phase-encode steps and still get a 512 resolution.

NO FREQUENCY WRAP (FREQUENCY OVERSAMPLING)

Mechanism

1. The echo is **oversampled**, thus assuring that the *Nyquist frequency* requirement is satisfied (e.g., 512 samples are obtained by the ADC even though Nx may read 256). Remember that the Nyquist Law requires that the sampling frequency ω_s be at least twice as high as the maximum frequency present in the signal (ω_{max}). Stated differently, at least two samples are needed per cycle corresponding to the highest frequency waveform.

2. Various low-pass filters (LPF) and band-pass filters (BPF) are also used to get rid of unwanted high frequencies in the signal.

Advantages

1. Avoids wraparound in the frequency-encode direction.
2. No increase in the scan time.

Disadvantages

1. May decrease SNR because, by increasing the number of samples, the sampling interval is reduced and thus the bandwidth is increased (remember BW = $1/\Delta$Ts and SNR $\propto \sqrt{1/BW}$).
2. This is done internally; i.e., the operator has no control over it.

Applications

1. Almost always automatically turned on during routine scanning

PHASE OFFSET RF PULSES
(Fig. 23-6)

Mechanism

1. Simultaneously excites two slices with two RF pulses that have a phase offset

Advantages

1. Doubles the number of slices per TR (without increasing time)
2. Can achieve more T1 weighting by reducing TR

Disadvantages

1. May increase wraparound artifact

Applications

1. When a short TR is desired, and a large area is studied
2. Gadolinium-enhanced studies in which shorter TR enhances paramagnetic effects of contrast

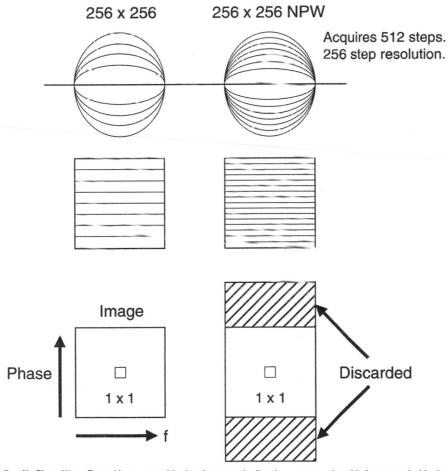

No Phase Wrap (NPW)

256 x 256

256 x 256 NPW

Acquires 512 steps.
256 step resolution.

Image

Phase

1 x 1

1 x 1

f

Discarded

Figure 23-5. No Phase Wrap. To avoid wraparound in the phase-encode direction, you can select this feature to double the FOV in that direction and automatically discard the unwanted portions at the end.

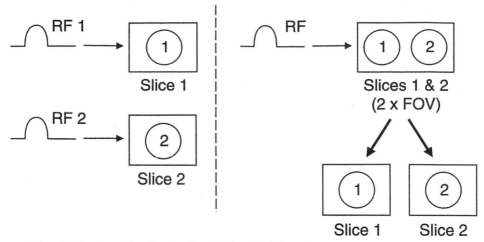

Figure 23-6. Phase-offset RF pulses. Two RF pulses with different phases excite two slices simultaneously.

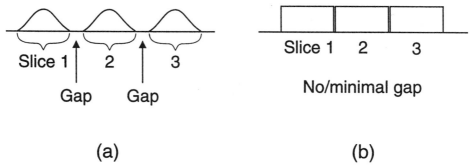

(a)   **(b)**

Figure 23-7. Contiguous slices can be achieved with an improved RF profile that better approximates a rectangle.

CONTIGUOUS SLICE OPTION (Fig. 23-7)

Mechanism

1. Employs longer RF pulses that have a more rectangular-shaped frequency transform, reducing cross talk
2. This eliminates/minimizes the need for interslice gaps

Advantages

1. Can achieve (almost) contiguous slices
2. Eliminates the need for interleaving (which doubles the scan time when correctly performed with two acquisitions)

Disadvantages

1. Increases TE (longer RF pulses)
2. Fewer slices per TR

Applications

1. When gaps are not desirable

3D ACQUISITION

Mechanism

1. Gradient echo (GRE) technique over a 3D volume
2. More recently, 3D FSE has become feasible

3. Requires a *phase*-encoding gradient along the slice select axis z
4. Contiguous slices (zero gaps)

Advantages

1. Increased SNR (due to acquisition from larger volume)
2. Allows thin high resolution contiguous slices
3. Allows for high-quality reformation in any plane

Disadvantages

1. May introduce wraparound artifacts at each end of the volume (end of the slab) caused by the presence of phase encoding in the z direction
2. Scan time now incorporates the number of phase encoding steps along the z axis (e.g. 28, 60) into the formula as well. That is to say,

Acq. Time (3D GRE)

$$= T(3D\ GRE)$$
$$= TR \cdot NEX \cdot Ny \cdot Nz$$
$$= Nz \cdot T(2D\ GRE)$$

but because TR is very short, this is acceptable. For 3D FSE, this formula becomes

Acq. Time (3D FSE)

$$= T(3D\ FSE)$$
$$= TR \cdot NEX \cdot Ny \cdot Nz/ETL$$
$$= Nz \cdot T(2D\ FSE)$$

where ETL can be chosen to be very large (see Chapter 27).

Applications

1. C spine
2. MR Angiography (e.g., circle of Willis)
3. Joints

SPATIAL SATURATION PULSES (SAT PULSES) (Fig. 23-8)

Mechanism (also see Chapter 24)

1. 90° saturation pulses are applied on either side of selected volume (can be applied in any direction: A/P, S/I, or R/L).

2. Sat bands are usually applied to suppress phase ghosts caused by flow-related phenomena.

Advantages

1. Minimizes phase ghosts
2. Minimizes flow artifacts

Disadvantages

1. May cause signal suppression in the remainder of the FOV
2. May lengthen TR, thus increasing the scan time

Applications

1. Imaging of the spine: saturation band is placed anterior to the vertebral bodies to suppress artifacts arising from the heart and great vessels.
2. MR Angiography: saturation pulses are placed at one end of a vessel to either suppress venous flow (to obtain MR Arteriography) or suppress arterial flow (to obtain MR Venography).
3. Abdominal imaging (minimizing artifacts from the aorta or IVC)
4. Brain (minimize artifacts from the internal carotid arteries and dural sinuses)

CHEMICAL (SPECTRAL) PRESATURATION (Fig. 23-9)

Mechanism (also see Chapter 24)

1. A frequency-selective presaturation pulse is applied before the RF excitation pulse, thus eliminating the longitudinal magnetization for a specific tissue.
2. The presaturation pulse is applied immediately before the 90° pulse of the SE. The tissue whose Larmor frequency matches the frequency of the presat pulse first sees a 90° spectral presat pulse that flips it into the x-y plane. A short time later, the longitudinal component M_z has really not had time to recover. Thus, the subsequent 90° excitation pulse that flips this minimal M_z into the x-y plane generates a minimal signal.

Application

1. To suppress fat or water by appropriate selection of the frequency

Advantages of Spectral Presaturation

1. It resolves tissues with similar T_1 values (such as fat and gadolinium-enhanced tumors).
2. This technique does not have any influ-

ence on the signal from tissues other than the one being suppressed (in contrast, IR affects the contrast of all tissues).

Disadvantages of Spectral Presaturation

1. Since this approach employs a frequency-selective technique, it suffers from sensitivity to magnetic field inhomogeneities.

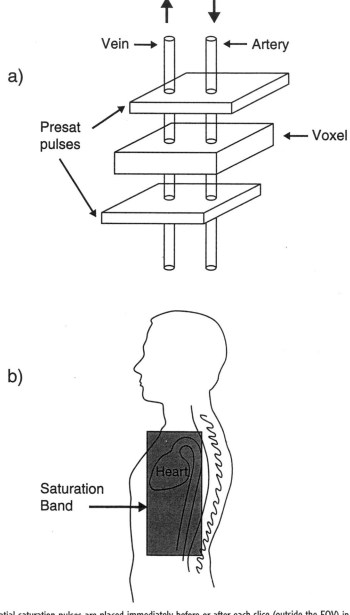

Figure 23-8. **(a)** Spatial saturation pulses are placed immediately before or after each slice (outside the FOV) in the case of flow imaging of arteries or veins. **(b)** Spatial saturation pulses are placed in front of the spine (within the FOV) to reduce artifacts from perivertebral vessels.

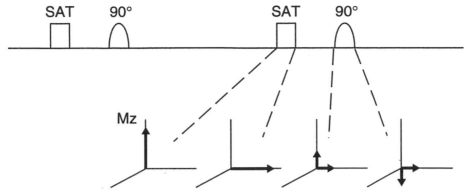

Figure 23-9. Chemical (spectral) presaturation pulses.

2. Requires extra time (thus lengthening TR and increasing the scan time).
3. Increases length of RF pulses causing extra RF heating.

LOW BANDWIDTH (VARIABLE BW)

Mechanism

1. On double echo SE sequence, the second echo has a lower BW

Advantages

1. Increases SNR (remember that SNR $\propto 1/\sqrt{BW}$) of second echo

Disadvantages

1. Increased chemical shift artifacts (to alleviate, use fat sat)
2. Decreases allowable number of slices (due to increased TE)

Applications

1. Any study requiring a higher SNR
2. Example: Dual SE of brain—a narrower BW is used on the second echo (to increase S/N, which is decreased because of T2 decay)

Key Points

Many new MR techniques were reviewed in this chapter. These, along with their major trade-offs, are summarized below.

1. To increase speed
   (a) Fractional NEX (*trade-offs*: ↓ SNR, ↑ artifacts)
   (b) FSE (*trade-offs*: ↓ coverage, ↑ contrast averaging)
   (c) Fast gradient echo techniques (*trade-off*: ↓ SNR)

2. To reduce TE
   (a) Fractional echo (*trade-off*: may ↑ artifacts)

   (b) Fractional RF (*trade-off*: may ↑ artifacts)

3. To increase resolution (without time penalty)
   (a) Asymmetric FOV (*trade-off*: ↓ SNR and ↑ potential for wraparound)

4. To reduce aliasing
   (a) No phase wrap (*trade-off*: may slightly ↑ scan time)
   (b) No frequency wrap (*trade-off*: may ↓ SNR)

5. To increase coverage
   (a) Phase offset RF pulses (*trade-off*: may ↑ wraparound)

6. To achieve contiguous slices
    (a) Contiguous slices (CS) (*trade-off*: may
    ↑ TE)
    (b) 3D acquisition (*trade-off*: ↑ scan time)

7. To achieve saturation
    (a) Spatial saturation
    (b) Spectral (chemical) saturation

8. To increase SNR
    (a) Low bandwidth (Variable BW)

Questions

23-1. Speed can be increased by:
    (a) FSE or GRE techniques
    (b) fractional NEX
    (c) reducing BW
    (d) all of the above
    (e) only (a)-(b)

23-2. An asymmetric FOV may result in all of
    the following EXCEPT:
    (a) reduced SNR
    (b) increased potential wraparound
    (c) increased resolution
    (d) increased scan time

23-3. A lower BW leads to all of the following
    EXCEPT:
    (a) reduces minimum TE
    (b) increased chemical shift artifacts
    (c) decreases coverage
    (d) increased SNR

23-4. T/F   The SNR is increased in 3D GRE.

23-5. T/F   Spatial saturation pulses are used
    to minimize phase ghosts and flow arti-
    facts.

23-6. T/F   Minimum TE can be reduced by
    using fractional NEX.

24 Tissue Suppression Techniques

INTRODUCTION

One of the beauties of MRI, especially with some of the new features, is the ability to image a body part while "suppressing" the signal coming from a certain selected tissue. This suppression allows perturbation of tissue contrast to enhance the signal coming from tissues of greater interest (such as a pathology). Two types of tissues are commonly suppressed in clinical practice: fat and water.

SUPPRESSION TECHNIQUES

Several suppression techniques are available, some of which are listed below.

1. Inversion recovery techniques
2. Chemical (or spectral) saturation or frequency-selective presaturation
3. Spatial presaturation in the FOV

Inversion Recovery (IR) Techniques

This technique was discussed at length in Chapter 7. The IR pulse sequence diagram (PSD) is shown in Figure 24-1. By appropriate selection of TI (time to inversion), we can nullify or suppress a certain tissue. In fact, as we saw in chapter 7, if

$$TI = (\ln 2) [T_1(\text{tissue x})] = 0.693\, T_1(\text{tissue x})$$

then tissue x is nulled. Thus, TI can be chosen to null fat or water or any other desired tissue depending on the application (Fig. 24-2).

STIR (SHORT TI INVERSION RECOVERY)

This is the IR technique that is used to suppress fat.

EXAMPLE 1:
What is the TI used in STIR? At 1.5 Tesla, T_1 of fat is approximately 200 msec. Then

$$TI = 0.693 \times 200 \cong 140 \text{ msec.}$$

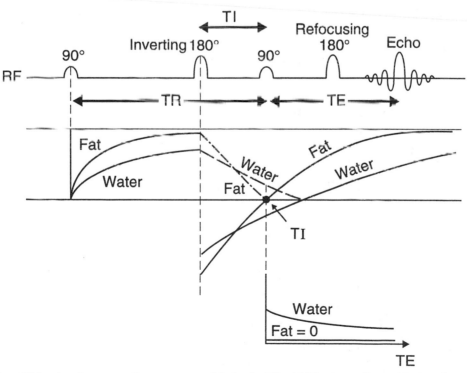

Figure 24-1. Inversion recovery. The recovery curves following the 90° and 180° pulses are illustrated for fat and water.

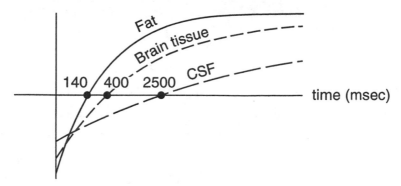

Figure 24-2.   TI required to null fat, brain, or CSF.

FLAIR (FLUID-ATTENUATED INVERSION RECOVERY)

This is an inversion recovery technique that nulls fluid. For example, this sequence is used in the brain to suppress CSF to bring out the periventricular hyperintense lesions, such as MS plaques.

EXAMPLE 2:

What is the TI used in FLAIR? At 1.5 Tesla, T_1 of CSF is approximately 3600 msec. Then

$$TI = 0.693 \times 3600 \cong 2500 \text{ msec.}$$

FAST FLAIR

This is a relatively new sequence that combines the FLAIR sequence with a fast technique, such as FSE, to achieve CSF suppression in a fast manner[a]. Figure 24-3 depicts a schematic representation for Fast FLAIR. In this scheme, the following parameters are used:

$$TR = 10,000 \text{ msec,}$$
$$TI = 2,500 \text{ msec,}$$
$$\text{FSE with ETL} = 8,$$
$$TE_{eff} = 112 \text{ msec}$$

In Figure 24-3, there are two packets of 15 slices each. During the first 5000 msec, 15 slice-selective 180° inverting pulses are followed 2500 msec (TI) later by 15 slice-selective FSE readout in 2500 msec. During the second 5000 msec, recovery occurs in the first 15 slices (for a total TR of 10,000 msec), and the process is repeated on the second set of 15 interleaved slices. In all, 30 slices are acquired.

---

[a] Hashemi RH, Bradley WG, et al. Suspected multiple sclerosis: MR imaging with a thin-section fast FLAIR pulse sequence. Radiology 1995; 196:505–510.

A TR of 10,000 msec allows almost complete longitudinal recovery of CSF. This relatively long time period also makes it possible to perform multislice interleaving during inversion and readout. The inversion "period" is the time during which 15 slice-selective 180° pulses are applied. It is the time TI (2500 msec in this case) from the first 180° inverting pulse to the 90° pulse at the beginning of the readout period. FSE readout takes 136 msec (8×17 msec) for each slice. The readout "period" is the time (also 2500 msec) during which 15 slice-selective readouts are performed. The recovery period is the time from the slice-selective 90° pulse beginning an FSE readout to the next slice-selective 180° inverting pulse, which is TR-TI (10,000 − 2500 = 7500 msec in this case).

The maximum number of slices that can be acquired in one TR is determined either by the time period TI or by (TR − TI), whichever is shorter. The longer the TR, the more complete recovery of magnetization will be before the next excitation. A long TR will also result in better S/N (signal to noise ratio) and increased C/N (contrast-to-noise ratio) between the lesion, gray matter, and white matter.

Unfortunately, when TR is increased, the TI necessary to null CSF does not increase to the same degree. This difference results in inefficient usage of time because (TR − TI) becomes larger and larger, and the number of slices is still limited by TI. Given the TR of 10,000 msec and the TI of 2500 msec used in this study, 5000 msec (i.e., 10,000 − 2 × 2500) would be "wasted" before the next cycle. To increase the efficiency, the sequence takes advantage of this dead time to acquire a second multislice inversion-readout slab.

FAST-FLAIR

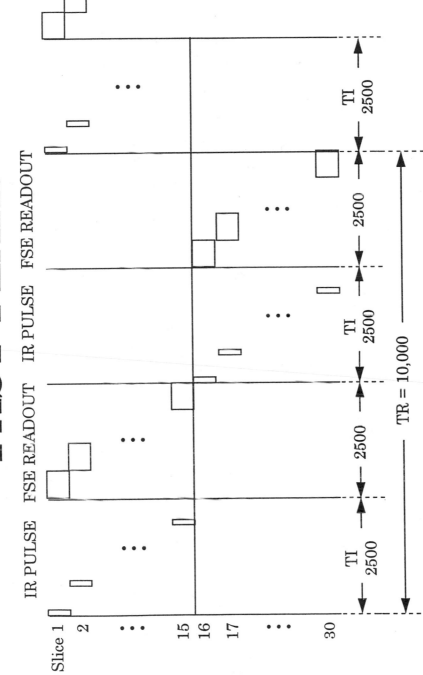

Figure 24-3. A schematic representation for Fast FLAIR. There are two packets of 15 slices each. During the first 5000 msec, 15 slice-selective 180° inverting pulses are followed 2500 msec (TI) later by 15 slice-selective FSE readout, in 2500 msec. During the second 5000 msec, recovery occurs in the first 15 slices (for a total TR of 10,000 msec) and the process is repeated on the second set of 15 interleaved slices. In all, 30 slices are acquired in 8 minutes.

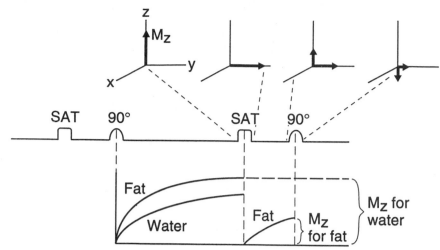

Figure 24-4. Spectral presaturation. A frequency-selective presaturation pulse is applied before the excitation pulse to eliminate longitudinal magnetization for a specific tissue such as fat or water.

In this arrangement, the number of slices acquired can be doubled in the same time duration with no dead time when the TR to TI ratio equals 4. As the ratio approaches 6, yet another multislice section can be added, and so on. This approach allows the flexibility to choose TR and TI with little concern for time efficiency.

Advantages of IR

1. No extra RF heating (like spectral presaturation—see later text)
2. No variability caused by magnetic field inhomogeneities (like spectral presaturation—see below)

Disadvantages of IR

1. Tissues with similar T_1 values are all suppressed and thus cannot be differentiated (e.g., fat and gadolinium-enhanced tumors)
2. Long acquisition times caused by long TRs
3. Low S/N

Chemical (Spectral) Presaturation

In this technique, a frequency-selective presaturation pulse is applied before the RF excitation pulse, thus eliminating the longitudinal magnetization for a specific tissue, e.g., fat. It can be used to suppress fat or water by appropriate selection of the frequency (based on the Larmor equation, keeping in mind that at 1.5 T, water protons precess 220 Hz faster than fat protons).

This scheme is illustrated in Figure 24-4. Here, the presaturation pulse is applied immediately before the 90° pulse of the SE. The tissue whose Larmor frequency matches the frequency of the presat pulse first sees a 90° spectral presat pulse that flips it into the x-y plane. A short time later, the longitudinal component M_z has really not had time to recover. Thus, the subsequent 90° excitation pulse that flips this minimal M_z into the x-y plane generates a minimal signal (Fig. 24-4).

Advantages of Spectral Presaturation

1. Resolves tissues with similar T_1 values (such as fat and gadolinium-enhanced tumors)
2. No influence on the signal from tissues other than the one being suppressed (in contrast, IR affects the contrast of all tissues)

Disadvantages of Spectral Presaturation

1. Suffers from sensitivity to magnetic field inhomogeneities because it employs a frequency- selective technique
2. Requires extra time (thus lengthening TR and increasing the scan time)
3. Increases length of RF pulses, causing extra RF heating

Spatial Presaturation

Spatial presaturation is done generally to reduce motion and flow-related artifacts of structures adjacent to—or actually within the FOV next to—the region of interest. Examples include:

1. Imaging of the spine: a saturation band is placed within the FOV anterior to the vertebral bodies to suppress artifacts arising from the heart and great vessels.
2. MR Angiography: saturation pulses are placed outside the FOV at one end of a vessel to suppress either venous flow

(for achieving MR arteriography) or arterial flow (for achieving MR venography).

Spatial presaturation is accomplished by applying an extra 90° pulse before the 90° pulse of the SE sequence. This additional Sat pulse saturates tissues, including moving structures, within the slice, eliminating signal (and thus associated artifacts). For more details, refer to the discussion on saturation in Chapter 23.

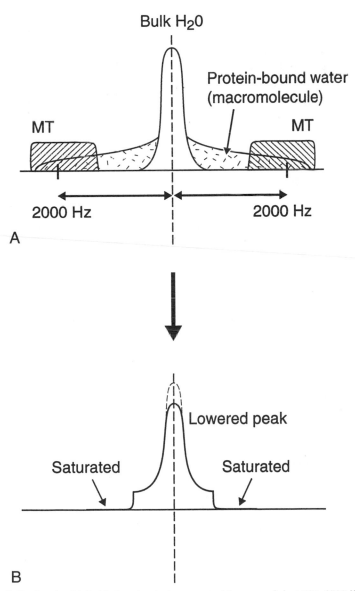

Figure 24-5. Magnetization transfer. **(a)** Protein-bound water has a resonant frequency of about 500–2500 Hz off that of bulk water. **(b)** Spectral saturation of these off-resonant frequencies will result in suppression of protein bound water. This technique is used, for example, in MRA for background suppression.

Magnetization Transfer (MT)

Magnetization transfer (MT) is a new technique that suppresses protein-bound water. The idea behind MT is that protons in protein-bound water exhibit a resonant frequency that is approximately 500 to 2500 Hz away from that of bulk water protons (Fig. 24-5). MT saturation pulses are simply off-resonant pulses with their center frequency 1000 to 2000 Hz removed from the Larmor frequency of protons and a bandwidth (BW) of several hundred to several thousand Hz, as shown in Figure 24-5a, thus allowing suppression of these protons. The result is shown in Figure 24-5b. Note that the off-resonant protein-bound water is saturated. Because the protein-bound protons and the bulk water protons are in rapid exchange, the saturation is transferred to the bulk phase protons. Thus, the peak amplitude of bulk water is reduced. MT is somewhat similar to spectral fat suppression techniques except that here, the off-resonant frequency is up to 2000 Hz (2 kHz) as opposed to 220 Hz in the case of fat suppression.

This technique is used, for example, in TOF (time of flight) MR angiography (see Chapter 26) as a means of suppressing the background brain tissue to enhance visualization of smaller, more peripheral vessels.

MAGNETIZATION TRANSFER EFFECT IN FSE

As discussed in Chapter 19, MT is inadvertently present in FSE because of the presence of multiple, rapid 180° pulses. These rapid 180° pulses have a broad BW that contains frequencies off the bulk water resonance frequency which tend to suppress protein-bound water.

A Few Clinical Applications of Fat Suppression
1. To differentiate between fat and methemoglobin.
2. *Musculoskeletal*: to minimize fat signal in the marrow to bring out the signal from marrow edema (e.g., due to bone contusion, tumor, infection, etc.).
3. *Orbits*: to suppress the retroorbital fat to allow detection of an enhancing retroorbital pathology on a contrast-enhanced study.
4. *Neck*: to suppress fat in order to detect, and better evaluate the extent of, a mass.

A Few Clinical Applications of Water Suppression
Brain: to suppress CSF to bring out periventricular high intensity lesions such as MS plaques, thus increasing their detectability.

Key Points

Tissue suppression is an important feature of MRI—it allows improved tissue contrast and enhanced lesion detectability. Generally, two tissues are subject to suppression: fat and water. The two major suppression techniques are inversion recovery (IR) and chemical (spectral) saturation. Each technique has its own advantages and disadvantages. The selection of the type of technique depends on the clinical application. Other tissues may be saturated (e.g., protein-bound water and flowing blood).

Major fat suppression techniques include:

1. STIR
2. Chemical (spectral) fat Sat

Major fluid suppression techniques include:

1. FLAIR
2. Fast FLAIR
3. Chemical (spectral) water suppression

Suppression of protein-bound water:

1. Magnetization transfer (MT) technique for background suppression
2. MT effect in FSE

Presaturation technique in the FOV:

1. Saturation bands reduce flow artifacts (e.g., in spine imaging)
2. Saturation pulses remove venous or arterial flow (e.g., in MRA or MRV)

Questions

24-1. In an IR sequence, the TI to null a tissue is given by:
(a) $0.693\ T_2$ (b) $0.693\ T_1$
(c) $(1/.693)\ T_1$ (d) $(1/.693)\ T_2$

24-2. The T_1 of CSF at 1.5 T is about 3600 msec. What is the approximate TI to null CSF?
(a) 2500   (b) 5000
(c) 140   (d) 249.48

24-3. T/F Protons in protein bound macromolecules have a resonant frequency that is about 220 Hz removed from that of bulk water.

24-4. T/F FSE demonstrates an inherent magnetization transfer property.

24-5. T/F Magnetization transfer techniques saturate the off-resonant protein-bound water protons.

24-6. Major fat suppression techniques include:
(a) STIR
(b) Spectral fat suppression
(c) FLAIR   (d) all of the above
(e) only (a)–(b)

24-7. Major water suppression techniques include:
(a) STIR
(b) Spectral water suppression
(c) FLAIR   (d) all of the above
(e) only (b)–(c)

25   Flow Phenomena

INTRODUCTION

Unlike CT (with or without contrast) where the appearance of flowing blood is predictable, the appearance of flowing blood in MRI is much more complicated. Flowing blood or CSF can appear dark or bright depending on numerous factors, including, but not limited to, the following:

1. velocity
2. pulse sequence (e.g., SE vs. GRE)
3. position of the slice containing the vessel relative to the rest of the slices
4. contrast (TR and TE)
5. echo number (even or odd)
6. slice thickness
7. flip angle
8. gradient strength and rise time
9. use of gradient moment nulling techniques, etc.
10. use of spatial presaturation pulse
11. use of cardiac gating
12. chance of cardiac gating (pseudogating)

TYPES OF FLOW

In Chapter 18 (MRI Artifacts), we discussed two types of motion: random and periodic. Blood and CSF flow have a periodic-type motion. Furthermore, flow of blood can be divided into the following:

1. Laminar flow
2. Plug flow
3. Turbulent flow
4. Flow (stream) separation/vortex flow

These types of flow are depicted in Figure 25-1. Let's discuss these separately.

Laminar Flow

This type of flow is seen in most normal vessels and has a parabolic profile. If the lumen radius is R, then the velocity v at position r would be

$$v(r) = V_{max}(1 - r^2/R^2)$$

where V_{max} is the maximum velocity in the center of the lumen. Therefore, the average velocity in the lumen is given by

$$V_{ave} = V_{max}/2$$

Plug Flow

This is an idealized type of flow in which the velocity across the lumen is constant, thus yielding a flat velocity profile:

$$v(r) = V_{max} = V_{ave} = constant$$

Turbulence

This phenomenon is observed in abnormal vessels (e.g., distal to stenosis) or at bifurcations during which a random motion of fluid elements is observed. **Vortex flow** and large scale recirculation zones (i.e., **eddies**) are other terms that refer to such random motions.

Flow (Stream) Separation

This phenomenon is observed near the wall of a vessel (e.g., in the proximal internal carotid artery) in which some of the flow is separated from the main streamline.

Question: What determines laminar versus turbulent flow?
Answer: A dimensionless number called the Reynolds number (Re) can predict the type of flow. It is given by

$$Re = (density \times velocity \times diameter)/viscosity$$

where density is in g/cm^3, velocity is in cm/sec, diameter is in cm, viscosity is in centipoise or g/cm-sec, and Re has no units. If Re < 2100, then flow is laminar. If Re > 2100, then flow is turbulent.

Question: What is a typical blood flow velocity?
Answer: It depends on the vessel. Here are some examples (Table 25-1).

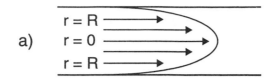

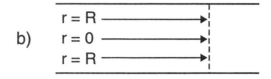

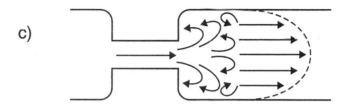

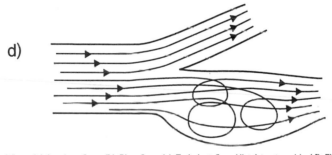

Figure 25-1. Types of flow: **(a)** Laminar flow. **(b)** Plug flow. **(c)** Turbulent flow (distal to stenosis). **(d)** Flow (stream) separation.

Table 25-1

Aorta	140 ± 40 cm/sec
Superficial femoral	90 ± 13 cm/sec
Vetebral	36 ± 9 cm/sec
Venous flow	<20 cm/sec

The blood velocity may be much higher in abnormal conditions, such as in an arterio-venous fistula (AVF).

Question: What is the difference between flow and velocity?

Answer: A mathematical relationship exists between bulk or volumetric flow in a vessel lumen and the velocity of flow:

$$v = Q/A$$

where v is the average velocity (in cm/sec), Q is the bulk or volumetric flow (in cm^3/sec), and A is the cross sectional area of the vessel (in cm^2).

Normal Appearance of Flowing Blood

Most flow effects can be attributed from one of the following:

1. Time of flight (TOF) effects
2. Motion-induced phase changes

TOF effects can lead to the following:

1. Signal loss ("high-velocity signal loss" or "TOF loss")

2. Signal gain ("flow-related enhancement" or FRE)

Flowing blood can appear bright or dark. Three main independent factors result in each case:

1. ↓ SI of flowing blood
   (a) high velocity
   (b) turbulent flow
   (c) dephasing
2. ↑ SI of flowing blood
   (a) flow-related enhancement (FRE)
   (b) even echo rephasing
   (c) diastolic pseudogating

Let's discuss each of these separately.

HIGH-VELOCITY SIGNAL LOSS

In SE imaging, the protons must be exposed to both a 90° and a 180° RF pulse to give off a signal. High velocity signal loss or **time-of-flight** (TOF) loss occurs when flowing protons do not remain within the selected slice long enough to be exposed to both RF pulses.

Figure 25-2 illustrates how the magnitude of signal loss is a function of the velocity. To see how this works, first recall the simple relationship between time, distance, and velocity:

$$\text{velocity} = \text{distance/time}$$

or

$$v = d/t$$

The distance each proton in flowing blood has to travel within a slice is the slice thickness Δz. The time between a 90° pulse and a 180° pulse is one-half TE.

Thus, if the velocity of flowing blood is

$$v = \Delta z/(\tfrac{1}{2}\ TE)$$

then protons flowing into the slice would be exposed only to the 90° pulse, and not to the 180° pulse, thus forming no signal or spin echo. Let's give this velocity an arbitrary name v_m, i.e.

$$v_m = \Delta z/(\tfrac{1}{2}\ TE)$$

However, if the velocity were 0 (i.e., for stagnant blood), then a spin echo would be formed. If the velocity falls in between, only a fraction of the protons would form a spin echo. The fraction of protons escaping the 180° pulse is

given by

$$v/v_m = v(\tfrac{1}{2}\ TE)/\Delta z$$

Thus, the fraction of protons receiving both RF pulses is

$$1 - v/v_m = 1 - v\ (\tfrac{1}{2}\ TE)/\Delta z$$

The signal intensity is, therefore, proportional to

$$I \propto (1 - v\ .\ TE/2\Delta z)$$

Figure 25-3 illustrates the linear relationship between signal intensity (I) and velocity v. It is clear from this graph that if the velocity of flowing blood is at least equal to v_m (i.e., $v \geq v_m$), then a flow void is observed.

EXAMPLE:

Suppose that the slice thickness $\Delta z = 1$ cm and TE = 25 msec. What is the velocity at which flow void is observed?

Using the above formula, the velocity should be at least

$$v_m = \Delta z/(\tfrac{1}{2}\ TE) = 1\ \text{cm}/(25\ \text{msec})$$
$$= 1000\ \text{cm}/25\ \text{sec} = 40\ \text{cm/sec}$$

which is seen in an artery.

Therefore, v_m is larger for thicker slices and smaller TEs, and vice versa.

N.B. Remember that TOF losses only apply to SE imaging and not to GRE imaging because, in GRE, the echo is formed via a single α RF pulse and refocussing gradients (without a 180° pulse).

TURBULENT FLOW

In turbulent flow (with Re > 2100), random flow exists that contains different velocity components (i.e., with different speed and direction of flow). Consequently, each of these components have different phases that tend to cancel each other out and result in no signal (flow void). This result can occur with low or high velocity flow.

DEPHASING

There are many causes of dephasing. One important cause is the so-called **odd-echo dephasing**. This phenomenon results in signal void on the first and other odd echoes. The protons in a voxel do not move at the same velocity across the lumen in laminar flow; thus, each precesses at a different frequency and accumu-

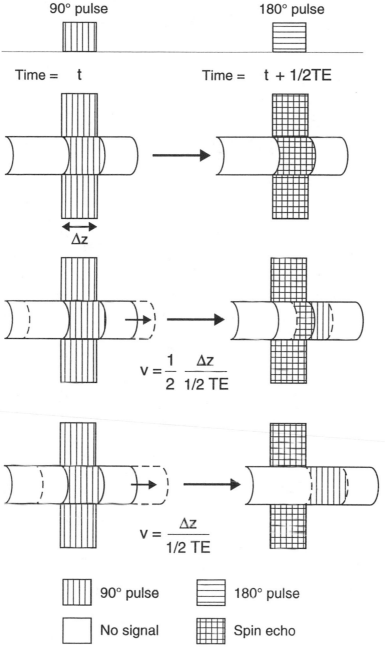

Figure 25-2. To form an echo, protons must be exposed to both a 90° and a 180° pulse. As velocity increases, a larger portion of flowing protons is exposed only to the 90° but not the 180° pulse, thus causing signal loss.

lates a different phase. (Also see the discussion below on even-echo rephasing.)

Another cause of dephasing is **intravoxel dephasing**. Because of laminar flow, different velocities may exist within a voxel, thus leading to phase dispersion (incoherence) and signal loss.

How to decrease intravoxel dephasing and increase SNR:

1. Decrease the voxel size (increase spatial resolution), either by increasing the matrix (*trade* off: will reduce SNR) or by reducing the FOV (*trade off*: may cause wraparound).

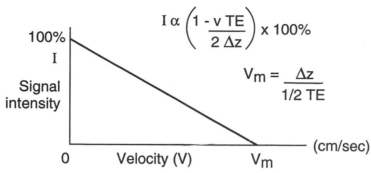

Figure 25-3. A plot of signal intensity versus velocity. The higher the velocity, the more the signal loss.

2. Reduce the TE (e.g., use a fractional echo).
3. Add flow compensation techniques (see below).

EVEN-ECHO REPHASING

This phenomenon is somewhat the opposite of odd-echo dephasing. It only occurs in SE imaging with symmetric echoes (i.e., when the second echo delay time is twice the first one, i.e. when $TE_2 = 2\ TE_1$; e.g., 30/60/90, 40/80/120, etc.). The result is higher signal intensity for even echoes compared with odd echoes. (We shall see later that in GRE or SE, flow compensation techniques basically yield "even-echo rephasing" on the first echo to minimize signal losses.)

To see how this works, we first need to learn about the relationship between phase and velocity. Recall that along the readout gradient,

$$\omega = \gamma\ B_x = \gamma\ G\ x$$

Now, for a constant velocity v, the position at time t is given simply by

$$x = v\ t$$

Thus, combining the above two, we get

$$\omega = \gamma\ G\ v\ t$$

Now, phase change $\Delta\phi$ and angular frequency ω are related by

$$\Delta\phi = \omega\ \Delta t$$

so that

$$\phi = \int \omega\ dt = \int (\gamma\ G\ v\ t)\ dt = \gamma\ G\ v \int t\ dt$$
$$= \gamma\ G\ v\ (t^2/2)$$

From this we can see the following:

1. Phase ϕ and velocity v are proportional.
2. A quadratic relationship exists between phase ϕ and time t, i.e., $\phi = k\ t^2$, where k is a constant ($k = \frac{1}{2}\ \gamma\ G\ v$).

On the contrary, for stationary tissue (with v = 0), the above relationship becomes

$$\phi = k'\ t$$

i.e., a linear relationship exits between phase and time for stationary tissues.

Now consider an SE sequence with symmetric echoes as shown in Figure 25-4. The phase changes over one cycle for both stationary tissues and flowing blood are plotted. This graph reveals that stationary tissues have zero phase on the first echo (TE) and the second echo (2TE). The situation for flowing blood, however, is different. On the first echo, the flowing blood has a positive phase. However, on the second echo, the phase is back to zero!

MATH: Let's try to prove the above fact mathematically. Assume that $\tau = \frac{1}{2}\ TE$. The phase gain at time TE/2 is $k\tau^2$, where k is a constant ($k = \frac{1}{2}\ \gamma Gv$). Right after the 180° pulse, the phase is $-k\tau^2$. Now, at time TE (i.e., at 2τ), the phase gain will be k $[(2\tau)^2 - (\tau)^2] = 3k\tau^2$. (The mathematically-oriented reader will recognize this as the integral of $\int 2k\tau$ from point τ to 2τ.) Thus, the net phase gain will be $3k\tau^2 + (-k\tau^2) = 2\ k\tau^2$. Similarly, at 3/2TE (or 3τ), i.e. at the second 180° pulse, the phase gain is k $[(3\tau)^2 + (2\tau)^2] = 5k\tau^2$, with a net gain of $5k\tau^2 + 2k\tau^2 = 7k\tau^2$. Immediately after this second 180° pulse, the phase will be $-7k\tau^2$. In a similar fashion, the phase gain at the time of the second echo (i.e., 4τ) will be $k[(4\tau)^2 - (3\tau)^2] = 7k\tau^2$. Therefore, the final net phase gain will be $7k\tau^2 + (-7k\tau^2) = 0$. That is to say, the net phase shift of flowing blood on the second echo is zero. This is illustrated in Figure 25-4 as well.

Thus, protons in flowing blood lose their coherence on the first echo (causing odd-echo dephasing) and subsequently regain coherence on the second echo (causing even-echo rephasing).

This pattern yields a higher signal of flowing blood on the second echo. It only works for symmetric echoes, not for asymmetric ones (interested readers can go through the previous math and prove this fact for themselves).

DIASTOLIC PSEUDOGATING

During a cardiac cycle, blood flow is more rapid during systole and slower in diastole. Thus, in diastole, a higher intravascular signal is observed (remember that higher flow results in more TOF losses). When **cardiac gating** is used, each slice is (theoretically) acquired at a fixed

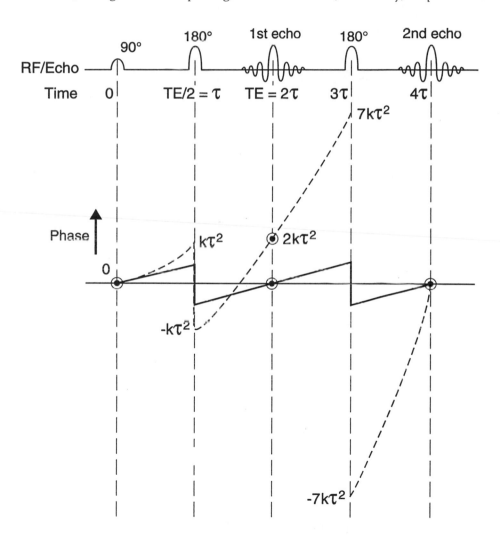

Figure 25-4. Phase accumulation for stationary and flowing protons.

point in the cardiac cycle (although different slices in a multislice acquisition are obtained at different points in the cycle). Consequently, a vessel traversing several slices will demonstrate varying signal intensities at different slices. In a cardiac-gated sequence, TR must be a multiple of the heart rate (HR). For example, if HR = 60 bpm (1 beat per second = 1 Hz), then TR = 1000, 2000, 3000, etc. In general,

$$TR = 1/HR$$

with appropriate units.

FLOW-RELATED ENHANCEMENT (FRE)

This phenomenon usually refers to the first slice that the flowing blood enters. Hence, FRE is also called the **entry phenomenon**. FRE is a type of TOF effect in which the fresh inflowing blood that enters the first slice is totally **unsaturated**, i.e. the protons within it have not as yet been subjected to any prior RF pulse and thus yield full magnetization, whereas the adjacent stationary tissue re-

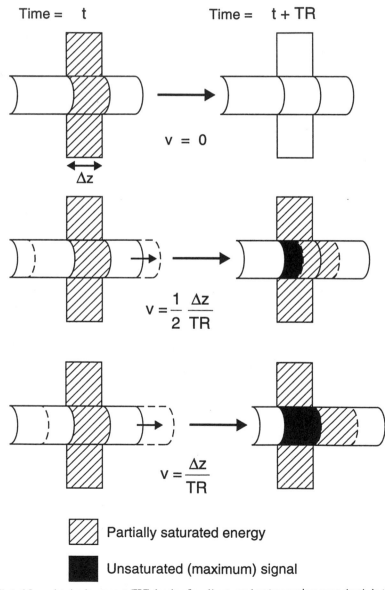

Time = t   Time = t + TR

$$v = 0$$

$$\Delta z$$

$$v = \frac{1}{2}\frac{\Delta z}{TR}$$

$$v = \frac{\Delta z}{TR}$$

▨ Partially saturated energy

■ Unsaturated (maximum) signal

Figure 25-5. Effect of flow-related enhancement (FRE) for slow flow. Unsaturated protons produce more signal. As the velocity increases, a larger portion of unsaturated inflowing protons will replace the previously partially saturated protons, thus increasing signal intensity.

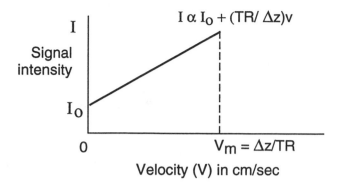

Flow-related enhancement (FRE)

Figure 25-6.   The plot of signal intensity versus velocity in FRE.

mains partially **saturated** because of prior RF pulses.

Figure 25-5 illustrates the relationship between FRE and the blood velocity. This diagram demonstrates that when v = 0 (i.e., stagnant blood), the protons are partially saturated. However, when the velocity is v = $\Delta z/TR$, then the unsaturated inflowing protons completely replace the previously partially saturated protons. Again, we shall give this velocity an arbitrary name v_M. The fraction of inflowing protons is then

$$v/v_M = v \, (TR/\Delta z)$$

Thus, the relationship between the intravascular signal intensity and velocity is

$$I \propto I_0 + (TR/\Delta z) \, v$$

where I_0 is the signal intensity of stagnant blood (i.e., at v — 0). This relationship is illustrated in Figure 25-6.

EXAMPLE:

At what velocity do you observe maximum FRE when Δz = 1 cm and TR = 1000 msec = 1 sec?

From the previous formula,

$$v_M = \Delta z/TR = 1 \; cm/1 \; sec = 1 \; cm/sec$$

which is consistent with a slow venous flow.

Why is Flowing Blood Bright on GRE Images?

You may have noticed that on most GRE images, vessels appear bright on all the slices. There are three main reasons for this:

1. GRE imaging is usually performed in a sequential mode (i.e., one slice at a time). Consequently, every slice is an entry slice. Thus, FRE applies to every slice in the volume.
2. Due to lack of a 180° refocusing pulse and the non-slice selectivity of the refocusing gradient, TOF losses are usually not significant in GRE imaging.
3. In GRE imaging, TE is usually very short, which minimizes signal losses caused by dephasing.

Question: *Is FRE only limited to the first (entry) slice?*
Answer: *The answer is no. If the velocity of flow is higher than $\Delta z/TR$ (but not too high for TOF losses to take place), then unsaturated protons can penetrate adjacent slices and yield FRE. Obviously, as these inflowing protons travel through the imaging volume, they are subjected to more and more RF pulses and become more and more saturated. Thus, FRE is always maximum at the entry slice and becomes gradually fainter in deeper slices (a good distinguishing point from an intraluminal thrombus). Now, how far FRE can penetrate the imaging volume has to do with the direction of flow and the direction of slice excitation.*

Cocurrent and Countercurrent Flow

The **slice excitation wave (SEW)** is the direction of successive 90° excitation pulses. If flow is perpendicular to the slices, then flow is either in the direction of the SEW (called **cocurrent**) or against it (called **countercurrent**). Intuitively, in a countercurrent setting, the flowing protons are subjected to fewer 90° pulses than in a cocurrent setting (Fig. 25-7). Consequently, FRE demonstrates deeper

penetration in a countercurrent setting (Fig. 25-8).

Combined Flow Phenomena

What would happen if very high velocity flow enters the entry slice? Although FRE affects the

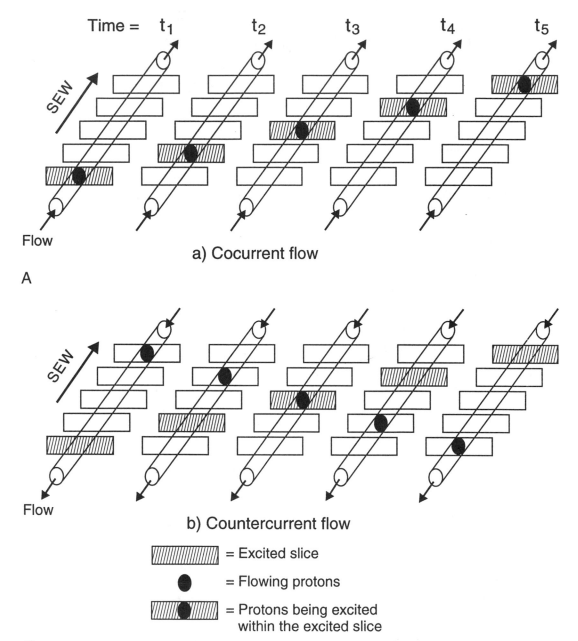

Figure 25-7. **(a)** Cocurrent flow. The flow and slice excitation wave (SEW) are in the same direction. **(b)** Countercurrent flow. The flow and SEW are in the opposite directions.

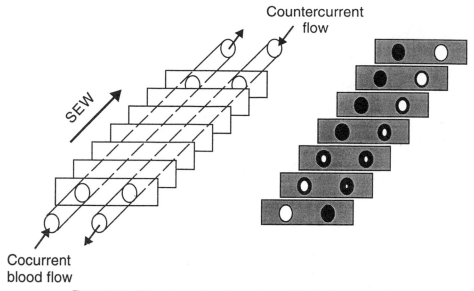

Figure 25-8.   FRE penetrates deeper in countercurrent flow than in cocurrent flow.

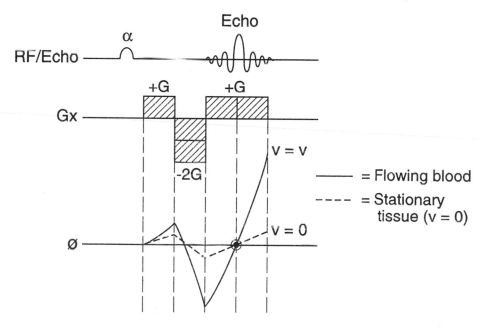

Flow Compensation in GRE

Figure 25-9.   Flow compensation in GRE. With this scheme, flowing protons (with constant velocity) are in phase (i.e., zero phase difference) at the center of the echo.

Table 25-2

Manufacturer	Acronym	Description
GE	FC	Flow Compensation
Picker	MAST	Motion Artifact Suppression Technique
Siemens	GMR	Gradient-Motion Rephasing

entry slice increasing intraluminal signal, TOF signal losses will also have an effect, thus somewhat offsetting FRE. In other words, in reality, flowing blood demonstrates a combination of flow phenomena, and the intensity of blood is, in

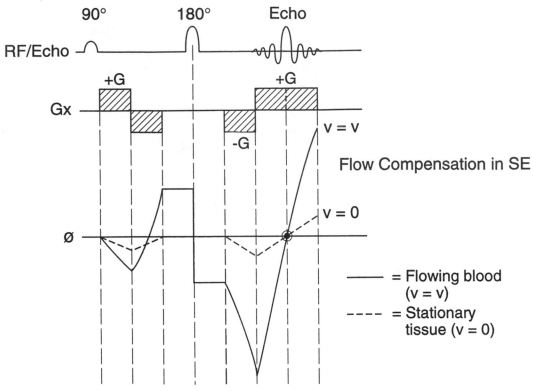

Figure 25-10.   Flow compensation in SE. With this scheme, flowing protons are in phase at the center of the echo.

Second-order (acceleration) Flow Compensation

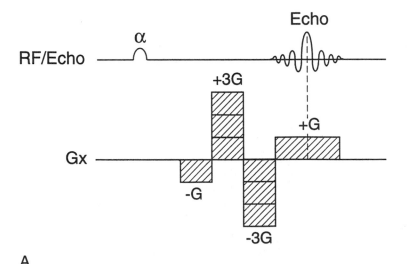

A

Figure 25-11.   **(a)** Second-order flow (acceleration) compensation. With this scheme, protons with second-order flow (i.e., acceleration) get in phase at the center of the echo. **(b)** Third-order flow (jerk) compensation. With this scheme, protons with third-order flow (i.e., jerk) get in phase at the center of the echo.

Third-order (jerk) Flow Compensation

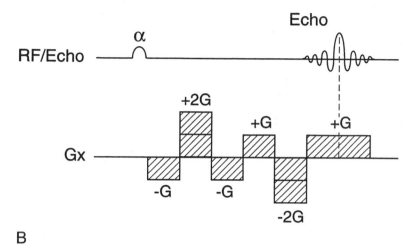

Figure 25-11. Continued.

the final analysis, determined by the phenomena that predominate.

GRADIENT MOMENT NULLING (FLOW COMPENSATION)

Gradient moment nulling (GMN) is one method of minimizing flow motion artifacts. It is based on the principle of even-echo rephasing. Even-echo rephasing is accomplished by adding extra gradient pulses to produce the even-echo rephasing effect on the first echo (thus eliminating first-echo dephasing). You can therefore achieve rephasing without having to use a double-echo sequence. There are several synonyms for GMN (Table 25-2).

Figures 25-9 and 25-10 demonstrate FC for both GRE and SE imaging. In both cases, protons in flowing blood will have a net phase of zero at the center of the echo. The mathematics is similar to the one for even-echo rephasing (see previous section), and the interested reader may wish to go through the exercise. The extra gradi-

ents associated with FC are referred to as gradient **lobes**. For instance, for GRE, the relative gradient strengths of these lobes demonstrate a ratio of $1:2:1$. Remember that this type of FC only corrects for first-order[a] (i.e., constant velocity) flow. To correct for higher-order motion (e.g., acceleration or jerk), additional gradient lobes are required (Fig. 25-11).[b] As you can see, the addition of these extra lobes lengthens the cycle thus lengthening TR and minimum TE (thus reducing the number of slices).

FC can be applied along each and all the three coordinates x, y, and z.

---

[a] Zero-order motion is stationary ($v = 0$). First order motion ($v = dx/dt = $ constant) is constant velocity. Second-order motion ($a = d^2x/d^2t$) is acceleration. Third-order motion ($j = d^3x/d^3t$) is jerk motion or pulsatility.

---

[b] For a more complete discussion, refer to Stark DO, Bradley WG, eds. Magnetic resonance imaging, Vol. 1. 2nd ed. St. Louis: Mosby, 1992.

Key Points

1. Several types of flow exist: laminar flow, plug flow, turbulent flow, and flow separation/vortex flow.

2. Intravascular flow is usually laminar, i.e. it has a parabolic profile.

3. Turbulent flow occurs distal to stenoses and on vessel turns.

4. The Reynolds number can predict laminar versus turbulent flow.

5. Most flow effects can be attributed to one of two phenomena: time of flight (TOF) or motion-related phase changes.

6. TOF can cause either signal loss (TOF loss) or signal gain (flow-related enhancement).

7. Causes of intravascular signal loss include high velocity, turbulent flow, and dephasing.

8. Causes of intravascular signal gain include flow-related enhancement (FRE), even-echo rephasing, and diastolic pseudogating.

9. Dephasing may be caused by intravoxel dephasing or odd-echo dephasing.

10. FRE is based on the entry phenomenon. FRE is the basis for TOF MR angiography (MRA).

11. FRE penetrates deeper slices when flow is countercurrent to the slice-excitation wave (SEW) rather than when it is cocurrent.

12. Even-echo rephasing causes bright intravascular signal on the second echo (when the echoes are symmetric).

13. Even-echo rephasing is the basis for flow compensation (gradient moment nulling). GMN, however, is accomplished via gradients that cause rephasing of flowing spins on the first echo and thus increased signal.

Questions

25-1. Normal intravascular flow is usually:
(a) plug flow   (b) laminar flow
(c) turbulent flow
(d) none of the above

25-2. T/F Turbulent flow is expected proximal to a stenosis.

25-3. T/F The Reynolds number (Re) can predict laminar vs. turbulent flow.

25-4. T/F Time-of-flight effects only cause signal loss.

25-5. Causes of intravascular signal loss include:
(a) high velocity
(b) turbulent flow
(c) dephasing
(d) all of the above
(e) only (a)–(b)

25-6. Causes of intravascular signal gain include:
(a) FRE
(b) even-echo rephasing
(c) diastolic pseudogating
(d) all of the above
(e) only (a) and (c)

25-7. T/F FRE is synonymous with the entry phenomenon.

25-8. T/F FRE penetrates deeper slices when flow is cocurrent rather than countercurrent.

25-9. T/F Given the parameters TR 2000, TE1 20, TE2 80, even-echo rephasing could be a potential source of artifacts.

25-10. T/F Even-echo rephasing is the basis for flow compensation techniques.

25-11. Laminar flow is given by the formula:
(a) $v(r) = V_{max} (1 - r^2/R^2)$
(b) $v(r) = V_{max} (1 - R^2/r^2)$
(c) $v(r) = (1 - r^2/R^2)/V_{max}$
(d) There is no formula for such a flow.

25-12. Flow effects include:
(a) time-of-flight (TOF)
(b) motion-induced phase changes
(c) both   (d) none of the above

25-13. TOF effects can lead to:
(a) signal loss   (b) signal gain
(c) both   (d) none of the above

25-14. T/F FRE is only observed in the first (entry) slice.

25-15. T/F Laminar flow has a parabolic profile.

25-16. Plug flow is given by the formula:
(a) $v(r) = V_{max} (1 - r^2/R^2)$
(b) $v(r) = V_{max} (1 - R^2/r^2)$
(c) $v(r) = \text{constant} = V_{ave}$
(d) none of the above

26 MR Angiography

INTRODUCTION

In this chapter, we will discuss the topic of **MR Angiography** (**MRA**). As in the last chapter, MRA may at first appear very complicated, but we'll try to present the major concepts in a simplified fashion. There are two main MRA techniques:

1. TOF (time-of-flight) MRA
2. PC (phase contrast) MRA

Each technique can be performed using two-dimensional Fourier Transform (2DFT) or three-dimensional FT (3DFT). Thus, there are a total of four different methods:

1. 2D-TOF MRA
2. 2D-PC MRA
3. 3D-TOF MRA
4. 3D-PC MRA

Each of these techniques lends itself to a different type of clinical application.

TOF MRA

TOF MRA is based on FRE (discussed in the previous chapter) in a 2D or 3D GRE technique. (Remember that in GRE imaging, TOF losses do not play an important role.) Usually, FC (Flow Compensation) is used perpendicular to the vessel lumen.

2D-TOF MRA

Figure 26-1 depicts a typical pulse sequence for 2D-TOF MRA. A presat (presaturation) pulse is applied above or below each slice to eliminate the signal from vessels flowing in the opposite direction. Usually a short TR (about 50 msec), a moderate flip angle (45°–60°), and a short TE (a few msec) are used.

3D-TOF MRA

Figure 26-2 depicts a PSD for a 3D-TOF MRA. Here, a slab of several cm (usually about 5 cm) is obtained which contains up to 60 slices.

2D-TOF MRA

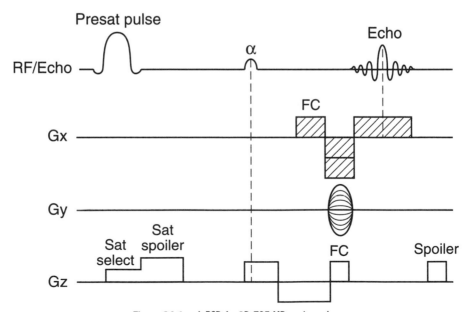

Figure 26-1. A PSD for 2D-TOF MR angiography.

3D-TOF MRA

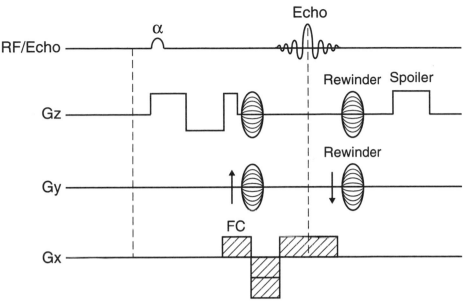

Figure 26-2. A PSD for 3D-TOF MRA.

Advantages of 2D-TOF MRA

1. Faster scanning
2. Maximized FRE because each slice is an entry slice

Advantages of 3D-TOF MRA

1. Higher SNR because signal is acquired from a larger volume
2. Improved spatial resolution

Disadvantages of 3D-TOF MRA

1. 3D techniques more susceptible to saturation effects (see below)
2. Less sensitive to slow flow

PC MRA

Phase contrast (PC) MRA is based on the fact that the phase gain of flowing blood through a gradient is proportional to its velocity (assuming constant velocity). We saw in the previous chapter that phase (ϕ) and velocity (v) are related by

$$\phi = \int \omega \, dt = \int (\gamma \, G \, v \, t) \, dt = \tfrac{1}{2} \gamma \, G \, v \, t^2$$

Therefore, knowing the phase at any point in time allows us to calculate the velocity.

The most common method for PC MRA is by the use of a **bipolar gradient** (Fig. 26-3a).

This process is called **flow encoding**. Because the two lobes in this bipolar gradient have equal area, no net phase change is observed by stationary tissues (Fig. 26-3b). However, flowing blood will experience a net phase shift proportional to its velocity (assuming a constant flow velocity). This is how flow is distinguished from stationary tissue in PC MRA. Figures 26-4 and 26-5 illustrate the PSD for 2D-PC and 3D-PC MRA, respectively.

There are several features unique to PC MRA, as the following discussions demonstrate.

Question 1: What are the "magnitude" image and the "phase" image?
Answer: As in PC MRA, you can not only get an image of the blood vessels (**magnitude image**), but also an image that shows you the direction of flow (**phase map**). The phase image would tell you whether the flow is right-left, superior-inferior, or anterior-posterior. An example is determination of centrifugal versus hepatopedal flow in the portal vein of a patient with cirrhosis.

Question 2: What is VENC?
Answer: VENC stands for velocity encoding. It is a parameter that is selected by the MR operator when using PC MRA. VENC represents

Bipolar Flow-encoding Gradient

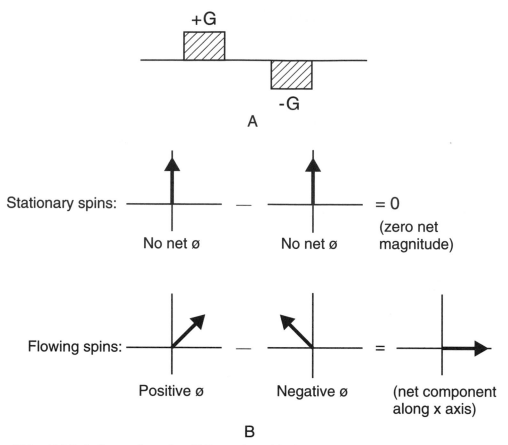

Figure 26-3. **(a)** A bipolar flow-encoding gradient. **(b)** Because the two lobes have equal areas with opposite polarities, no phase change is observed by stationary spins. However, flowing spins will yield a net phase change proportional to their velocity, which is the principle behind PC MRA.

2D-PC MRA

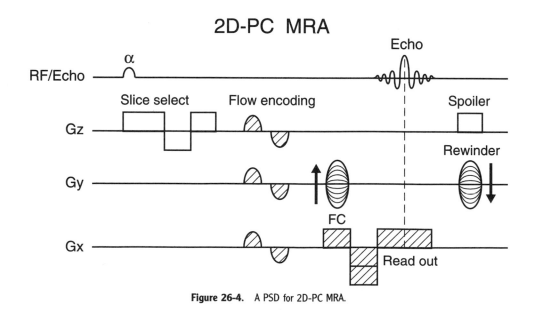

Figure 26-4. A PSD for 2D-PC MRA.

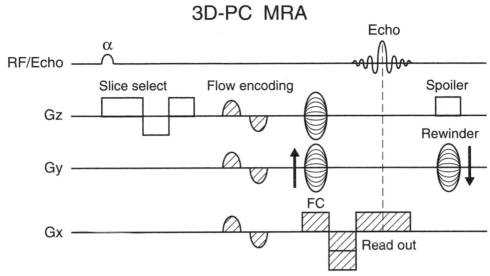

Figure 26-5.   A PSD for 3D-PC MRA.

the maximum velocity present in the imaging volume. Any velocity greater than VENC will be aliased according to the following formula:

$$aliased\ velocity = VENC - actual\ velocity$$

For instance, if VENC = 30 cm/sec, then a vessel with a flow velocity of 40 cm/sec will be represented as a flow of

$$v = 30 - 40 = -10\ cm/sec$$

i.e., a flow of 10 cm/sec in the opposite direction. A smaller VENC is more sensitive to slow flow (venous flow) and to smaller branches, but causes more rapid (arterial) flow to get aliased. A larger VENC is more appropriate for arterial flow. Sometimes you may image the same thing with two different VENCs—a small VENC and a large VENC—to accurately image all the flow components (an example is imaging an AVM or an aneurysm).

Advantages of PC MRA

1. The capability to generate magnitude and phase images
2. Superior background suppression
3. Less sensitive to intravoxel dephasing or saturation effects

Disadvantages of PC MRA

1. Takes longer to do
2. More sensitive to signal losses caused by turbulence and by dephasing on vessel turns (e.g., carotid siphon)
3. The need to guess the maximum flow velocity in order to select an optimum VENC

2D versus 3D PC-MRA

1. 2D techniques are faster
2. 3D techniques have better SNR

Table 26-1 contains a summary of some of the major clinical applications of the four methods of MRA discussed above.

MAXIMUM INTENSITY PROJECTION (MIP)

We can finally explain how we can image just the blood vessels (in a way that looks three dimensional) and not the stationary tissue. This imaging is accomplished via an algorithm called **maximum intensity projection (MIP)**. MIP can be used as a noun, verb ("the raw data are mipped"), or adverb ("mipped image"). Mipping is done as follows: because flowing blood in MRA techniques has high intensity, the intensity of a pixel in a slice is compared with the corre-

Table 26-1

2D-TOF MRA	Carotid and vertebral arteries in the neck
	Venous structures (due to slow flow)
3D-TOF MRA	Intracranial vasculature (circle of Willis)
	Intracranial vascular malformations and aneurysms
2D-PC MRA	Portal vein
	CSF flow study
	Localizer for determining VENC
3D-PC MRA	Intracranial vasculature
	Intracranial vascular malformations and aneurysms

Maximum Intensity Projection (MIP)

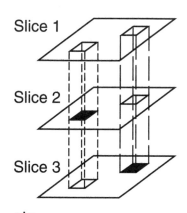

etc.

Figure 26-6. Maximum intensity projection (MIP). A channel of similar pixels in every slice is selected, and the pixel with the maximum intensity (provided its intensity is above a certain threshold) is projected onto an image. This process is repeated for all the pixels to form an image.

sponding pixels in all the other slices (as in a channel), and the one with maximum intensity is selected. For example, pixel (1,1) in slice 1 is compared to pixel (1,1) of all other slices. This process is repeated for all the pixels in the slice. In other words, the high intensity dots in space are connected to generate an MRA image. Thus, the mipped image represents the highest intensities (hopefully all caused by flowing blood) in the imaging volume. This image is illustrated in Figure 26-6. Obviously, a certain *internal* threshold is used, below which no pixel in the channel falls.

DISADVANTAGES OF MIP

The major drawback of MIP is that bright structures other than flowing blood may poten-

tially be included in the mipped image. Examples are fat, subacute hemorrhage, and the posterior pituitary gland. This problem is mainly with TOF MRA and not with PC MRA (the latter is a subtraction technique based on velocity-induced phase shifts rather than on tissue T1 and T2).

SATURATION EFFECTS

Saturation effects refer to the gradual loss of longitudinal magnetization caused by repeated excitation RF pulses. This, in turn, leads to loss of signal (and thus reduced SNR). This problem usually arises in a 2D acquisition in which flowing blood has to travel within (rather than through) a slice or in a 3D acquisition in which the blood travels through a thick imaging volume (or slab). In such a situation, saturation effects may cause the distal portion of a vessel not to be included in the image.

There are two main causes of saturation effects:

1. Decreasing TR
2. Increasing α

Decreasing TR

As shown in Figure 26-7, a shorter TR causes less recovery of longitudinal magnetization from one cycle to the next, causing gradual loss of the Mz component. This effect is less pronounced with a longer TR.

Increasing α

Next consider the case of a large α. A larger α causes more loss of longitudinal magnetization. Therefore, for a given TR, there is more gradual loss of Mz with a larger α than with a smaller one (Fig. 26-8).

In GRE, saturation effects become problematic because very short TRs are used. The use of small flip angles counteract this effect. These saturation effects become especially important in 2D- or 3D-in plane flow or in 3D imaging in which volume imaging is performed over a slab, and signal losses might be significant from one end of the slab to the other. Multislice GRE techniques that use longer TRs decrease these saturation effects and allow for larger flip angles (which improves the SNR).

Parenthetically, there is another way of reducing these saturation effects: using a paramagnetic contrast agent, such as gadolinium. The use of this agent causes T1 shortening of blood. Consequently, the T1 recovery is faster with less saturation effects (Fig. 26-9).

Two newer techniques are also now available to reduce saturation effects: MOTSA and TONE.

Multiple Overlapping Thin-Slab Acquisition (MOTSA)

MOTSA (Multiple Overlapping Thin-Slab Acquisition) is a combination of 2D-TOF and 3D-TOF techniques for the purpose of reducing the saturation effects associated with a *thick* slab. In this method, multiple *thin* slabs are used, which are overlapping by 25–50% (Fig. 26-10). The final imaging volume is created by extracting the central slices of each slab and discarding the peripheral slices (which are more affected by saturation effects). The main drawback of this technique is the potential for "**Vene-**

Saturation Effects (TR variable, α fixed)

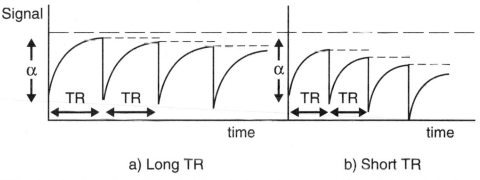

a) Long TR b) Short TR

Figure 26-7. Saturation effects. A longer TR (for a fixed flip angle α) causes better recovery of longitudinal magnetization, thus reducing saturation effects.

Saturation Effects (α variable, TR fixed)

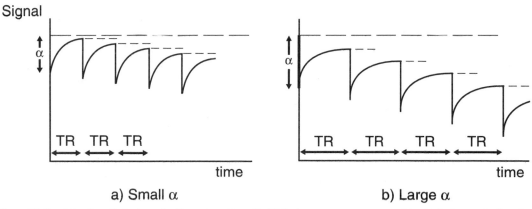

a) Small α b) Large α

Figure 26-8. Saturation effects. A smaller flip angle α (for a fixed TR) also causes more recovery of longitudinal magnetization, thus leading to reduced saturation effects.

Saturation Effects (use of Gadolinium)

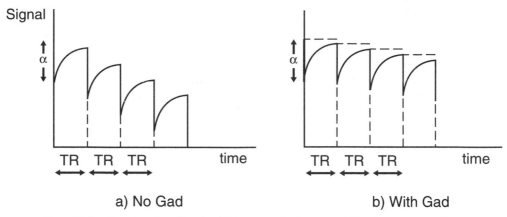

a) No Gad   b) With Gad

Figure 26-9. Saturation effects. Use of gadolinium causes T1 shortening, which reduces saturation effects.

MOTSA

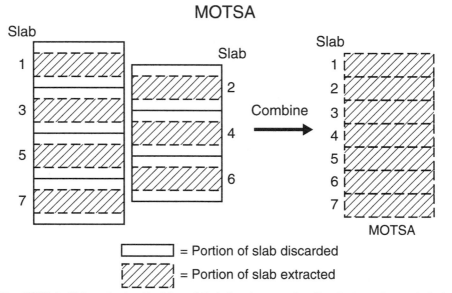

☐ = Portion of slab discarded

▨ = Portion of slab extracted

Figure 26-10. MOTSA (multiple overlapping thin-slab acquisition). To reduce saturation effects in deeper slices, multiple thinner slices are processed (in this example, 7). Next, the peripheral slices in each slab are discarded and the remaining slices are extracted and combined to form an image.

tian blind" artifact at the points where the slabs overlap.

Tilted Optimized Non-saturating Excitation (TONE)

In this scheme, the flip angle α is increased progressively as the flowing spins move into the imaging volume by using increasing RF pulses. Recall that a larger α yields a higher SNR. Thus, increasing α counteracts saturation effects of slowly-flowing blood in deeper slices. This

allows better visualization of distal vessels and slow-flowing vessels. This scheme is illustrated in Figure 26-11 in which a **ramped** flip angle excitation pulse is used. In this example, the center flip angle is 30° and the flip angle at each end varies by 30% (i.e., 20° at the entry slice and 40° at the exit slice).

There are five main ways of reducing saturation effects:

1. *Decreasing the flip angle α*
2. *Increasing the repetition time TR*

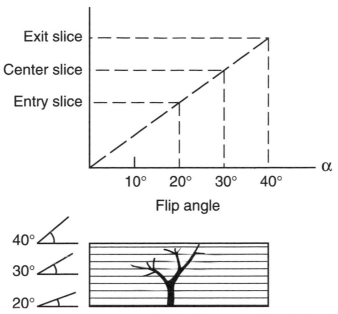

Figure 26-11. TONE (tilted optimized nonsaturating excitation). In this scheme, a ramped flip angle is used, which is larger in deeper slices. Because a larger α yields a larger transverse component in the x-y plane, this scheme would improve S/N in deeper slices, counteracting the saturation effects of slow-flowing blood.

3. Using a paramagnetic contrast agent, such as a gadolinium chelate
4. MOTSA
5. TONE

Question: How does magnetization transfer (MT) affect MRA?
Answer: Magnetization Transfer (MT) saturation was discussed in Chapter 24. MT is based on suppression of the off-resonant protein-bound water protons (e.g., brain tissue). This technique, combined with TOF MRA, helps to suppress the background signal (e.g., it can reduce the signal from brain parenchyma by about 30%), increasing conspicuity of small and distal branches, vessels with slow flow, and aneurysms. MT can also be combined with TONE for further visualization of small vessels.

Question: Why do MRA techniques overestimate the degree of stenosis?
Answer: Because accelerated flow through the stenotic area leads to dephasing during TE. To reduce this effect, use a shorter TE. Also, turbulent flow and vortex flow (flow eddies) as well as stream separation distal to stenosis and at vessel turns (e.g., carotid siphon) may cause de-
phasing and flow void, overestimating the length of stenosis (in the case of post stenosis) or mimicking stenosis (in the case of vessel turns).

BLACK BLOOD MRA

Black blood MRA is another technique for MR angiography in which flowing blood appears dark rather than bright. It is *not* just a photo negative of bright blood MRA. Rapidly flowing blood (arterial flow), as discussed in the previous chapter, demonstrates TOF signal losses. Slow flowing blood (venous flow) has higher intensity. Various flow presaturation pulses and dephasing methods via gradients are employed in this technique to render flowing blood black. Note that the maximum intensity projection is replaced by a ***minimum* intensity projection** algorithm.

Advantages of Black Blood MRA
1. This technique does not overestimate the degree of stenosis as much as bright blood TOF MRA.
2. Dephasing in vessel turns that mimic stenosis with bright blood TOF MRA is not a problem here.

Disadvantages of Black Blood MRA
1. Calcified plaques may also be dark and therefore invisible. Thus, this technique may *underestimate* the degree of stenosis.

2. Other black materials (such as air or cortical bone or calcification) may mimic flow.

Key Points

1. Two main MR angiography (MRA) techniques exist: time-of-flight (TOF) and phase contrast (PC).

2. Both TOF and PC MRA can be performed in 2D or 3D.

3. TOF MRA is based on FRE.

4. PC MRA is based on velocity-induced phase changes.

5. PC MRA techniques allow acquisition of magnitude and phase images.

6. Phase images provide information regarding the direction of flow (not provided by TOF MRA).

7. VENC (velocity encoding) is a parameter that needs to be input by the operator when doing PC MRA. It represents the maximum flow velocity before aliasing occurs.

8. If VENC is too low, aliasing is more likely to occur. If VENC is too high, slow flow and small vessels are not well visualized. Therefore, low VENC is good for visualization of slow (venous) flow and small branches. High VENC is good for high-velocity (arterial) flow.

9. MIP (maximum intensity projection) is an algorithm used in MRA in which the highest intensity dots in space are connected to generate a three-dimensional looking image of the vessels.

10. 3D imaging is subject to saturation effects (as blood enters deeper slices).

11. Saturation effects can be minimized by several methods: (a) decreasing the flip angle, (b) increasing TR, (c) using gadolinium, (d) MOTSA, (e) TONE.

12. MOTSA (multiple overlapping thin-slab acquisition) uses several overlapping thin slices to reduce saturation effects. A potential problem is Venetian blind artifacts.

13. TONE (tilted optimized nonsaturating excitation) uses a ramped RF flip angle (small α at the entry slice and larger α at the exit slice) to reduce saturation effects.

14. TOF MRA tends to overestimate the degree of stenosis (due to dephasing effects).

15. Black blood MRA is based on TOF signal losses. Instead of maximum intensity projection, a minimum intensity projection algorithm is used. This technique overcomes the problem of overestimating the degree of stenosis.

Questions

26-1. The main MRA techniques include:
    (a) TOF MRA   (b) PC MRA
    (c) both   (d) none

26-2. The parameter VENC must be set for:
    (a) TOF MRA   (b) PC MRA
    (c) both   (d) none

26-3. Match:
    (i) more sensitive to slow flow
    (ii) aliasing
    (iii) poor visualization of small branches

(iv)   arterial flow
with
(a)   low venc   (b)   high venc

26-4.   T/F   In the MIP algorithm, the pixel with the highest intensity is selected for each slice.

26-5.   Saturation effects can be reduced by:
(a)   decreasing the flip angle
(b)   increasing TR
(c)   using a gadolinium chelate
(d)   MOTSA
(e)   all of the above
(f)   only (a)–(c)

26-6.   T/F   MT allows better visualization of smaller vessels with slow flow in the brain.

26-7.   T/F   TOF MRA is based on FRE.

26-8.   Match:
(i)   MOTSA   (ii)   TONE

(iii)   aliasing
(iv)   countercurrent flow
(v)   PC MRA
with
(a)   ramped RF
(b)   Venetian blind artifact
(c)   deeper FRE
(d)   magnitude and phase images
(e)   low VENC

26-9.   T/F   TOF MRA may underestimate the degree of stenosis.

26-10.   Compared with conventional bright blood MRA, black blood MRA
(a)   uses a minimum intensity projection algorithm
(b)   does not overestimate the degree of stenosis as much
(c)   both (a) and (b)
(d)   none of the above

27 High Performance Gradients

INTRODUCTION

This chapter briefly discusses the new technology of high performance gradients. As you know by now, gradients have many purposes, including slice selection, spatial encoding, flow compensation, spoiling, rewinding, and presaturation. It should be fairly obvious that every time you use a gradient, you are lengthening the pulse cycle (thus increasing minimum TE).

Consider the two gradients in Figure 27-1a and b. The gradient in Figure 27-1a has half the strength of the one in Figure 27-1b but twice the duration. Thus, both these gradients have the same area (shaded area). They both achieve the exact same result (e.g., phase shift) on *stationary* spins, but the second

one is twice as fast and allows reducing the echo delay time TE. Therefore, the first requirement of a high performance gradient is a higher maximum strength.

When we discuss high performance gradients, we want to not only achieve a stronger magnitude or strength, but we want the maximum strength to be achieved in as short a time as possible (i.e., a short rise time) to minimize the duration of the gradient. Therefore, the second issue is how fast a gradient can reach its plateau (Fig. 27-2). The ratio of the maximum gradient (G_{max}) to the **rise time** (t_R) is called the **slew rate** (SR):

$$SR = \text{slew rate} = G_{max}/t_R \text{ (in mT/m-msec)} \quad \text{(Eqn. 27-1)}$$

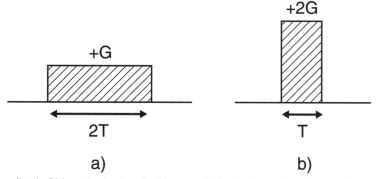

Figure 27-1. The gradient in **(b)** has twice the strength of the one in **(a)** but half the duration. Consequently, they both have the exact same area and thus achieve the same results for stationary spins. However, the one in **(b)** has the advantage of being faster, a condition that is required for fast scanning.

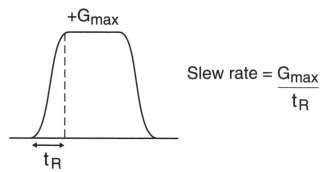

Figure 27-2. In reality, it takes a certain amount of time (t_R) for a gradient to rise to its plateau G_{max}. The ratio G_{max}/t_R is called the slew rate (in mT/m-msec).

Flow Compensation

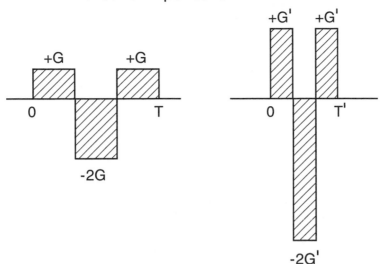

Figure 27-3. With high-performance gradients, flow compensation can be accomplished faster (again because by increasing the strength and reducing the duration, the same area can be achieved).

The requirements for high performance gradients are the following:

1. *high gradient strength (G_{max})*
2. *short rise time (t_R)*

i.e., a high slew rate (G_{max}/t_R).

Early gradients had a G_{max} of 3–6 mT/m and t_R of 1.5–2 msec (i.e., SR of 1.5 to 4 mT/m-msec). In the mid 1980s, GE introduced shielded gradients with G_{max} of 10 mT/m and t_R of 675 μsec = 0.675 msec (i.e., SR of 15 mT/m-msec). The new high performance systems (Siemens' VISION, GE's EchoSpeed, Picker's EDGE, Philips' ACS-NT, etc.) have G_{max} as high as 27 mT/m and t_R of 180 μsec with SR as high as 120 mT/m-msec.

Advantages of High Performance Gradients

1. Shorter cycles are possible. As discussed previously, a stronger gradient can be applied over a shorter duration. Consider the example of flow compensation (FC). Figure 27-3 demonstrates two FC gradients that achieve the same thing, but the second one has higher strength ($G' > G$) and is thus applied over a

shorter period ($T' < T$). (As an aside, because of the quadratic nature of phase accumulation for flowing spins, no linear relationship exists between $G/G' : T/T'$—i.e., if G is doubled, the duration is not halved.) Higher-order motion (e.g., acceleration, jerk) requires the addition of even more gradient lobes. You can see how high performance gradients can save a lot of time during each cycle allowing for shorter TEs (reducing dephasing) and TRs (for fast scanning).

2. Smaller FOVs are possible. As we saw in Chapter 15, an inverse relationship exists between the gradient strength along one axis and the field of view (FOV):

$$FOV = BW/(\gamma \cdot G)$$

where G is the gradient strength, BW is the bandwidth defined as

$$BW = 2 f_{max}$$

where f_{max} is the **Nyquist frequency** (Chapter 12). Thus, increasing G allows us to reduce the FOV, leading to higher spatial resolution (an example is high resolution imaging of a small part such as the pituitary gland). That is,

$$FOV_{min} = BW/(\gamma \cdot G_{max})$$

Because spatial resolution is defined as the FOV divided by the number of encoding steps:

$$spatial\ res. = FOV/N$$

then minimizing FOV (while keeping N fixed) results in improved spatial resolution.

EXAMPLE:

For a standard high field system, the BW = 32 kHz ($\pm$16 kHz) and G_{max} = 10 mT/m. Then

$$FOV_{min} = 32\ kHz/(42.6\ MHz/T$$
$$\times\ 10\ mT/m) \cong 7.5\ cm$$

Now if G_{max} is increased to 25 mT/sec, then

$$FOV_{min} = 32\ kHz/(42.6\ MHz/T$$
$$\times\ 25\ mT/m) \cong 3\ cm$$

If you reduce the BW to 16 kHz ($\pm$8 kHz), then the minimum FOV will be reduced even further to about 1.5 cm.

3. Faster imaging is possible, including faster FSE (fast spin echo), **GRASE** (**gradient and spin echo**), and EPI (echoplanar imaging).
4. 3D FSE is possible (useful for 3D T2W imaging in brain and spine).
5. Detection of very slow flow (blood or CSF) is possible via PC techniques.
6. PC MRA can now be performed in a reasonable acquisition time with in-

creased sensitivity to slow flow (the duration of flow-encoding gradient can be reduced, allowing for a shorter TR).

7. High-resolution imaging of CSF flow in small shunts is possible.
8. Ultra high-resolution MRA is possible (1024 $\times$ 1024 matrix over 22 cm FOV resulting in 250 μ resolution!)
9. High-resolution (both spatial and temporal) dynamic MR techniques are possible because, by shortening the TE and TR, a larger matrix can be employed at a given FOV in the same acquisition time. Thus, both spatial and temporal resolutions can be improved. One application is dynamic MR study of breast cancer (TurboFLASH sequence with TR = 7 msec, TE = 3 msec, 128 $\times$ 128 matrix, acq. time = 7 $\times$ 128 = 896 msec $\cong$ 0.9 sec).
10. The minimum TE can be reduced, thus minimizing dephasing and increasing T1 contrast. For example, high performance gradients can provide high-dose gadolinium performance with the use of a single dose of gadolinium, or, alternatively, provide single dose performance with only half a dose of gadolinium.

Diffusion imaging is possible by the addition of diffusion-sensitizing gradient pulses to any pulse sequence. Possible clinical applications include early detection of cerebrovascular accidents (CVA) and monitoring thermal ablation of brain tumors.

Key Points

High performance gradients have revolutionized MR imaging. In short, a higher magnetic strength allows a shorter duration, thus reducing the cycle time. This in turn reduces the minimum TE and TR, which shortens the acquisition time. In summary, high performance gradients allow many new and improved features, including: faster scanning (including EPI, GRASE, 3D-FSE, etc.), improved spatial and temporal resolution, smaller FOV, high-resolution MRA (both TOF and PC) with improved visualization of small vessels and slow flow, and improved imaging of CSF flow, just to name a few.

Questions

27-1. High performance gradients require:
(a) high gradient strength (G_{max})
(b) long rise time (t_R)
(c) both (d) none

27-2. The slew rate is defined as:
(a) t_R/G_{max} (b) G_{max}/t_R
(c) $\gamma \, G_{max}/t_R$
(d) none of the above

27-3. Advantages of high performance gradients include all of the following EXCEPT:
(a) faster scanning

(b) smaller FOV without experiencing aliasing
(c) reduced chemical shift
(d) diffusion imaging

27-4. T/F Two gradients with different profiles but the same area (Fig. 27-1) will have the same effects (i.e., phase changes) on
(a) stationary spins
(b) flowing spins
(c) both (d) none

Answers

Chapter 1

1-2. $e^{i(x+y)} = e^{ix} \cdot e^{iy}$. So cos $(x + y)$ + i sin $(x + y)$ = (cos x + i sin x) . (cos y + i sin y)
= (cos x . cos y − sin x . sin y) + i (cos x . sin y + sin x . cos y)

1-3. sinc (0) = sin (0)/0 = $\lim\limits_{x \to 0}$ d/dx (sin x/x) = $\underset{(@x=0)}{\cos x/1}$ = cos 0/1 = 1/1 = 1.

1-4. (a) e^{-1} = 0.37   (b) e^{-2} = 0.14   (c) e^{-1} = 0.37

1-5. (a) d/dt $(Ae^{-t/T})$ = A $(-1/T)$ $e^{-t/T}$, which is $-A/T$ at t=0. This is the slope of the line tangent to the curve at t = 0 which crosses the t-axis at t = T.

1-6. ln (e^x) = x = ln 4 = ln 2^2 = 2 ln 2 = 2 × 0.693 = 1.386.

Chapter 2

2-1. (a) 14.9 MHz   (b) 21.3 MHz   (c) 42.6 MHz   (d) 63.9 MHz   (e) 85.2 MHz

2-2. T   2-3. F (only mobile protons)   2-4. F   2-5. T   2-6. F (speed of light)

2-7. T   2-8. F   2-9. F   2-10. T   2-11. T

Chapter 3

3-1. T   3-2. F   3-3. T   3-4. T

Chapter 4

4-1. (a) T   (b) F   (c) F   (d) T

4-2. c   4-3. d   4-4. F (by T_2^*)   4-5. b

Chapter 5

5-1. (a) 1.56 (b) 90 msec   (c) 0.72 and 1.05   (d) 1.28 , 50 msec, 0.88 and 1.28   (e) 2.10

5-2. H_2O/fat = 0.25 and 1.63; CSF/GM = 0.41 and 1.40   5-3. c   5-4. a

5-5. (a) N(H) $e^{-TE/T2}$ (i.e., ideal T2W)   (b) N(H) $(1 - e^{-TR/T1})$ (i.e., ideal T1W)   (c) N(H) (i.e., ideal PDW).

Chapter 6

6-1. T   6-2. (i) c   (ii) a   (iii) d   (iv) a   6-3. T

Chapter 7

7-1.   Setting $1 - 2e^{-t/T1} = 0$, we get $e^{-t/T1} = 1/2$ so $-t/T1 = ln\,(1/2) = -0.693$ so $t = 0.693\ T1$

7-2. $S \propto N(H)\ (1 - 2e^{-TI/T1})\ (1 - e^{-TR/T1}) = N(H)\ (1 - 2e^{-TI/T1} - e^{-TR/T1} + 2e^{-(TR+TI)/T1}) \cong N(H)\ (1 - 2e^{-TI/T1} - e^{-TR/T1} + 2e^{-(TR)/T1}) = N(H)\ (1 - 2e^{-TI/T1} + e^{-TR/T1})$

7-3.   (i)   a   (ii)   b

Chapter 8

8-1.   (a) $N\ (1 - e^{-TR/T1})\ e^{-TE1/T2}$ and $N\ (1 - e^{-TR/T1})\ e^{-TE2/T2}$ (b) $N\ (1 - e^{-TR/T1})\ e^{-TE1/T2^*}$ (c)   0.61 and 0.37

8-2.   (i)   a   (ii)   b   (iii)   d   8-3.   F (not that due to spin-spin interactions)

Chapter 9

9-1.   T   9-2.   (a)   F   (b)   F

Chapter 10

10-1.   (a)   4.7 mT/m   (b)   1 mm   10-2.   f

Chapter 11

11-1.   (i)   a   (ii)   c   (iii)   b   11-2.   T   11-3. $360°/128 = 2.8°$ 11-4.   (i)   d   (ii)   a

Chapter 12

12-1.   b   12-2.   c   12-3.   F   12-4.   F $(1/\sqrt{BW})$ 12-5.   d

Chapter 13

13-1.   T   13-2.   F (phase encode gradient)   13-3.   T   13-4.   T   13-5.   F (frequency domain)

13-6.   F   13-7.   F (there is a *conjugate* symmetry)

Chapter 14

14-1.   b, c, e   14-2.   (a)   768 sec = 12 min, 48 sec.   (b)   7680 sec = 128 min = 2 hrs, 8 min!

Chapter 15

15-1.   (a)   20 cm (reduces the minimum FOV)   15-2.   b   15-3.   61°   15-4.   d   15-5.   F (increases)

Chapter 16

16-1.   T   16-2.   (a)   T   (b)   F (cycles/cm)   16-3.   T   16-4.   d   16-5.   (a)   T   (b)   T

Chapter 17

17-1. (a) 256 sec = 4 min, 16 sec   (b) 2560 sec = 42 min, 40 sec   (c) 4 min, 16 sec

17-2. (a) 10 slices   17-3. (a) SNR is increased by $\sqrt{2}$ (b) Chem shift is doubled
       (c) coverage is reduced since Ts = Nx/BW is doubled.   17-4. c   17-5. b   17-6. a

17-7. g   17-8. f   17-9. d   17-10. c   17-11. c   17-12. e   17-13. a   17-14. e

17-15. d   17-16. d

Chapter 18

18-1. e

18-2. (i) In terms of number of pixels

	.2 T	.5T	1.0T	1.5T
50kHz	0.15	0.38	0.76	1.15
10kHz	0.76	1.91	3.82	5.73
4kHz	1.91	4.77	9.54	14.31

(ii) In terms of mm

	.2 T	.5T	1.0T	1.5T
50kHz	0.14	0.36	0.72	1.07
10kHz	0.72	1.79	3.58	5.37
4kHz	1.79	4.48	8.95	13.43

(iii) The narrower the BW or the stronger the main magnetic field, the greater the chemical shift.

18-3. (a) 51.2   (b) 256/51.2 = 5   (c) fewer ghosts   18-4. b   18-5. d

18-6. F (the other way around)   18-7. a   18-8. T   18-9. d

18-10. (a) 48 pixels or 7.5 cm   (b) 2 ghosts   18-11. c   18-12. c   18-13. d

18-14. F (55°)   18-15. a   18-16. b   18-17. e

Chapter 19

19-1. d   19-2. (a) 25 min, 36 sec   (b) 3 min, 12 sec   19-3. F (decreased coverage)   19-4. d

19-5. d   19-6. c   19-7. 8 min, 32 sec

Chapter 20

20-1. F   20-2. T   20-3. T   20-4. T   20-5. T   20-6. F (more T1W)

20-7. (a) 7.7 sec   (b) 92 sec = 1 min, 32 sec   20-8. F (the opposite)   20-9. F   20-10. b

Chapter 21

21-1. d   21-2. f   21-3. T   21-4. T

Chapter 22

22-1. T   22-2. F   22-3. d   22-4. F   22-5. F   22-6. T   22-7. b

Chapter 23

23-1. e   23-2. d   23-3. a   23-4. T   23-5. T   23-6. F

Chapter 24

24-1. b   24-2. a   24-3. F   24-4. T   24-5. T   24-6. e   24-7. e

Chapter 25

25-1. b   25-2. F (*distal* to a stenosis)   25-3. T   25-4. F   25-5. d   25-6. d   25-7. T

25-8. F   25-9. F   25-10. T   25-11. a   25-12. c   25-13. c   25-14. F

25-15. T   25-16. c

Chapter 26

26-1. c   26-2. b   26-3. (i) a   (ii) a   (iii) b   (iv) b   26-4. F   26-5. e

26-6. T   26-7. T   26-8. (i) b   (ii) a   (iii) e   (iv) c   (v) d   26-9. F

26-10. c

Chapter 27

27-1. a   27-2. b   27-3. c   27-4. a

References

1. Budinger TF, Margulis AR, eds. Medical magnetic resonance—A primer. Society of Magnetic Resonance in Medicine, Inc., 1988.
2. Chun Y, Udo SP, et al. Three-dimensional fast spin-echo imaging: pulse sequence and in vivo image evaluation. JMRI 1993;3:894–899.
3. Edelman RR, Wielopolski P, Schmitt F, et al. Echo-planar MR imaging. Radiology 1994;192(3):600–612.
4. Elster AD. Questions and answers in magnetic resonance imaging. Chicago: Mosby, 1994.
5. Erickson SJ, Cox IH, Hyde JS, et al. Effect of tendon orientation on MR imaging signal intensity: a manifestation of the "magic angle" phenomenon. Radiology 1991;181:389–392.
6. Hashemi RH, Bradley WG, Chen D-Y, et al. Suspected multiple sclerosis: MR imaging with a thin-section fast FLAIR pulse sequence. Radiology 1995;196:505–510.
7. Henkelman RM et al. Why fat is bright in RARE and fast spin-echo imaging. J Magn Reson Imaging 1992; 2(5):533–540.
8. Hennig J et al. RARE imaging: a fast imaging method for clinical MR. Magn Reson Med 1986;3:823–833.
9. Horowitz AL. MRI Physics for radiologists—a visual approach. 2nd ed. New York: Springer-Verlag, 1992.
10. Kapelov SR, Teresi LM, Bradley WG, et al. Bone contusions of the knee: increased lesion detection with fast spin-echo MR imaging with spectroscopic fat saturation. Radiology 1993;189(3):901–904.
11. Lufkin RB. The MRI Manual. Chicago: Mosby, 1990.
12. Oppenheim AV. Signals and systems. Prentice-Hall, 1983.
13. Thomsik-Schröpfer D, ed. Siemens magnetom insights. The Siemens news for magnetic resonance professionals 3:1–11.
14. Signa advantage application guides, Vol. 1-5, GE Medical Systems.
15. Stark DD, Bradley WG, eds. Magnetic resonance imaging. 2nd ed., Vol. 1-2. Chicago: Mosby, 1992.

Index